Therapeutic Recreation Service principles and practices

RICHARD KRAUS, Ed.D.

Professor and Coordinator of Recreation Curriculum
Department of Health, Physical Education and Recreation
Herbert H. Lehman College
City University of New York
Bronx, New York

1973

W. B. SAUNDERS COMPANY
PHILADELPHIA LONDON TORONTO

W. B. Saunders Company: West Washington Square
Philadelphia, Pa. 19105

12 Dyott Street
London, WC1A 1DB

833 Oxford Street
Toronto 18, Ontario

Therapeutic Recreation Service: Principles and Practices   ISBN 0-7216-5506-8

Print No.:   9   8   7   6   5   4   3   2   1

TO S.S.M.

Preface

This book is designed to serve as a text for college and university courses dealing with the provision of recreation programs for the ill and disabled in both institutional and community settings. Its purpose is twofold: (a) to provide a theoretical rationale for the development of therapeutic recreation services for such groups as the physically disabled, mentally ill, mentally retarded, socially deviant, or dependent aging persons, and (b) to offer practical guidelines for the operation of such programs, including detailed examples of activities and leadership methods.

Over the past two decades, therapeutic recreation has become a rapidly growing and dynamic field. It has shifted its focus from the hospital setting—where it was too often regarded as a diversionary rather than a truly rehabilitative service—to a total concern with the disabled, in both institutional and community settings. Today, recreation specialists work closely with medical and other rehabilitation specialists in providing a total continuum of service. In order to provide a comprehensive picture of therapeutic recreation today, the author has drawn information from a variety of sources:

1. A considerable bulk of material regarding contemporary concepts and professional development of therapeutic recreation service has been excerpted from such publications as journals, conference reports, research surveys and similar documents.
2. Hundreds of hospitals, training schools, municipal recreation departments and similar agencies were asked to submit printed materials, such as program schedules, leadership manuals, annual reports or similar documents. While it is not possible to list all such contributors, a number of the agencies that responded generously include:

Athens, Ohio, Mental Health Center
Blythedale Children's Hospital, Valhalla, New York
Brainerd, Minnesota, State Hospital
Chicago, Illinois, Park District
Children's Village, Dobbs Ferry, New York
Chillicothe, Ohio, Correctional Institute
Coldwater State Home and Training School, Coldwater, Michigan
Detroit, Michigan, Department of Parks and Recreation
Downey, Illinois, Veterans Administration Hospital
Dutchess County, New York, Psychiatric Day Care Center
Evansville, Indiana, Psychiatric Children's Center
Flint, Michigan, Department of Recreation and Parks
Illinois State Training School for Boys, at St. Charles
Illinois State Training School for Girls, at Geneva
John Umstead Hospital, Butner, North Carolina
Junction City, Ohio, Treatment Center
Karl Holton School for Boys, Stockton, California
Keystone Training and Rehabilitation Residence, Scranton, Pennsylvania
Lafayette Clinic, Detroit, Michigan
Lima State Hospital, Ohio

Mansfield State Training School and Hospital, Connecticut

Mt. Sinai Hospital, New York, New York

Muscatatuck State Hospital and Training Center, Butlerville, Indiana

National Institutes of Health Hospital, Bethesda, Maryland

National Wheelchair Athletic Association, Woodside, New York

New Haven, Connecticut, Department of Parks and Recreation

New Lisbon State School, New Jersey

New York Association for the Blind, New York

Northern Minnesota Therapeutic Camp, Brainerd, Minnesota

O. H. Close School for Boys, Stockton, California

Ohio Reformatory for Women, Marysville, Ohio

Ontario School for the Blind, Brantford, Ontario, Canada

Parsons State Hospital and Training Center, Parsons, Ohio

Plymouth State Home and Training School, Northville, Michigan

Porterville, California, State Hospital

Rainier State School, Buckley, Washington

Recreation Center for the Handicapped, San Francisco, California

Rockland County Mental Health Association, New York

San Antonio, Texas, State Hospital

San Bernardino, California, Young Women's Christian Association

Souris Valley Hospital, Weyburn, Saskatchewan, Canada

Spring Grove State Hospital, Catonsville, Maryland

Springview Hospital, Springfield, Ohio

Toledo, Ohio, Mental Health Center

Traverse City State Hospital, Traverse City, Michigan

Washington, D.C., Department of Recreation

In particular, useful materials were received from such practitioners or state consultants as: William P. Dayton, Office of Mental Health, State of Pennsylvania; Richard Endres, Brainerd State Hospital, Brainerd, Minnesota; Dorothy G. Mullen, Office of Public Health, State of Connecticut; Janet Pomeroy, Director of the Recreation Center for the Handicapped, San Francisco, California; Richard Stracke, Veterans Administration Hospital, Kansas City, Missouri; and Byron Welker, Muscatatuck State Hospital and Training Center, Butlerville, Indiana.

3. The author expresses his appreciation of Dedra Hauser and Henry Dunow, both of Bennington College, who assisted him in carrying out research for the book. The author also relied heavily on his own direct experience in the field of therapeutic recreation. While his chief professional role over the past twenty years has been that of university professor, he has also served as a recreation leader in a large private psychiatric hospital in New York State, coordinator of senior citizens' events for a county recreation department, activities leader in a private nursing home in New York City and program specialist with retarded children and deaf teen-agers and adults. He has also conducted numerous workshops for professional organizations in the field of therapeutic recreation service.

It is the author's hope that this textbook will be of real value not only to those who are preparing to enter this career field but also to those currently employed in it. If this goal is achieved, major credit is due to those practitioners in the United States and Canada who had a vision of the potentiality of recreative experience in meeting the needs of the disabled in our society, and in promoting their total rehabilitation. As individuals, and as members of such organizations as the National Association of Recreation Therapists, the Hospital Recreation Section of the American Recreation Society and, today, the National Therapeutic Recreation Society, their contribution has been immense. Thanks to their efforts, the lives of millions of Americans, young and old, have been enriched.

RICHARD KRAUS

Contents

Chapter 1

Therapeutic Recreation Service: Past and Present

In a large state-sponsored school for retarded children and youth, extensive programs of sports, hobbies, social activities, art and music are provided. Elderly residents in a nursing home enjoy hobbies, discussion groups, entertainment, bingo, singing and crafts. In the psychiatric ward of a municipal hospital, patients are involved in a variety of individual and group activities, including creative dancing, cardplaying, cooking, games and outings. Orthopedically disabled children in the community visit a children's zoo as part of a weekly trip program.

In thousands of settings around the United States and Canada today, groups of children and adults with varying kinds of disability are being provided with specially planned and directed *therapeutic recreation service*.

Exactly what does this term mean? How did it come into being? What are its goals? Who is served by it? Who provides it? What does it consist of? It is the purpose of this textbook to provide answers to these questions.

In a broad sense, recreation provides important therapeutic benefits for all human beings. It offers the opportunity for physical activity, emotional release, social involvement and creative expression that is essential for healthy personal adjustment and well-rounded, happy living. However, in a narrower sense, the term therapeutic recreation service is used to describe those activities or leisure-related experiences which are provided for individuals who have special impairments, such as chronic illness or physical, mental or social disability. Such persons have intensified needs for constructive and enriching recreational outlets, and specially-designed programs must be provided, both to contribute to their rehabilitation and recovery and to make their lives as full and happy as possible.

In the past, several other descriptive terms were applied to this field of service, including: *hospital recreation, medical recreation* and *recreation for the ill and handicapped*. For a variety of reasons, these terms are no longer fully descriptive.

Hospital recreation implies that recipients of service must be residents or patients in an institutional treatment center. However, therapeutic recreation programs are provided in many community-based settings. The term *medical recreation* suggests that programs must be carried on under direct medical supervision. Obviously, many individuals who are mentally retarded, aged or physically disabled may require specially designed recreation programs; however, these need *not* be under medical direction. Similarly, the term *recreation for the ill and handicapped* is no longer widely used today because of its emphasis on the word "handicapped." Today it is believed that, while many individuals have disabilities, they need not be significantly handicapped. Indeed, it is the task of therapeutic recreation service, along with other rehabilitation services, to minimize the functional limitations of those it serves.

In some settings, the term *recreational therapy* has been used to describe this field of service. For example, in a manual describing programs offered in its Physical Medicine and Rehabilitation Service, the Veterans Administration states:

> Recreational therapy is a professional and integral part of Physical Medicine and Rehabilitation Service. . . . The role of recreation in patient treatment becomes greatly expanded in the rehabilitation of long-term, chronically ill, and psychiatric patients. Recreation helps the patient accept and utilize constructively a prolonged period of hospitalization. Recreation activities develop interpersonal relationships, resocialization, relieve anxieties and tensions, and promote the patient's ability to more fully participate in society.[1]

Ball suggests that, in order to define recreational therapy, the meaning of its components must be examined. *Recreation,* in her view, consists of those experiences in which individuals participate for the sake of pleasure, and to meet other fundamental human needs. *Therapy* is defined as the "act of healing, remedial." Putting the two together, she defines recreational therapy as "pleasing recreation that is remedial."[2]

Although there has been considerable pressure to define the field as a specific therapy, comparable to physical therapy or occupational therapy, this position has been challenged by a number of authorities. Knudson writes:

"*Is* recreation *therapy?*" Since the word therapy has different meanings for different

people, the answer requires a distinction. If therapy is defined as prescribed or medically guided participation of the team mobilized for a potential therapeutic attack on illness, then most assuredly recreation is frequently therapy. But recreation cannot be labeled as therapy in the sense of a precise cure for a specific ailment.[3]

This point of view, which was strongly supported by Haun (see pp. 36–37), has prevailed throughout the field. It reflects the growing concern of medical practitioners with not only curing disease but also helping to restore the total person by preventing disability and helping him realize his maximum potential as a human being. While recreation may not be specifically helpful in curing an illness, it is therapeutic in that it contributes to the patient's constructive outlook while in the hospital, and to his healthy socialization and overall recovery. Shivers, for example, states that the term "therapeutic" implies a process designed to assist in the total recuperation or rehabilitation of a patient. It connotes:

> . . . activities which appear to support the morale, physical reconditioning, and mental outlook of those who are undergoing medical treatment. The term is also used to identify those activities which provide psychological stimulation and physical involvement to those individuals for whom medical treatment is no longer necessary, for whom custodial care is pertinent, for those afflicted by permanent disability, and for those who are either home-bound, handicapped, or confined to institutions.[4]

The emphasis on using recreation as a specific modality in treatment is reflected in a statement of the Public Health Service: "Therapeutic recreation is the specific use of recreational activity in the care, treatment and rehabilitation of ill,

[1] *Manual on Physical Medicine and Rehabilitation Service.* Washington, D.C.: Veterans Administration, Manual M–2, July, 1966, pp. 4–6.

[2] Edith L. Ball: "The Meaning of Therapeutic Recreation," *Therapeutic Recreation Journal,* November, 1970, p. 17.

[3] A. B. C. Knudson: "Concepts of Recreation in Rehabilitation." *In The Doctors and Recreation in the Hospital Setting.* Bulletin No. 30. Raleigh, North Carolina, North Carolina Recreation Commission, 1962, p. 40.

[4] Jay S. Shivers: "One Concept of Therapeutic Recreation Service." *Therapeutic Recreation Journal,* 2nd Quarter, 1971, p. 51.

handicapped and aged persons with a directed program."[5]

Another definition sees therapeutic recreation as:

> . . . a process which utilizes recreation services for purposive intervention in some physical, emotional, and/or social behavior to bring about a desired change in that behavior and to promote the growth and development of the individual.[6]

Summing up, then, therapeutic recreation service may be perceived as a form of professional service which provides recreational and related activities which are specially designed to meet the needs of individuals suffering from some significant degree of illness or disability. It may be provided in an institutional setting, where its primary purpose is to contribute to the process of overall recovery and to facilitate successful return to the community. It may also be a continuing service for those with permanent disability, intended to enrich the quality of their lives, and provide psychological, physical and social benefits. As a later section of this text will make clear, it may be carried on as a carefully prescribed activity, in which the participant is expected to take part in an obligated, instructional program. It may also be carried on in essentially free time, on a fully voluntary basis.

Goals of Therapeutic Recreation Service

The goals vary widely, according to the setting in which they are carried on, those who are performing the service and, most important, the individuals or groups being served. The author has written elsewhere:

> Basically, the aim of therapeutic recreation, like that of the overall rehabilitation pro-

cess, is to help the ill, disabled, aged, or retarded individual help himself to live the fullest physical, mental, social, psychological and economic life possible, as an individual and as part of a family or community, that is possible within the limits of his illness or disability. The goal within a treatment center is to return a happier, more productive, and better adjusted individual to community living, or, short of this, to help him live as fully as possible in some type of sheltered environment. . . .[7]

The constructive use of leisure is an important element in the lives of all human beings. Recreation has become recognized as a key aspect of healthy living particularly in this era in which leisure has become increasingly available for the great mass of the population. Luther Terry, formerly Surgeon General of the United States Public Health Service, supports this view strongly, pointing out that a modern concept of health is concerned with man's capacity for coping with or adapting effectively to all the physical, emotional, intellectual, social and economic demands of his environment. Life, writes Terry, is a dynamic process involving a variety of stimulus-response relationships:

> Meaningful activity is important to health throughout the life span. In order to mature—physically, intellectually, emotionally and socially—a child must be exposed to appropriate stimuli. And so too must the adult if he is to remain at his peak. Today, people are increasingly involved in leisure activity. . . . More and more people have time on their hands. Moreover, the injudicious use of leisure time is a characteristic feature of both maladjusted teen-agers and adults, and of retired, elderly persons. Too often, because of ignorance, indifference, or inertia, we are faced with the time-consuming and difficult task of reestablishing a human capacity which need never have been lost. Recreation has an important—and an increasing—role in rehabilitation.[8]

[5] *Health Resource Statistics—1968.* Washington, D.C., Public Health Service, 1968, p. 185.

[6] Statement formulated at Ninth Southern Region Institute of Therapeutic Recreation, University of North Carolina, 1969. *In* Virginia Frye and Martha Peters: *Therapeutic Recreation: Its Theory, Philosophy, and Practice.* Harrisburg, Pennsylvania, Stackpole Books, 1972, p. 41.

[7] Richard Kraus: *Recreation Today: Program Planning and Leadership.* New York, Appleton-Century-Crofts, 1966, p. 304.

[8] Luther Terry: Preface to *Recreation in Treatment Centers.* September, 1965, p. 3.

An excellent statement of purpose has been developed by the Veterans Administration which might generally serve to describe the goals of recreation in most chronic disease or psychiatric treatment settings:

1. To facilitate the patient's adjustment to hospital life and to make him more receptive to treatment.
2. To facilitate the patient's early physical, mental and social rehabilitation, recovery and discharge.
3. To assist in minimizing the risk of unnecessary readmission, by aiding in the patient's transition to his community, following discharge.
4. To improve his morale and sustain it at a high level.
5. To encourage the formation of habits and attitudes which will permit his confident participation in normal activities.
6. To compensate for his disabilities and limitations while inspiring him to fulfill his potentialities.
7. To channel his aggressive drives into appropriate outlets.
8. To encourage his desire to remove or overcome the physical or mental barriers that stand between him and a normal life.
9. To stimulate new or dormant interests and talents, as well as to reestablish old ones.[9]

In institutional settings, program activities for *psychiatric* patients are generally designed to promote the resocialization of patients, and to bring them face to face with reality situations and encourage maximum participation. Recreation activities for patients suffering from *cardiac* or *pulmonary* disease are limited to participation of a physically passive or only mildly active nature. In settings for the rehabilitation of those who have suffered severe *physical* trauma, such as strokes resulting in paralysis or other serious loss of function, paraplegia or amputation, the emphasis is on helping the patient learn to live with his residual powers, gain new recreation skills and become able to travel easily and take part in community-based recreational events.

When there is no serious physical limitation and when the person to be served is living in the community, the goal of therapeutic recreation service may be chiefly to help him enjoy his leisure to the fullest and to be accepted within community groups. Avedon, for example, describes the purposes of sociorecreative programming for the *retarded* as:

1. Providing recreation education and information which will develop the individual's capacity for meeting his own leisure needs.
2. Using recreation to improve the general health, minimize atypical appearance, and modify behavior to help retardates become more socially acceptable in community settings.
3. Offering a variety of recreational and social experiences to help individuals learn and practice needed skills.
4. Counseling retarded youth and adults about recreational resources in the community and arranging opportunities for involvement.
5. Acting as a liaison between the community and the retarded individual and his family to assure acceptance of retarded persons in community programs and facilities.
6. Coordination of community wide efforts to meet the vocational, educational, social and recreational needs of the retarded.[10]

Role of the Therapeutic Recreation Specialist

The role of the therapeutic recreation specialist does not consist solely of providing activities for ill and disabled persons in institutional or community settings. He may also serve as a counselor to patients or clients, as a community educator, as an organizer, a researcher, a consultant, or in a variety of other roles.

---

[9] C. C. Bream, Jr.: "Rehabilitative Recreation in V.A. Hospitals." *Recreation,* May, 1964, pp. 224–225.

[10] For a detailed statement, see: Elliott M. Avedon, and Frances B. Arje: *Socio-Recreative Programing for the Retarded, a Handbook for Sponsoring Groups.* New York, Teachers College, Columbia, Bureau of Publications, 1964, pp. 4–6.

Nesbitt describes the extremely diversified tasks that a typical therapeutic recreation specialist might undertake:

Therapeutic recreation specialists perform many roles and functions in the course of a week, during a work day, within any given hour. They move quickly and easily from role to role. In a short period of time a therapeutic recreation specialist will set up a day room for the evening . . . arrange for a large group of patients to participate in a community recreation program . . . set up a special party for a small group of patients not yet ready to go into the community or act on their own . . . and sit down for one-to-one counseling with a patient having problems socializing with other people. . . . The therapeutic recreation specialist performs many roles—therapist, administrator, supervisor, leader and consultant among others. . . .[11]

Therapeutic recreation includes a wide variety of social situations, and deals with an extremely broad range of disabilities. The specialist may be working in any of the following types of situations:

1. A community recreation situation (either a voluntary agency or a program operated by a public recreation or park department) in which mildly disabled individuals may mingle and take part in a fully integrated way.
2. A community recreation situation, as described in number one, in which disabled individuals with somewhat more severe disability—such as the orthopedically disabled child with limited mobility—may take part in some activities that are integrated with the nondisabled, but also may be involved in some activities or groups that are designed specifically *for* groups of disabled children.
3. A community recreation situation in which the only participation by physically or mentally disabled individuals is within specially organized, separate groups which do *not* mingle with other participants.

4. The therapeutic recreation specialist may also be employed in a community agency that does not provide direct service, but acts in a promotional, advisory or organizational role, to assist and encourage other groups in providing recreation for the disabled, as well as other social services.
5. Within institutional settings, the recreation specialist may be responsible chiefly for providing mass activities with little direct therapeutic purpose—seen chiefly as leisure time programs—like films, entertainment, informal sports, bingo.
6. He may provide program activities that are designed to meet the needs of groups of patients, or of individuals, in terms of deliberately prescribed programs that consciously serve treatment goals.
7. He may provide a program that operates on several levels: (a) prescribed individual or small group activity, of an instructional or carefully supervised nature; (b) large group activity, which patient groups are required to attend, but in which their actual participation becomes more or less voluntary; (c) programs involving complete free choice, whether concerned with participation in mass events, or small-group or individually oriented programs.

Therapeutic recreation specialists normally have close working relationships with individuals in a variety of other disciplines. The recreation worker must be able to relate closely to occupational therapists, physical therapists or corrective physical educators, nursing personnel, doctors, vocational counselors, ward personnel, nurses, volunteers and a host of other individuals. Within the community setting, he is likely to have close contact with the parents or relatives of disabled individuals, with regular program participants, with administrators and supervisors of community recreation programs, with social workers and school teachers and others concerned with helping the disabled.

His role, then, is a complex one. It is also a highly challenging and emotionally satisfying one, because the need for constructive and enjoyable recreational activity on the part of most disabled individuals is so strong.

[11] John A. Nesbitt: "The Mission of Therapeutic Recreation Specialists: To Help and to Champion the Handicapped." *Therapeutic Recreation Journal,* 4th Quarter, 1970, pp. 2–4, 41–42.

The Scope of Therapeutic Recreation Service

What, specifically, are the settings in which therapeutic recreation service is carried on? They fall under several major headings.

HOSPITALS OF ALL TYPES. These include hospitals under varied sponsorship, such as Veterans Administration, military, public health, state, county, municipal, voluntary, sectarian and proprietary hospitals. They serve many types of patients: general, psychiatric, pediatric, chronic disease, geriatric and others; some are long-term, while others involve short patient stays.

NURSING HOMES. These generally are regarded as extended-care facilities for ill or disabled aging persons, although they may also include persons of middle age who have suffered from heart attacks or strokes, who cannot live independently.

SCHOOLS OR RESIDENTIAL CENTERS FOR THOSE WITH SPECIFIC DISABILITY. There are thousands of such institutions throughout the country, which house, either permanently or for a period of years, the physically disabled (blind, deaf, orthopedically or neurologically impaired) or the mentally retarded or emotionally disturbed. As in the case of hospitals, they operate under a wide variety of auspices: voluntary agency, sectarian, municipal, county or state-sponsored.

SPECIAL SCHOOLS OR TREATMENT CENTERS FOR THE SOCIALLY DEVIANT. These include adult penal institutions, such as prisons, jails or other detention centers, as well as work camps, reformatories and special schools for youth who have been committed by the courts for delinquent behavior. These may also include special schools or shelters for emotionally disturbed children and youth, or those from broken families or families incapable of providing adequate care. In some cases, these include custodial treatment centers for alcoholics or drug addicts.

HOMES FOR AGED PERSONS. There are increasing numbers of residential centers for aged persons who cannot live independently or with their families, but who do not require intensive nursing or medical care, and can meet some of their own needs independently. These may include municipal, county or state homes for aged persons, residential centers sponsored by sectarian agencies or service organizations, or even low-income housing projects with special units for the aged.

CENTERS FOR PHYSICAL MEDICINE AND REHABILITATION. These are treatment centers for those who have suffered serious physical disability, but are no longer under treatment for the acute phase of their illness or injury, and are being given varied forms of physical, psychological, vocational and social rehabilitation to facilitate their return to their families and to community life.

PROGRAMS OPERATED BY PUBLIC RECREATION AND PARK DEPARTMENTS. Such agencies have traditionally concentrated their efforts on serving the nondisabled population of all ages with recreational activities and facilities. However, in recent years, many have initiated programs to serve the disabled—particularly the mentally retarded and physically handicapped.

PROGRAMS OF VOLUNTARY AGENCIES. A number of national organizations have been established to promote services for specific groups of handicapped children, youth or adults, such as the blind, deaf, cerebral palsied, physically handicapped or mentally retarded. Usually operating through county or local chapters, many of these organizations sponsor recreation programs specially designed to meet the needs of the disabled.

AFTER-CARE CENTERS AND SHELTERED WORKSHOPS. Particularly in the fields of mental illness, mental retardation and drug addiction, many organizations have established after-care centers, sheltered workshops, drop-in centers and similar facilities to provide multiservice programs to meet the needs of those who have been institutionalized and who need assistance in adjusting to the demands of community life. Frequently, such programs include recreational and social activities.

It is the function of all of these different types of agencies or institutions to provide therapeutic recreation service to meet the needs of the physically, mentally and socially disabled in our society.

Numbers and Types of Disabled in the United States

There have been varied attempts to classify and measure the number of disabled or handicapped persons in the United States. In 1966, the Social Security Administration carried out a study of noninstitutionalized, disabled adults. They found that there were 18 million people between the ages of 18 and 64 with some work limitation as a result of health conditions. The National Society for Crippled Children and Adults has estimated that one out of seven persons in the United States has a permanent physical disability. The total number of all persons who are chronically ill or disabled, or who suffer from emotional problems which prevent their successful functioning, has been calculated in excess of 40 million.

Drawn from several authoritative sources, the following statistics of populations in need of therapeutic recreation service are presented.[12] Obviously, in some categories, only a percentage of the overall population is in need of specially designed services, while in others, all of the individuals suffering from a particular disability are limited to the degree that they cannot function independently.

Aging	20,000,000
Mentally retarded	6,000,000
Mentally ill	9,000,000
Blind or visually impaired	1,000,000
Epilepsy	1,500,000
Orthopedically disabled	590,000
Cerebral palsy	600,000
Multiple sclerosis	500,000
Muscular dystrophy	200,000

[12] See, among others: *Annual Report of Title WI-A of the Elementary and Secondary Education Act for 1968.* Washington, D.C., Bureau of Education for the Handicapped, U.S. Office of Education, April, 1969; Helen Jo Mitchell and William A. Hillman, Jr.: "Disability and the Disadvantaged." *In* John A. Nesbitt, Paul D. Brown, and James F. Murphy, (eds): *Recreation and Leisure Service for the Disadvantaged.* Lea and Febiger, Philadelphia, 1970, pp. 190–198; and Ralph Treifel: *Rehabilitation of the Disabled.* Washington, D.C., Social Security Bulletin, Office of Research and Statistics, March, 1971, p. 3.

These are conservative estimates. In some sources, the number of mentally ill has been calculated at 18 million, and the number of those with cardiovascular disability as high as 10 million. There are other major categories which undoubtedly include large numbers of persons who are seriously disabled, either physically or socially, and who might require specially planned and guided recreation programs. These include those suffering from alcoholism, estimated at 6.5 million, and those with arthritis, estimated at 11 million persons. In many cases, individuals suffer from multiple disability. In a high percentage of cases in which there is a serious physical disability, the individual also has severe psychological problems as well, stemming from or relating to the other disability.

Although a high proportion of those with mental illness or social disability are institutionalized, the majority of those with physical disabilities or mental retardation live in the community with their families. A study carried on by the Social Security Administration revealed that only about seven per cent of all severely disabled persons in the United States were residents of long-term hospitals, special schools or homes.

Activities in Therapeutic Recreation Service

The provision of enjoyable leisure activities is *not* the sole focus of therapeutic recreation service. Obviously, there are elements that involve counseling, referral, a variety of other forms of personal assistance, and efforts with respect to developing community programs and cooperative arrangements among institutional and community groups. In many situations, the emphasis is not so much on *providing activities* as on developing a *social climate* or living situation in which the patient or disabled person can function with satisfaction and increasing social capability.

Pattison, for example, describes the "milieu therapy" approach, found in many psychiatric treatment settings today, in the following terms:

The thrust of milieu therapy is not to unlock specific psychodynamic conflicts but rather to provide integrating, guiding, rehabilitating social experiences. This begins with those socializing activities that the most regressed patients can participate in, then on to social activities requiring more ego control and personal-relatedness, and finally to reality-oriented social functions that are part and parcel of everyday living. Seen in this perspective, the adjunctive therapies are experiences in socialization and social interaction. The task of the adjunctive therapist is not that of individual therapist or extension thereof, but that of a social systems specialist.[13]

Similarly, in many community-based treatment centers or halfway houses that serve discharged mental patients, those attending day clinics, and others with psychiatric problems, recreation serves particularly as a means of helping individuals regain social competence and confidence. For example, in one halfway house:

. . . the club provides opportunities for mental patients, discharged patients, and persons under psychiatric care to participate in social rehabilitation programs, recreation, and other activities. Through this means, they can make social contacts, reestablish social adequacy, reorient social status, regain lost skills, and restore lost self-confidence . . . to make the gradual readjustment back into the mainstream of community life . . . .[14]

However, in the majority of settings that provide therapeutic recreation service, there is a strong emphasis on offering activities that *will* capture the interest of patients or other disabled persons, in which they can gain strong satisfactions and feelings of achievement, develop personal skills, spend time pleasurably and

benefit in the ways described earlier. Some of the major categories of activities include:

Social activities: parties, cards, discussion groups, bingo, clubs, informal game room or lounge programs.

Sports and active games: dual sports, such as golf, tennis, badminton, bowling, shuffleboard, horseshoes; team sports, such as basketball, volleyball, softball; and individual activities, such as skating, swimming or archery.

Entertainment: professional entertainment, or programs presented by community theatre groups, bands, orchestras or dance clubs; watching television, listening to radio, listening to records; films; patient talent shows.

Hobbies: various types of collections, such as stamps, coins or matchbooks; creative writing; ham radio; construction activities; bird-watching; cooking.

Arts and crafts: drawing, painting, sculpture; ceramics, leathercraft, weaving, print-making, jewelry work, macramé.

Performing arts: dramatics, instrumental music (learning to play instruments or taking part in bands or orchestras), choral music, ballet and modern dance.

Service activities: in a large hospital situation, being on the staff of a hospital radio station or newspaper, or assisting in the conduct of the recreation program.

Outdoor recreation: swimming and other water sports, picnicking, camping, nature study and group travel.

Motor activities: gymnastics, stunts and tumbling and other motor learning activities, particularly of a developmental nature, especially for the retarded or those with perceptual motor problems.

Special events: barbeques, carnivals, holiday celebrations, scavenger hunts, treasure hunts or progressive contests.

These and many other specialized activities may be found in therapeutic recreation programs. In hospitals with several hundred patients or more, the range of activities may be extremely diverse. By contrast, in nursing homes with only a small number of patients (many of whom may be in wheelchairs or confined to their beds), program activities are likely to be extremely limited.

[13] E. Mansell Pattison: "The Relationship of the Adjunctive and Therapeutic Recreation Services to Community Mental Health Programs." *Therapeutic Recreation Journal,* 1st Quarter, 1969, pp. 19–20.

[14] Jerry S. Hong, and Ralston S. Bauer: "Have You a Halfway House Program?" *Parks and Recreation,* November, 1966, p. 914.

History of Therapeutic Recreation Service

It is helpful, in analyzing the present role of therapeutic recreation service, to examine its historical background. Undoubtedly, prehistoric man discovered for himself, at an early point in his history, certain crude forms of treatment for his ills. Krusen writes that, at some time prior to the Paleolithic Age, probably before the year 7000 B.C.,

> . . . the first primitive man who crawled into the sunshine to receive benefit of its warmth and vitalizing effect unwittingly started the practice of heliotherapy; the first man who bathed a wound in some woodland stream unknowingly instituted the practice of hydrotherapy; and the first man who rubbed a bruised muscle unconsciously introduced massage.[15]

In most primitive societies, the approach to the treatment of illness was based on magical belief in the supernatural. Prehistoric man believed that everything in nature was alive with invisible forces and possessed supernatural powers. Disease was caused by evil spirits that entered the body, and many techniques were used to drive out these demons. Primitive man often sacrificed animals or human victims to heal the ill. He wore amulets to guard against evil spirits, and medicine men or witch doctors carried out detailed rituals intended to cure victims of disease.

Often, art, music, dancing, chanting and other expressive activities were used in this healing process. As an example, among the American Indian tribes of the Southwest, medicine men conduct an elaborate ceremony which goes on for days in a special medicine hut, involving chanting, the use of herbs, incense and the making of sand paintings with colored sand and crushed minerals—all as part of a highly secret process intended to cure the diseased.

In a sense, such elaborate rituals carried on by primitive and prehistoric man represented an early form of therapeutic recreation service. They demonstrate a fundamental truth—that many forms of illness are psychosomatic in nature rather than organic—and that many forms of treatment which have no medical base can be highly effective in healing illness.

Therapeutic Recreation in Pre-Christian Societies

History has recorded a number of references to the early use of therapeutic recreation in ancient societies.

For example, in ancient China, varied forms of medical gymnastics and massage were used as far back as 3000 B.C. These included free exercises which were combined with breathing, sitting, kneeling and lying and standing positions. The Chinese healing arts often included such magical practices as making sacrificial offerings, and frightening evil spirits by beating gongs and shooting off firecrackers. Avedon states that an ancient Chinese surgeon is reported to have used recreational activities for a variety of purposes. "In one instance he operated on a poisoned arrow wound in the arm of General Kuan Kung, while encouraging the General to use the unaffected hand in a table game."[16]

As early as 2000 B.C., Egyptian temples were established to treat the mentally ill by providing games and other pastimes. Priests were said to have been aware that healing was promoted by the beauty of the temple and its surrounding gardens, and the songs and dances of temple maidens. One source reports that:

> Patients . . . were required to walk in the beautiful gardens which surrounded the temples, or to row on the majestic Nile. . . . Dances, concerts, and comic representations were planned for them . . . .[17]

Similarly, in the Indian province of Kashmir during the second century B.C., a physician named Charaka is said to have advocated the use of toys and games to divert patients and promote their re-

---

[15] Frank H. Krusen: *Physical Medicine.* Philadelphia, W. B. Saunders, 1941, p. 9.

[16] K. C. Wong, et al.: *History of Chinese Medicine.* Tientsin, China, Tientsin Press, 1932, p. 37.

[17] W. A. F. Browne: *What Asylums Were, Are, and Ought to Be.* Edinburgh, A. and C. Black, 1837, pp. 141–142.

covery. Dock and Stewart describe Indian "professional musicians and storytellers who cheered and diverted patients by singing and by reciting poetry."[18]

In ancient Greece, the use of recreation became a more highly recognized technique in the treatment of the ill. The Greeks named their health temples Asklepiadas, after the highly revered god of healing, Asklepia. One of these temples was at Epidaurus, and was similar to a fashionable modern health resort. The temple was an architectural masterpiece, built on a high hill with an outstanding view. Under medical supervision, patients enjoyed scenic walks and exercise and massage in a gymnasium, diet, bathing in mineral waters, an outdoor theater and an extended program of treatment similar to that in a modern spa.

The Romans developed an elaborate system of therapeutic exercise under the leadership of the pioneer physician Galen, who lived in the second century A.D. He developed and classified exercises that improved muscle tone, such as digging, diving, carrying weights and rope-climbing, as well as others involving sparring, punching ball play and other movements. The Roman baths represented a remarkable advance in treatment approaches. The Baths of Caracalla in ancient Rome were tremendously expensive:

> . . . covering acres of land, they accommodated thousands of persons in the most grandiose manner. The spacious interior had high arched ceilings and was beautifully ornamented with marble and exquisite inlaid mosaics. There were auditoria, gymnasia, reading rooms, patios with cool foundations, soft music, and swimming pools to delight the patrons and provide diversional therapy.[19]

Therapeutic Recreation in the Middle Ages

Following the fall of the Roman Empire, the treatment of the mentally ill,

mentally retarded, crippled or other disabled persons tended to be extremely cruel and punitive.

It was thought that persons who suffered from such disabilities had been cursed by the gods. The mentally ill in particular tended to be treated like animals, chained and manacled, beaten and tortured to drive out their madness, or subjected to such devices as revolving beds or whirling cages to calm them.

Most institutions during the Middle Ages and well into the Renaissance period served chiefly to confine the seriously ill or disabled, and did little to uplift the spirits of patients. In a few hospitals, such as St. Catherine of Siena, or St. John's Hospital in Bruges, beautiful frescoes or paintings were displayed to provide diversion and improve the morale of the plague sufferers or lepers who were receiving care. However, well into the 18th century, most hospitals were dark, dismal and lacking in rehabilitative services.

Therapeutic Recreation in the 18th and 19th Centuries

Early in this period, most hospitals provided little real care; often they were little more than prisons. Dolan describes Newgate Prison of East Granby, Connecticut; this institution with a pathetic history of torture was the first colonial prison in Connecticut:

> Prisoners were not segregated according to sex, type of crime or mental condition; the mentally ill and mentally retarded shared quarters with the most vicious criminal. Screams were heard for quite a distance from the dungeons to which all inmates had to descend every night.[20]

Gradually, however, medical pioneers began to introduce new and innovative services. Dr. Benjamin Rush, a leading American physician who was on the staff of the Pennsylvania Hospital in Philadelphia in the 1780s, and who was shocked by the lack of care or comfort for the "lunatics" in this setting, fought for better

---

[18] Lavinia L. Dock, and Isabel M. Stewart: *A Short History of Nursing.* New York, G. P. Putnam and Sons, 1938, p. 26.

[19] Josephine A. Dolan: *The History of Nursing.* Philadelphia, W. B. Saunders Co., 1969, p. 59.

[20] *Ibid.,* p. 176.

hospital conditions and services. Dolan writes:

> . . . he called attention to the need for diversional therapy for psychiatric patients; for suitable companions to listen sympathetically to patients . . . for a plan for recreation and amusement; for personnel to direct these activities; and, lastly, to separate the mentally ill from those who were convalescing. . . .[21]

By the early 1800s, varied forms of therapeutic recreation had been introduced in a number of hospitals—particularly those serving psychiatric patients. In a description of the York Retreat, an English mental hospital in 1819, physicians were urged to involve patients in "regular employment" and "bodily exercise," and to interest them in activities that would confront them with reality and involve their emotions:

> . . . every effort should be made to divert the mind of melancholiacs by bodily exercise, walks, conversations, reading, and other recreations. Those who manage the insane should sedulously endeavor to gain their confidence and esteem, to arrest their attention and fix it on objects opposed to their delusions. . . .[22]

In other hospitals for the mentally ill in America and abroad, such activities were provided as: checkers, chess, backgammon, bowling, swinging, gardening, reading and writing. Mental patients were permitted to dance and engage in or listen to music, to take part in outdoor sports, to use "airing courts," rocking horses and a variety of other pastimes or forms of equipment.

One of the best examples of therapeutic recreation in a psychiatric setting was found in the Brattleboro, Vermont, Retreat, founded in 1836 as the Vermont Asylum for the Insane. An early description of this hospital made clear that "due provision has been made for the exercise, amusement, and employment of the pa-

tients." In addition to gardening and farming, there were many pastimes:

> Battle-door, chess, draughts, and the like amusements will be afforded. The females will be employed in knitting, needlework, painting, etc. Carriages will be provided for the daily riding of the patients in suitable weather, and they will also take daily walks with nurses and attendants. A small and select library . . . and several periodicals will be furnished for the purpose. . . .[23]

In addition to mental hospitals, other forms of treatment or custodial institutions gradually came into being in the United States during this period. Institutions were provided for the deaf in 1817, the blind in 1832, the mentally retarded in 1850, the crippled in 1867 and the epileptic in 1890. In many of these settings, varied forms of diversional activities began to be provided.

In military hospitals, a strong impetus was given to recreation by the great nursing pioneer, Florence Nightingale. In her text on nursing, published in 1873, she urged that nurses should pay attention not only to the patient's body but also to his mind and morale. She urged that music and conversation be encouraged, that beautiful objects be placed in patient wards, that the family be encouraged to visit and that patients keep small pets. Florence Nightingale was the first to introduce innovations such as furnished classrooms and instruction for soldiers, reading rooms, day rooms and recreation huts which have become an accepted part of military life. Under her leadership, so-called bedside occupations were introduced in military hospitals to cheer up injured soldiers.

The United States in the 20th Century

Soon after the entrance of the United States into World War I, the Red Cross began to provide recreation programs in

[21] *Ibid.,* p. 159.

[22] "Description of the York Retreat, 1819." Taken from *Biennial Report for 1950–52,* California State Department of Mental Hygiene.

[23] Ardis Stevens: "Recreation in Community Mental Health." *Therapeutic Recreation Journal,* 1st Quarter, 1971, p. 14.

hospital wards and convalescent homes. Recreation leaders were employed in a growing number of military and veterans' hospitals during the 1920s. It became more widely recognized that recreation— among other innovative rehabilitative techniques—was of value in reducing the length of the patient's stay in the hospital, and the extent and duration of his disability.

Gradually, federal laws, such as the Federal Vocational Rehabilitation Act of 1920, the Social Security Act of 1936 and the Barden–La Follette Act of 1942, provided for improved rehabilitation services for both children and adults in the United States.

Typically, during the 1920s public school systems began to offer special classes for disabled children, with special transportation. By 1929, there were a number of special public schools for the blind. In institutional settings during the 1920s and 1930s, the custodial approach to caring for disabled children shifted to a stronger emphasis on reeducation and reintegration of the disabled into community life.

Varied forms of rehabilitative services came into being. More and more, recreation emerged as one of these services. As a single example, at the Lincoln State School Colony in Illinois, a recreation department was established in June, 1929, in order to ". . . conduct a program of activities, consistent with the interests and abilities of mentally handicapped children . . . to serve as a substitute for former repressive measures of control." Increasingly, experiments were carried on with the mentally retarded, using various forms of play and play equipment, and more and more state and private institutions began to develop extensive recreation programs.

A number of national organizations took the lead in developing such services. For example, the Association for the Aid of Crippled Children began as early as 1900 to provide services for disabled children in their homes, in schools and in hospitals. It operated camps and summer programs for the disabled, and brought occupational therapy and similar modali-

ties into the homes of crippled children as a demonstration service, and as a means of parental education.

The growing recognition of the need for recreation for the disabled was demonstrated in the so-called Bill of Rights for the Handicapped that was drawn up at the White House Conference on Child Health and Protection in 1932. This statement called for:

> . . . a life on which his handicap casts no shadow, but which is full day by day with those things which make it worth while, with comradeship, love, work, play, laughter and tears—a life in which those things bring continually increasing growth, richness, a release of energies and joy of achievement.[24]

During World War II, there was a marked acceleration in the hospital recreation movement. Red Cross hospital recreation personnel increased to a high total of 1809 at the end of World War II, and, following the war, recreation programs in hospitals became a permanent part of peacetime Red Cross services to the armed forces. In 1945, the Veterans Administration founded a Hospital Social Services Division. This included Recreation Service, along with Canteen, Library, Chaplaincy and Voluntary Services; recreation personnel were assigned to all hospitals.

Extent of Therapeutic Recreation Service Today

During the 1950s, and 1960s, there was a steady expansion of therapeutic recreation services throughout the United States. While there has been no overall, comprehensive survey of the exact number of institutions or agencies providing services, several surveys *have* been carried out that give a picture of key aspects of the field.

1959 REPORT ON RECREATION IN HOSPITALS.   At the request of the Council for

---

[24] *The Handicapped Child, Report of the White House Conference on Child Health and Protection.* New York, D. Appleton-Century, 1933, p. 3.

Table 1–1. *Percentages of Responding Institutions Providing Recreation*[25]

BY AUSPICES	PERCENTAGE	BY TYPES OF SERVICE	PERCENTAGE
Veterans Administration	98.8	General	26.7
Military	81.7	Chronic disease	69.7
Public Health	49.0	Tuberculosis	90.7
State	89.3	Mental illness	98.0
County	32.0	Mental retardation	84.8
Municipal	24.6	Miscellaneous	64.7
Voluntary (nonsectarian)	35.0		
Voluntary (sectarian)	32.4		
Proprietary	27.0		
Miscellaneous	24.1		

the Advancement of Hospital Recreation, the National Recreation Association sponsored a national study on hospital recreation. This study gave a picture of the types of hospitals which provided recreation service, the number of personnel employed, the activities offered and similar information. Overall, it found that 42.4 per cent of the 3507 hospitals responding to the questionnaire had organized recreation programs.

Larger hospitals tended to have organized recreation programs, while smaller ones did not. Typically, 88.4 per cent of hospitals with 500 to 999 bed capacity offered recreation service, while only 48.7 per cent of hospitals with between 100 and 499 beds offered it. The study explained the pattern of varying recreation sponsorship among types of hospitals by pointing out:

. . . in these institutions, particularly in the state institutions devoted largely to mental illness and tuberculosis, the patients tend to stay for longer periods of time and, therefore, are in greater need of organized recreation activities. The higher percentage in the Veterans Administration hospitals is due to the fact that recreation is an integral part of the VA program and is established as one of the professional services in each hospital. The low percentage of organized recreation programs in municipal, propri-

etary and miscellaneous hospitals is probably due, at least in part, to the fact that most of these hospitals treat acute conditions. Patients remain in these institutions for a relatively short period of time, and the need for organized recreation programs is therefore not as obvious as in the institutions where the length of stay is longer.[26]

Many hospitals provided swimming pools, gymnasiums, auditoriums, athletic fields and special recreation rooms, although wards, solariums and day rooms were also used heavily for recreation. The most popular activities were: passive or mental activities, such as reading, radio, television-watching and movies (found in 86.4 per cent of the hospital); arts and crafts (72.5 per cent); social activities (61.0 per cent); musical activities (47.6 per cent); active games and sports (47.0 per cent); service activities (43.4 per cent); and nature and outing activities (33.2 per cent).

SURVEY OF COMMUNITY RECREATION SPONSORSHIP. In 1964, the National Recreation Association and the National Association for Retarded Children assisted Marson in carrying out a survey of 2000 community recreation departments to determine what community services were being provided for the mentally or physically disabled.[27] The 427 responding agencies indicated that they provided either recreation facilities or programs for the

[25] John E. Silson, Elliott M. Cohen, and Beatrice H. Hill: *Recreation in Hospitals: Report of a Study of Organized Recreation Programs in Hospitals and the Personnel Conducting Them.* New York, National Recreation Association, 1959, pp. 22–23.

[26] *Ibid.,* p. 20.
[27] Ruth Marson: *In* Morton Thompson: "The Status of Recreation for the Handicapped, as Related to Community and Voluntary Agencies." *Therapeutic Recreation Journal,* Vol. III, No. 9, pp. 20–23.

disabled. However, only 202 departments responded to a follow-up survey which sought fuller information.

In 139 communities, the mentally retarded were served separately in such facilities as playgrounds, community recreation centers, parks, swimming pools and day camps. In 164 cases, the physically handicapped were served separately, in similar facilities.

Program activities provided for disabled groups—chiefly children—consisted of activities very much like those enjoyed by the nonhandicapped: arts and crafts, games, picnicking, spectator sports and music. However, the variety of programs offered was quite limited. Only about one-third of the responding groups provided transportation assistance to disabled participants, and many special programs were supported financially by fees or contributions from parents or interested community groups. Marson concluded:

> Despite the tremendous growth of recreation, new developments in medical science and increased leisure for Americans, there has been a great lag in developing recreation services for the handicapped by community recreation departments. We believe that the next few years will show a marked increase in this service by communities.[28]

PLAY IN PEDIATRIC HOSPITALS. In 1968, Williams carried out a survey to determine the status of therapeutic play activities in pediatric hospitals or children's units in general hospitals.[29] Her questionnaire covered such elements as the extent of programs, nature of personnel responsible for them, activities offered and techniques used. Of the 48 hospitals surveyed, 46 (96 per cent) replied. Of these, 30 hospitals (65 per cent) indicated that they offered some form of supervised play programs.

In general, the responding hospitals indicated that they felt there was a need to provide play sessions to help relieve children of the anxiety associated with hospitalization—particularly in the preoperative period. However, the findings indicated that therapeutic play in children's hospitals was generally quite limited, and that there was a need to develop this field further and provide specialized training for workers in this field.

NATIONAL SURVEY OF SENIOR CENTERS. In 1969, the Institute for Interdisciplinary Studies of the American Rehabilitation Foundation published the report of a study of Senior Centers carried out by Anderson.[30] This survey was funded by the Administration on Aging, of the United States Department of Health, Education and Welfare. The final study report was based on findings from 1002 senior centers that responded to a long-form questionnaire, covering such topics as: the clientele served, types of programs and other services, budgets, facilities, staffing patterns, size of membership and relations with other community social or health agencies.

Anderson found that, despite the widespread attention recently given to the need for developing social and recreation programs for older Americans, these programs tended to be quite limited. First, it was apparent that, even if the active membership of these centers averaged as high as 150 to 200 active members each, this would mean that less than one per cent of the population in this age group throughout the country was actually served by senior centers. Fewer than half of the centers reported having full-time directors. Generally, their facilities were inadequate, and they operated with annual budgets that averaged $27,000—certainly not enough to provide the varied services needed by aging citizens in many communities.

In Section 304 of the Older Americans Act, Congress gave its strong support to:

> . . . the establishment of new or expansion of existing centers providing recreational and other leisure time activities, and information, health, welfare, counseling and re-

---

[28] *Ibid.,* p. 23.

[29] Yvonne Barnthouse Williams: "Therapeutic Play Services in Children's General Hospitals in the United States." *Therapeutic Recreation Journal,* 2nd Quarter, 1970, pp. 17–21.

[30] Nancy N. Anderson: *Senior Centers: Information from a National Survey.* Minneapolis, Minnesota, Institute for Interdisciplinary Studies, American Rehabilitation Foundation, 1969.

ferral services for older persons and assisting such persons in providing volunteer community or civic services. . . .[31]

The Anderson report makes clear the need to give stronger support to the development of multiservice senior centers throughout the country in order to meet these goals.

RECREATION SERVICE TO DISABLED CHILDREN. In 1971, Berryman, Logan and Lander, of the New York University School of Education, published a comprehensive report on recreation services provided to meet the needs of disabled children in a sampling of large metropolitan areas throughout the United States.[32] The findings were based on a three-year study

Table 1–2. *Percentage of Categories of Responding Agencies Providing Recreation for Children and Youth*[33]

AGENCIES	PERCENTAGE
Commercial and Proprietary Businesses	81
Churches, Libraries and Museums	82
County and Municipal Recreation and Park Departments	94
Fraternal and Service Organizations and Miscellaneous	87
Hospitals and Residential Schools	100
All Health Organizations	87
Private and Parochial School Districts	96
U.S. Department of Agriculture, County Extension Service, 4-H Clubs	92

financed by the Children's Bureau of the United States Department of Health, Education and Welfare. It explored several thousand potential sponsors of recreation services for disabled children and youth; a high percentage of these agencies were reported as providing such services.

An in-depth field study was carried out on 616 of these agencies. It was found that 88 per cent provided some recreation services to handicapped children and youth, although it was not made clear how extensive such services were. In general, those who were not serving the disabled felt that this was not expected of their agency, and that the lack of trained staff, or poorly designed facilities, would limit their effectiveness.

This extensive study of potential resources for serving disabled children pointed out: (a) the need to develop more programs integrating the disabled with the nondisabled; (b) the need to eliminate architectural barriers that keep the disabled from participating in community programs; and (c) the need for more specialized programs in hospitals and residential schools. Based on this Children's Bureau report, it is clear that many potential resources exist, but that program services need to be developed more fully.

RECREATION SERVING THE DISABLED IN MAJOR CITIES. In 1971, the Community Council of Greater New York carried out a study of administrative problems in recreation and parks, involving a sample of 80 cities with populations of 150,000 or over, throughout the United States.[34]

Table 1–3. *Percentage of Responding Municipal Recreation and Park Departments Offering Recreation for Disabled Groups*[35]

TYPES OF PROGRAMS OFFERED	PERCENTAGES OFFERING SERVICE
Programs for Aging Persons	89
Programs for Physically Disabled	67
Programs for Mentally Retarded	64
Drug Addiction Programs	19
Programs for Homebound Persons	8

[31] See *Older Americans Act of 1965* (Public Law 89-73), Section 304.

[32] Doris L. Berryman, Annette Logan, and Dorothy Lander: *Enhancement of Recreation Service to Disabled Children.* New York, New York University School of Education, Report of Children's Bureau Project, 1971.

[33] *Ibid.,* p. 16.

[34] Richard Kraus: *Urban Parks and Recreation: Challenge of the 1970's.* New York, Community Council of Greater New York, 1972.

[35] *Ibid.,* pp. 28–29, 81–82.

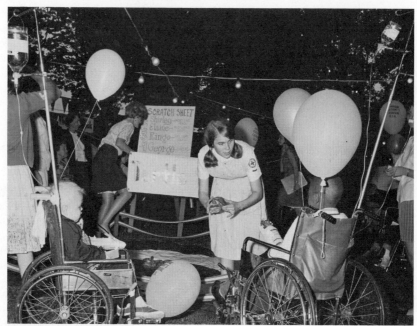

Children enjoy the annual patients' carnival at the National Institutes of Health Clinical Center, in Bethesda, Maryland.

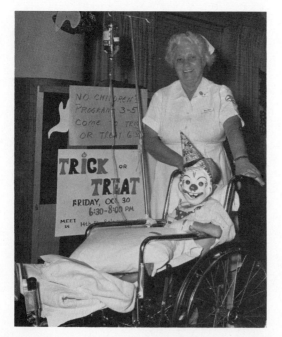

Halloween is party time for youngsters at the same institution.

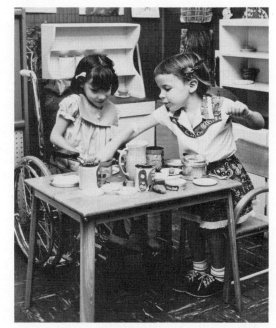

Children take part in creative play, with "pots and pans" . . .

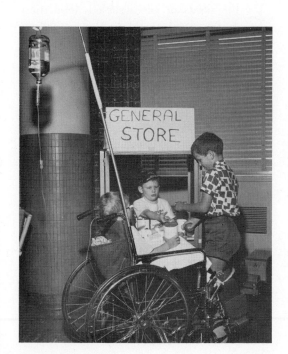

. . . and a "general store," at the federal hospital in Maryland.

Forty-five cities (56.2 per cent of the sample) participated in the study. A high proportion of these cities provided one or more forms of recreation service for special populations suffering from physical, mental or social disability.

The examples of such programs offered by large cities included: day camps for the mentally retarded, busing programs for the blind and aging, resident summer camps for the physically disabled, a "meals on wheels" program for the homebound, physical development and social activities programs for various disabled groups, after-care programs for discharged mental patients, and many similar types of services.

Despite these encouraging findings, it is apparent that therapeutic recreation service still needs to be developed much more fully, if it is to meet total community needs. In 1970, David Park wrote:

> If the public recreation program is to provide adequate recreation programs and resources for the *total population,* we must realize that there are significant numbers in our communities who will require special programs and it is the communities' responsibility to provide special programs for these special groups.[36]

A key problem in this area is that there is a marked communication gap between therapeutic recreation specialists and community recreation and park administrators. For example, Richard Stracke reported in 1969 the findings of a survey of 500 community recreation administrators in 40 states.[37] His report showed that only 18 per cent of the administrators had frequently worked or cooperated with therapeutic recreation specialists in providing services for the disabled. Seventy-four per cent of them felt that therapeutic recreation should *not* be confined to hospitals or institutions, and 84 per cent felt

that their communities had inadequate programs serving the disabled.

Overall, although a substantial proportion of municipal and county recreation and park departments now serve the disabled, it is clear that only a small proportion of those needing special services actually receive them. It has been estimated, for example, that public recreation and park departments in California provide services for only 3000 of the state's 130,000 disabled children. Undoubtedly, similar situations prevail elsewhere throughout the country. Indeed, no comprehensive studies have been done to determine the number or type of recreation programs in community mental health centers, correctional institutions and similar agencies. However, it would appear that such programs are few in number and limited in scope.

Promoting Therapeutic Recreation Service

What steps need to be taken to improve the provision of therapeutic recreation service, in both institutional and community settings?

AROUSING PUBLIC CONCERN. The great mass of people tend to be unaware of the needs of the disabled population, until they are brought to their attention. In some cases during the past few years, when budget cuts have resulted in inadequate programs in state institutions for the mentally retarded—with newspaper and television coverage of neglected children and adults in filthy, crowded wards—public concern has compelled immediate state action in restoring needed funds and hiring personnel for such institutions.

However, such efforts to arouse public concern and support must not be keyed only to crisis situations. There must be a fuller recognition of the needs of the mentally and physically disabled of all ages and in all settings. Every effort must be made to help those living in the community lose their fear or resentment of the disabled, and to accept them as human beings. In past centuries, the crippled and deformed or mentally ill were

---

[36] David C. Park: "Therapeutic Recreation: A Community Responsibility." *Parks and Recreation,* July, 1970, p. 25.

[37] Richard Stracke: "The Role of the Therapeutic Recreator in Relation to the Community Recreator." *Therapeutic Recreation Journal,* 1st Quarter, 1969, pp. 26–29.

shut up in custodial institutions—away from the public eye or conscience. Today, however, we have accepted the principle of total rehabilitation and involvement in community life, where possible, for the disabled. This implies the need for fuller social acceptance by the nondisabled, an area in which recreation and park services play a vital role.

DEVELOPING MORE EFFECTIVE PROGRAMS. There is a need for improved research and professional efforts to develop models of effective service, as well as the need to improve communication with related disciplines, such as medicine, social work or other rehabilitation fields.

Timothy Nugent points out the need for more therapeutic recreation professionals to become cooperatively involved in such large-scale programs as the National Wheelchair Games, which serve many thousands of disabled persons with track and field, archery, swimming, bowling and other forms of sports competition—all under the direction of laymen. More unified efforts with the general public, and with other recreation and park professionals, are vital to promoting the broad field of therapeutic recreation service, in Nugent's view.[38]

IMPROVING THERAPEUTIC RECREATION CURRICULA. A closely related area of concern is the need to develop more sharply defined programs of professional education in therapeutic recreation service in colleges and universities throughout the United States and Canada. Although a number of colleges now offer majors in therapeutic recreation service, the content in such programs varies widely, as do the opportunities for meaningful clinical experience or field placement, or the standards of training.

In the fields of occupational therapy or physical therapy, professional training is carried on in close cooperation with medical authorities or educators, and with the certification of practitioners approved on a statewide level under standards approved by medical societies. Although the

question of the degree of medical knowledge or orientation required by therapeutic recreation specialists is not fully resolved, it is clear that a more precise definition should be developed concerning the nature of required preparation for professionals in this field.

Closely attached to this area is the problem of upgrading Civil Service or other employment requirements in this field, and the elimination of nonqualified personnel in professional recreation positions.

DEVELOPING WORKING RELATIONSHIPS BETWEEN THERAPEUTIC AND COMMUNITY RECREATION PERSONNEL. In the past, when the bulk of therapeutic recreation was carried on in hospital settings, the need for improving the relationship between therapeutic recreation specialists and community recreation and park administrators was not as pressing as it is today. With the trends toward breaking up large state hospitals and other institutions and developing new, community-based, smaller facilities, and providing a variety of rehabilitation services within communities themselves, the relationship becomes more crucial. Under the present concepts of rehabilitation, in which every effort is made to keep individuals active within the community rather than hospitalize them, it is essential that community programs to serve the disabled or hospital-discharged individual be established.

Throughout the country, strong efforts have been made in this direction. Many state recreation and park societies include branches or sections concerned with therapeutic recreation service. Presently, many municipal recreation and park departments not only provide services for the disabled, or cooperate with other agencies that do, but also have employed therapeutic recreation specialists to head up their own programs.

EXPANDING GOVERNMENT SUPPORT OF THERAPEUTIC RECREATION SERVICE. Inevitably, it is more difficult and expensive to serve the disabled child, youth or adult than it is to serve nondisabled persons. The requirements of expanded or specially trained staff, modified or special facilities and transportation arrangements mean that the cost of providing thera-

---

[38] Timothy J. Nugent: "Research and Demonstration Needs for the Physically Handicapped." *Journal of Health, Physical Education and Recreation*, May, 1969, pp. 47–48.

peutic recreation is higher than that of meeting the needs of nondisabled participants.

Since this is the case, both the federal government and the individual states have contributed significantly in promoting therapeutic recreation programs on the local level. Typically, states have established demonstration programs, formed task forces to develop statewide plans, supported research and provided financial aid to meet the needs of disabled persons.

The federal government has been active in providing financial support for therapeutic recreation service, particularly in areas relating to mental retardation, the physically handicapped and, more recently, aging persons. For example, William Hillman points out that the President's Panel on Mental Retardation issued a report in October, 1962, that expressed considerable support for the recreation and leisure needs of the retarded, along with other high priority topics such as education, vocational preparation or institutional care. Whereas, in the past, recreation had been viewed as a "fringe" benefit, now, through the experiences of special educators and vocational counselors:

> . . . it was observed that failure to provide the retarded individual with adequate leisure skills often resulted in his failure to adjust in the community setting.[39]

As a consequence, subsequent federal legislation included numerous specific programs of financial support for recreation programs serving the retarded. The Division of Educational Services of the Bureau of Education for the Handicapped, of the United States Office of Education, provided substantial assistance to state-related

schools to enhance services to the disabled. The Division of Mental Retardation, now part of the Rehabilitation Services Administration of the Department of Health, Education and Welfare, has supported numerous recreation programs, including daytime activity centers for mentally retarded adults.

The Division of Training Programs of the Bureau of Education for the Handicapped has initiated a program, authorized by Public Law 90-170, for the training of physical educators and recreational personnel to work with mentally retarded and other disabled children. Other federal support has been given to universities exploring the role of play in the lives of the disabled, to demonstration programs, comprehensive state planning for the disabled, information centers on recreation for the disabled and a number of special college programs for training therapeutic recreation specialists. The Administration on Aging has given substantial support to university departments preparing administrative personnel for multi-service centers, consultants and researchers concerned with aging. Conferences have been held and publications issued to promote the modification of architectural barriers to permit use by the disabled. In numerous other ways, federal support has been given to therapeutic recreation service.

Obviously, it is not enough. As succeeding chapters will show, although there has been a tremendous growth in this field, with many outstanding programs now in operation throughout the country, great numbers of disabled individuals are still unserved. The entire field needs a sharper focus, a clearer identity, improved professional preparation and stronger processes of selection, and finally, a stronger level of local, state and federal support. This can only be accomplished when the rationale for therapeutic recreation service is thoroughly developed and understood.

---

[39] William A. Hillman, Jr.: "Federal Support of Recreation Services Related to Mental Retardation." *Therapeutic Recreation Journal,* 3rd Quarter, 1969, pp. 6–12.

Suggested Topics for Class Discussion, Examinations or Student Papers

1. Develop a meaningful definition of contemporary therapeutic recreation service, outlining its basic elements and the goals it seeks to accomplish.

2. Describe three distinctly different types of settings for therapeutic recreation service, showing how its objectives and program content vary according to the nature of the setting and the population group being served.
3. Propose several steps that need to be taken to strengthen therapeutic recreation service today, including such elements as public understanding and support of the field, the role of federal, state and municipal governments and professional preparation.

Chapter 2

The Rationale for Therapeutic Recreation Service

This chapter presents in detail a number of the underlying concepts, goals and values of therapeutic recreation service. It also clarifies its role within the total structure of rehabilitation service to the disabled today, and contrasts it with other treatment modalities.

It should be stressed that recreation is *not* solely of value to the emotionally or physically disabled. *All* persons have important needs for release, expression and involvement that may be met through satisfying leisure activity. Therefore, recreation must be viewed as therapy for the total range of the population, and as a vital preventative of illness, in that it helps to minimize emotional strains and keep the individual functioning in a healthy way. However, the focus of this text *is* on the use of recreation with persons suffering a significant degree of disability, who therefore have acute unmet needs and special problems.

In examining the use of recreation in institutional or community programs serving the disabled, the question of its value arises immediately. In past centuries, the United States has been so work-oriented in its prevailing philosophy of life, that we have paid little attention to recreation and leisure needs as a society. It is true that we have built a vast network of public and voluntary recreation agencies, and that we spend well over $100 billion a

year on recreational pursuits as a nation. However, we tend not to invest our play with an awareness of its serious social purpose.

Therefore, it is important to ask—as we examine the rationale for therapeutic recreation service—what support there is for this field. Do medical practitioners fully support recreation as part of the total treatment procedure?

These are particularly crucial questions because it is often difficult to determine precisely the effect of recreation service. Unlike surgery or drug treatments, which have measurable and predictable effects, recreation contributes to recovery, or to the individual's well-being, in more subtle and less tangible ways.

Views of Medical Practitioners

The strongest support to recreation as a form of rehabilitative service has come from psychiatrists who have seen diversional activities as useful in arousing the interest and improving the morale of the mentally ill. Over the past several decades, leading psychiatrists have given eloquent support to this field.

Dr. Menninger, codirector of the Menninger Clinic in Topeka, Kansas, Chief of Army Neuropsychiatric Services during World War II and past President of the

American Psychiatric Association, has vigorously supported the use of recreation. In a speech before the National Recreation Congress in 1948, he stated:

> It has been the privilege of many of us practicing medicine in psychiatry to have had some very rewarding experiences in the use of recreation as an adjunctive method of treatment. Along with direct psychological help, hydrotherapy, shock and insulin therapy, many of us have, for years, used various forms of education, recreation and occupation in the treatment of our patients. Within the American Psychiatric Association—a national organization of approximately 4,500 psychiatrists—we have a standing committee on leisure time activities (based on) the assumption that professional recreation experience can contribute to psychiatric practice, and psychiatrists can add to the knowledge of professional recreation workers.[1]

Menninger stressed the value of recreation, not only in the treatment program of mental patients but also in helping former patients to remain well. He outlined three key psychological needs that can be met for many individuals through recreation: (a) competitive games as an outlet for instinctive aggressive drives; (b) creative activities in art, music or literature as a release for erotic drives; and (c) entertainment activities as a means of providing relaxation and vicarious involvement.

He pointed out also that a conspicuous symptom of many persons who are mentally ill is their inability to feel comfortable with others, or to identify with and belong to a social unit. The process of gradually helping a patient become re-socialized is readily carried on within group recreational activities, such as parties, ball games, square dances or dramatic productions. Menninger wrote:

> Some very concrete evidence of the relation between avocations and mental health was revealed in a survey made at our clinic some years ago. A group of well-adjusted individuals was surveyed as to the type,

number and duration of their hobbies. The findings we compared to those from a similar survey of a group of psychiatric patients. In the well-adjusted group, both the number and the intensity of the pursuit of hobbies was far in excess of those of the patients. This cannot be interpreted to mean that, because the individual has a hobby, it necessarily keeps him well. It does mean, however, that a well-adjusted individual learns how to play and does include play as an important feature of his life, much more frequently than does the average maladjusted person.[2]

A second leading psychiatrist and former President of the American Psychiatric Association, Alexander Reid Martin, took a deep interest in the relationship between leisure behavior and mental health. He pointed out that many otherwise highly successful individuals are unable to deal effectively with leisure in their private lives. Often, they are compulsively driven by work. Martin wrote:

> Psychiatry has an extensive and intensive interest in leisure because, in most instances of psychoses and neuroses, the earliest and most unamenable signs and symptoms are disturbances in natural recreative functioning. They include sleeplessness, inability to relax, so-called nervous and mental tension, fear of leisure, and the compulsive need to keep going. Furthermore, the *first signs of recovery are shown in a return to natural recreative functioning.* Improvement is never revealed as clearly in the patient's attitude toward work as it is in his attitude toward leisure and relaxation and in the free play of his body, mind, and feelings, that is, in the free play of his whole personality.[3]

Probably the most eloquent spokesman of the need for recreation in promoting mental health generally, as well as in the treatment of psychiatric patients, has been Paul Haun. Haun was a leading authority on hospital design, both for the Veterans

---

[1] William C. Menninger: "Recreation and Mental Health." *Recreation,* November, 1948, p. 340.

[2] *Ibid.,* p. 343.

[3] Alexander Reid Martin: "Professional Attitudes and Practices." *In Recreation for the Mentally Ill.* Washington, D.C., Conference Report, American Association for Health, Physical Education and Recreation, 1958, p. 15.

Administration and a number of major state mental health systems, and taught psychiatry in a number of outstanding universities and medical colleges. His view of play was that it represented an essential aspect of healthy life, and constituted a natural rhythmic alternative to work.

In making a "medical case" for recreation, Haun wrote:

> It provides patients and appropriate staff members with many familiar social roles through which pleasant and accustomed expressive interaction can occur. It affords the patient a physiological escape from somatic pain and disruptive emotional experiences. It capitalizes upon and supports the non-pathological elements of his personality. It constitutes a path by which he may return from the malignant equilibrium of defensive withdrawal, first to the make-believe universe of the play world and then, after finding this tolerable, to the yet tighter existence of prosaic day-to-day existence. It offers a gratifyingly wide opportunity for instinctual discharge in socially acceptable channels without the need for complicated sublimations.[4]

Haun concluded that, when competently administered and skillfully presented in a hospital environment, recreation was able to encourage the timid patient, disarm the aggressive, motivate the lethargic, calm the restless and divert the melancholic. For these reasons, he supported it strongly as an important element in psychiatric treatment.

A similar statement of support was made by Robert H. Felix, a leading psychiatrist for over 30 years and Director of the National Institute of Mental Health. He commented that the problem of filling leisure with satisfying activity is particularly acute in many mental hospitals simply because many patients have so much free time. However, beyond this, Felix believed that recreation serves as a "great healing force" in providing a means by which leisure can be molded to promote physical and psychological well-being:

> The greatest value of recreation is that it can be prescribed as a definitive therapeutic treatment. Particularly in the field of psychiatry . . . recreation plays a positive role in the care and treatment of the mentally ill. Because the activities included in recreation programs usually require some degree of skill and concentration, recreation allows the patient to lose himself in the activity at hand, giving his mind a rest from the mental and physical problems that beset him. It provides a controlled outlet for the release of tensions that otherwise might be directed inward or toward others. It offers a means whereby the patient can acquire and put into practice new knowledge about himself. And recreation helps morale by giving the individual a feeling of satisfaction and accomplishment at having mastered some small skill or compensated for a handicap.[5]

Felix stressed that recreation provides the individual with an opportunity to function independently, while at the same time encouraging him to function in harmony with other human beings. He concluded that recreation contributes significantly to the "more rapid physical, mental and social rehabilitation of the patient" and thus has come to be recognized as a clinically-oriented discipline, acknowledged by other branches of the medical and health professions.

A leading heart research specialist, Dr. Joseph B. Wolffe, formerly president of the American College of Sports Medicine and Medical Director of the Valley Forge Medical Center and Heart Hospital, reported on the specific contribution of recreation in the treatment of patients suffering from acute thrombosis, congestive heart failure and allied illnesses:

> A survey of 1,000 patients has shown that carefully selected recreation to suit the patient's problem and personality resulted in reduction both in drug requirements as well as length of hospital stay, when compared to the control group in the institution without the program.[6]

[4] Paul Haun: *Recreation: A Medical Viewpoint.* New York, Teachers College, Columbia, Bureau of Publications, 1964, p. 52.

[5] Robert H. Felix: Preface to *Recreation in Treatment Centers,* September, 1962, p. 3.

[6] Joseph B. Wolffe: *The Doctors and Recreation in the Medical Setting.* Raleigh, North Carolina, North Carolina Recreation Commission, 1962, p. 19.

It was found that a special activity program resulted in lessening drug requirements for various types of patients from 30 to 50 per cent, and actually shortened their hospital stay by approximately 15 per cent. As an example, Wolffe points out that in the treatment of neurocirculatory asthenia, a reduction of 35 per cent in the need for sedatives and tranquilizers was noted, as a consequence of a carefully planned patient recreation program.

The value of therapeutic recreation in the field of physical medicine and rehabilitation has been affirmed by Dr. Howard A. Rusk, Director of the Institute of Physical Medicine and Rehabilitation of the New York University-Bellevue Medical Center in New York City. An internationally known authority in the rehabilitation of the physically disabled, Rusk stressed the need for patients to become involved in their own rehabilitation, and in achieving greater emotional, vocational and social self-sufficiency. He asked:

> What good does it do for a chronically disabled person to learn to walk again if he is so withdrawn and fearful that he will not leave his home? For a handicapped child to realize his highest potential for physical functioning if his emotional and social growth is stunted in the process? For a post-psychiatric patient to be vocationally rehabilitated but unable to make further progress toward healthy social interaction with others?[7]

Rusk pointed out that in rehabilitation centers disabled children spend a great deal of time following directions for ambulation and self-care exercises. Often, the recreation session gives them their only opportunity for independent action, with a minimum of adult direction, that will be helpful in achieving social and emotional maturity. Rusk was one of the first authorities to stress the need for providing recreation counseling that would help discharged patients achieve full social independence following their return to community life.

Summarizing these statements, it is apparent that leading medical practitioners strongly recognize and support the need for recreation in hospital settings. There *is* continuing disagreement among some doctors as to whether recreation ought to be regarded as a specific form of therapy and, therefore, provided on an individualized, prescriptive basis—a controversy discussed later in this chapter. However, there is widespread agreement that it does contribute significantly to the total process of recovery.

In part, this recognition comes from an awareness of the value of recreation as an important element in the healthful living of *all* persons.

Recreation's Contribution to Healthful Living

Increasingly, we have come to recognize that all people need a degree of release, and the opportunity to fulfill certain fundamental drives, if they are to function effectively. The very concept of health implies far more than physical well-being alone. The Preamble to the Constitution of the World Health Organization states: "Health is a state of complete physical, mental and social well-being and not merely an absence of disease or infirmity."

To attain this state of well-being, it is necessary to achieve a harmonious relationship between work and recreation. Recreation represents the opportunity for refreshment of mind, body and spirit. Meyer points out that it is the time we pause, change our pace and recover our energies, in order to face the strains and demands of a mechanized and competitive society. He writes:

> The physiological concept of "stroke" and "glide" for the harmonious performance of any body organ applies equally to the total body operating as a synchronized machine in the execution of any task requiring the expenditure of energy. The "stroke" is the thrust, the "glide" the recovery. Our whole life is a continuous "stroke" and "glide" and psychologically the "stroke" is our work phase, our vocational pursuit, and the "glide" our recreation, our recovery. The harmonious relationship between work and

---

[7] Howard Rusk: "Therapeutic Recreation." *Hospital Management,* April, 1960, pp. 35–36.

recreation is essential for . . . good mental health.[8]

This does not mean that recreation provides only relaxation. Particularly for those workers whose job is boring or monotonous, or makes few physical demands, recreation may provide a challenge that is far more demanding or exciting than work. For example, many individuals become far more involved and committed in their play than in their jobs. Few individuals would accept, as part of their job, the physical training and self-discipline required of college varsity swimmers or crew members, or put up with the weekly battering that a football player receives. Even the commitment of spectators in many forms of entertainment is often so great that it is not uncommon for sports fans to have cardiac seizures at major sports events. Few office workers get heart attacks because of the strain of their day-by-day jobs.

Hans Selye, a physician who has done outstanding research and written extensively on the concept of stress, points out that it is a mistake to assume that rest and relaxation are necessarily desirable:

> . . . simple rest is no cure-all. Activity and rest must be judiciously balanced, and *every person has his own characteristic requirements for rest and activity.* To lie motionless in bed all day is no relaxation for an active man. . . . Many a valuable man, who could still have given numerous years of useful work to society, has been made physically ill and prematurely senile by the enforcement of retirement at an age when his requirements and abilities for activity were still high. This psychosomatic disease is so common that it has been given a name: *retirement disease.*[9]

Selye points out that one of the most fundamental laws regulating the activities of complex living beings is that no one part of the body must be disproportionately overworked for a long period. Stress serves as an equalizer of activities within the body; it helps to avoid one-sided exertion. It is necessary to achieve balance in the full range of activities, if sound health is to be maintained.

Recreation can make an important contribution in helping individuals meet their total psychological and social needs. There have been many analyses of these needs, and they have been widely described in the literature.

In a study of personality drives, Abraham Maslow suggested that human needs begin at a basic level related to maintaining existence or survival, and that when these needs are satisfied, the individual moves on to progressively newer and higher levels of need. For example, the primary needs are for *physiological* well-being, based on maintaining adequate nutrition, freedom from the elements, avoidance of illness and similar threats to health. The second level of human need is based on the need for *safety,* which Maslow characterizes as security, stability, freedom from fear or chaos—the need for structure, order and law. People normally prefer a safe, orderly, predictable and organized world.

Maslow points out that when both physical and safety needs are fairly well met, the individual will next require love and *affection:*

> He will hunger for (affectionate) relations with people in general . . . and will strive with great intensity to achieve this goal. He will feel sharply the pangs of loneliness, of ostracism, of rejection, of friendlessness, of rootlessness.[10]

On the next level, most people in society have a need or desire for a stable, firmly based and high evaluation of themselves, which Maslow refers to as *self-esteem.* This is closely related to the desire for strength, adequacy, a sense of mastery and competence, the capacity for independent action and recognition or appreciation from others. Following the satisfaction of the physical, safety, love and esteem needs, Maslow contends that there

[8] Martin W. Meyer: "The Rationale of Recreation as Therapy." *Recreation in Treatment Centers,* September, 1962, p. 23.

[9] Hans Selye: *The Stress of Life.* New York, McGraw-Hill Book Co., 1956, p. 265.

[10] Abraham Maslow: *Motivation and Personality.* New York, Harper and Row, 1970, pp. 35–50.

are significant needs for individual *self-actualization,* for satisfying the urge to *know and to understand* and, finally, *aesthetic needs.*

Within this context, it is easy to see how recreation provides a varied and rich opportunity to meet significant human psychological needs. Within our society, there are numerous examples of how such needs are not being met, and how their deprivation causes serious effects on individual well-being.

The problem of human loneliness offers one such example. Even in a crowded society, many individuals lead lives of great loneliness. An Ohio State professor of psychiatry, John Whieldon, has found that loneliness is not so much an active phenomenon as a void—the incapacity to develop meaningful relations with others. He writes:

> One of the basic processes of childhood is to resolve one's loneliness. To do this, everyone must learn to make meaningful emotional contact with others.[11]

The lonely person, Whieldon believes, has never learned to do this, or has lost the capacity for it. As a consequence, he falls back on a variety of defenses, such as sexual promiscuity, daydreaming, tantrums, narcissism, hyperactivity or the "last defense"—schizophrenia. Numerous studies with laboratory animals have indicated the damaging effects of social isolation. Monkeys and dogs which have been deprived of mothering or of social companionship at an early age typically become unable to relate to others and are highly neurotic in their behavior. Typically, in one study, puppies which were raised in complete isolation wound up as either withdrawn and indifferent, or overactive, snapping viciously, screaming hysterically and pacing aimlessly.

The obvious value of recreational pursuits in overcoming the problem of loneliness and isolation is clear. Most leisure activities are carried on in group settings and, from earliest childhood, it is possible to encourage participation in play groups, clubs, teams or musical or theater organizations that help youngsters develop the capacity for relating to others.

Tension, strain and boredom are also important characteristics of modern life. Recent research has indicated that about one person out of every four in the United States is using sedatives or tranquilizers today. In some occupational groups or social classes today, the incidence of strain and tension is such that serious social and familial breakdown occurs at a high rate of frequency. In the aerospace industry, for example, although workers have all the accouterments of success, such as prestigious jobs, high salaries and fine homes, there is a great sense of rootlessness, job insecurity, a lack of involvement in community life or meaningful social relationships and a high rate of both alcoholism and marital break-up. Some have predicted that these problems will become increasingly widespread throughout our society as it becomes more and more technologically oriented.

The challenge to American family structure is becoming more and more acute. Margaret Mead asks: "Can the family survive? Students in rebellion, the young people living in communes, unmarried couples living together, call into question the very meaning and structure of the family unit as our society has known it."[12] One of every four American marriages now ends in divorce, and in some West Coast communities, the rate is running as high as 70 per cent.

While there are many causes for this accelerating breakdown, such as the reduction in meaningful roles assigned to the family in our society, one important factor seems to be the lack of opportunity for families in urban and suburban communities to share meaningful social contacts and group involvements. Urie Bronfenbrenner, a noted psychologist and authority on family life, comments:

> We just do not try hard enough to involve the different ages with each other. When

[11] John Whieldon: *In* "A Study of Those 'Blues' That Start in Loneliness." *New York Post,* June 5, 1964, p. 77.

[12] Margaret Mead: *In* "The American Family: Future Uncertain." *Time,* December 28, 1970, p. 34.

an American architect plans a housing project, he puts the playgrounds here so that the noise doesn't bother, and the parents have another park there. The European architect does it the other way. He plans the playgrounds so that the children can run over and see the parents and the parents can watch them. Or look at different societies in terms of their games. I'm for the revival of potato-sack racing because anyone can do it, and if Grandpa beats the three-year-old it's a great victory. . . .[13]

What all this suggests is that many of our psychosocial problems in modern society stem from a sense of lack of involvement and physical release, from boredom and from the unfulfilled need for meaningful social contact. Boredom in modern life is an important and enduring problem. Sociologists have pointed out that people who have to work for long periods at repetitive tasks often complain of being bored and dissatisfied with their lives; frequently their performance declines sharply. Excessive boredom, induced experimentally, results in irritability, blank periods, lost of memory and even hallucination.[14]

As a single example of the kinds of social problems that may arise because of the unmet need for meaningful involvement and personal expression, one might point to the high incidence of alcoholism cited earlier. In a study of motivations for drinking, Riley, Marden and Lifshitz found that Americans drank for such reasons as: "to be sociable," "because all of our friends drink" or "to be a good sport." They conclude that drinking, at least until the point where it becomes a compulsive and destructive act, is carried on "for relaxation or for euphoric effect . . . as an escape from worries, responsibilities and frustration. . . ."[15]

Indeed, many forms of play or leisure activity represent self-destructiveness or harmful release of neurotic drives. Paul Haun has written extensively on so-called pathological play.[16] In one form, an individual whose hate is self-directed may strive desperately *not* to win, and may seek defeat, failure or even physical injury as a deserved punishment for feelings of guilt or personal crime. Beyond this, Haun saw play being distorted as a means of blotting out or resisting reality.

He described a number of forms of play which are extremely violent or dangerous, and which afford almost completely unsublimated release for primitive drives, lending themselves "with exceptional ease to sadistic, masochistic, and compulsive distortion by the participant." Some of these types of play occupy a kind of twilight zone, slipping back and forth between pathology and wild adventure, such as speedboat and automobile racing, reckless mountain climbing, bullfighting or fencing with unprotected weapons. Others are completely pathological in their self-destructive potential:

> . . . the most notorious example being that of "Russian Roulette," which is played by spinning the cylinder of a revolver containing a single round of live ammunition, placing the muzzle of the gun at one's temple and pulling the trigger. Another example is the game of "Chicken," in which two contestants drive their automobiles toward each other at the highest possible speed on the same highway lane. The first to weaken and swerve out of the path of certain destruction is said to lose in this singular display of immaturity—and is accordingly labeled "chicken". . . .[17]

Such examples reveal the ways in which play may serve as a release for harmful or self-destructive drives. In contrast, there are many forms of play that serve as a healthy and constructive means of maintaining emotional balance and preventing neurosis. As a single example which has become increasingly popular in recent years, one might cite the hobby of "back-packing" in the wilderness set-

---

[13] Urie Bronfenbrenner: *In* "The American Family: Future Uncertain." *Time,* December 28, 1970, p. 37.
[14] Woodburn Heron: "The Pathology of Boredom." *Scientific American,* January, 1957, pp. 52–56.
[15] John W. Riley, Jr., Charles F. Marden, and Marcia Lifshitz: *In* Eric Larrabee, and Rolf Meyersohn: *Mass Leisure.* Glencoe, Illinois, The Free Press, 1958, pp. 327–333.

[16] Paul Haun: *op. cit.,* p. 26.
[17] *Ibid.*

ting. This has become an enthusiastic interest of great numbers of Americans of all ages and walks of life; it has been estimated that, in recent years, no fewer than 20 million Americans have taken up this hobby. In part, the interest in wilderness hiking stems from a desire to get away from the artificiality and tension of city life. In part, it comes from the need to meet direct physical challenge, and to find out what one is capable of doing and not doing.

Supreme Court Justice William O. Douglas has commented:

> Hiking or walking is man's most natural exercise. We were biological beings before our intellectual or spiritual powers matured. The cells and protoplasm, the blood vessels and tissues, the muscular and circulatory systems have not changed since the days of the cave man. The veneer of progress and civilization is a thin one. The intellectual man and spiritual man can dominate the animal man. But the animal man needs constant renewal. His health is indeed a prerequisite to complete well-being. . . . The subconscious carries a heavy burden of our worries, concerns and problems. On a long hike it functions free of additional tensions and pressures. And somehow or other it seems to unravel many a tangled skein of problems during a six-to-eight hour hike. The process is a mystery, though I have experienced it again and again.[18]

It is apparent that for many persons who are not ill or disabled in any serious or permanent way, recreation serves to meet important psychosocial and physical needs. It may be constructively used, or, when not understood and dealt with intelligently, may provide an outlet for harmful or dangerous drives that can result in great damage to the individual. For these reasons, it is essential that *all* individuals be aware of their leisure needs and behavior, and that full opportunity be provided in the community at large for varied, creative and constructive recreational participation.

However, this problem is obviously far more acute for the ill or handicapped person than for those who do not suffer from any form of disability.

Recreational Needs of the Disabled

As indicated earlier, the term "disability" is today regarded as preferable to "handicap," because it stresses the concept of disability, which is a reality and may be overcome, rather than that of handicap, which has a negative connotation in our society. In this text, the term "disability" is used throughout, except in quotations from the past, or titles of organizations or projects which continue to make use of the term "handicap."

A statement formulated by the 1960 White House Conference on Children and Youth defines the "handicapped" child as one who ". . . cannot play, learn, work or do the things other children his age can do; or is hindered in achieving his full physical, mental and social potentialities; whether by a disability which is initially small but potentially handicapping, or by a serious impairment involving several areas of function with the probability of life-long impairment."[19]

Disability may be mild or total, single or multiple, and may affect persons of every age, socioeconomic condition, race, religion or region. As described in Chapter One, it has been estimated that as many as 40 million persons suffer from some fairly severe disability in American society. When one recognizes that for each such person, there is also a family unit involved in the problem, it is apparent that meeting the total needs of disabled persons and helping them fit as successfully as possible into the total society represent crucial concerns in the United States and Canada today.

During the past several decades, there has been a radical shift in public concern about the disabled. Social work agencies today provide a variety of welfare services in community settings, youth houses, hos-

[18] William O. Douglas: "Animal Man Needs to Hike." *New York Times Magazine,* March 21, 1965, pp. 34–35.

[19] *Conference Proceedings.* White House Conference on Children and Youth. Washington, D.C., p. 381.

pitals and residential centers for the disabled. The accent today has shifted to constructive, rehabilitative approaches in many of the most enlightened states.

To a large degree, the public has also shifted in its attitudes toward the disabled in society. In past centuries, the physically or mentally disabled were often seen as persons who had been cursed by the gods. Often they were cruelly rejected, hidden, ridiculed or even, in some cases, disposed of. We have not *totally* overcome these attitudes, either in the United States or elsewhere in the world. In a three-year study of attitudes toward the disabled, two German psychologists, Jansen and Esser, questioned several thousand adults and school-age children regarding their feelings toward disabled persons. They found a high incidence of continuing prejudice and aversion. Ignorance appeared to be a major obstacle to social contact with the disabled; those questioned did not seem to know how to approach them, or deal with them realistically.

Jansen and Esser summarized their findings:

> Although many of those questioned spoke sympathetically of their attitudes toward the handicapped . . . often they felt revulsion . . . few wished to be friends with them, or to marry one . . . most (63 per cent) thought that severely disabled persons should be kept out of sight in institutions; while none recommended that they deserved to die, openly, actually some spoke carefully of the merits of euthanasia. . . .[20]

It is apparent that many prejudices toward the disabled have not totally disappeared. Many people still have feelings that range from excessive pity (which overprotects the disabled person and makes him less likely to make independent efforts in his own behalf) to outright rejection and even fear.

However, by and large, the view is becoming more widely accepted that disabled persons are in many ways like everybody else, with important physical, social and emotional needs that must be met if they are to reach their fullest potential as human beings. In many ways, the federal and state governments have moved vigorously to promote total rehabilitation of the disabled.

Programs of vocational rehabilitation expanded steadily in the 1960s. Federal support was given to research and personnel training, and to the development of new facilities to serve the disabled. Demonstration projects were widely supported, dealing at first with the physically disabled and later extended to retardation, mental illness, alcoholism, drug addiction, public offenders and disabled persons who are socially and culturally disadvantaged. According to Joseph Hunt, Commissioner of the Rehabilitation Services Administration (established in 1968 under the newly organized Social and Rehabilitation Service of the Department of Health, Education and Welfare), over 207,000 persons were rehabilitated in a single year, 1968, with over 680,000 persons being served by various federal programs.[21] Within this total context, recreation has become an increasingly recognized area of service for the disabled.

What is the specific justification for providing special therapeutic recreation service in community life? The answer is twofold.

1. Like all people, the disabled have a right to self-expression, social involvement, creative experience and the other important values that can be provided by recreation. They are human beings, and they and their families are taxpayers; thus, they should be served fully by public agencies in this field of service. This principle is illustrated by a statement in the "credo" of the American Recreation Society, about the obligation of professional recreators:

> That recreation is of, and for, all the people; and that therefore the purpose of [this] profession should be to administer Recreation as a public trust, so as to multiply

---

[20] "Hostility to the Handicapped." *Time,* Dec. 20, 1971, p. 67.

[21] Joseph Hunt: "A Decade of Progress." *Journal of Rehabilitation,* January-February, 1969, p. 9.

opportunities for happiness regardless of age, race, sex, creed, or condition in life.[22]

2. The second principle is that many disabled individuals find most aspects of "normal" life, such as the opportunity to complete their education, marry and have a family, enter a profession and earn a livelihood or travel freely, closed to them. For this reason, recreation represents a particularly crucial need. If it is not provided, their lives are cruelly barren and empty. The author has pointed out elsewhere:

> Those who suffer from disability . . . frequently find difficulty in meeting their recreative needs in constructive and varied ways, in part because serious physical handicaps obviously limit the extent of participation. . . . Much recreative deprivation of the disabled is, however, caused by the reluctance of society to permit them to engage in activity to the extent of their real potential. Sometimes communities or recreation agencies do not make the kinds of adaptations in the design of facilities needed for disabled persons to use them fully. Sometimes recreational and park agencies actively bar disabled persons from their programs because they feel that to serve them would require specialized leadership to a degree they could not afford.[23]

Frequently, park and recreation administrators fear that the presence of blind, retarded or orthopedically handicapped individuals might be distasteful to the public at large. Sometimes parents or relatives shelter disabled people excessively, and sometimes they are barred from recreational participation by their own lack of skill or fear of rejection by others. Whatever the reason, many disabled persons are therefore unable to make use of available community recreation resources.

The problem of acceptance in community life is particularly difficult for those who are visibly disabled. Those who suffer from a severe physical disability or crippling deformity are acutely aware of the reactions of others, the threat of social isolation and the direct limitations that are imposed, in terms of one's capability for full and varied social involvement. Wright points out that while physical limitations themselves may cause frustration or suffering, the more serious deprivation comes from the attitudes of others:

> One of man's basic strivings is for acceptance by the group, for being important in the lives of others, and for having others count positively in his life. As long as physical disability is linked with shame and inferiority, realistic acceptance of one's position and one's self is precluded.[24]

The task of gaining acceptance for the disabled in community settings is primarily a matter of helping the public come to grips with its own attitudes about the disabled, and to perceive them in a more accurate light. Wright points out that people with disabilities are frequently considered to be compensating when they are merely interested in an activity; they may be regarded as showing a sense of inferiority, when they are merely hesitating before committing themselves to an activity because of a realistic awareness of their own limitations. Thus, it becomes extremely important that our attitudes in general about the disabled be based on an intelligent comprehension of their needs and capabilities rather than on stereotyped and distorted attitudes.

This is particularly true with respect to the attitudes of families toward disabled members of the family unit. As pointed out earlier, relatives frequently tend to be overprotective, and unconsciously limit the extent to which such individuals may strike out independently. A study carried out at the University of Pennsylvania, under a grant from the Social and Rehabilitation Service of the Department of Health, Education and Welfare, suggested that society sometimes has a vested interest in having its members remain disabled:

[22] "Credo for the Recreation Profession." American Recreation Society.

[23] Richard Kraus: *Recreation and Leisure in Modern Society.* New York, Appleton-Century-Crofts, 1971, pp. 364–365.

[24] Beatrice Wright: *Physical Disability: A Psychological Approach.* New York, Harper and Row, 1960, p. 14.

The disabled handicaps the family unit in many ways, most obviously economically and socially. Within the unit, the members attempt, with varying degrees of success, to "negotiate" a satisfying relationship. . . . Despite the sympathy that such a setup might draw from society . . . the interplay of dependent and helper often satisfies the deeper psychological needs of each individual, often retarding the handicapped person's rehabilitation.[25]

In this study, it was found that the disabled person typically was not an independent entity but rather the hub of a complex set of family relationships that in effect creates a "disabled family." It was found that both the family and the larger society "use" the disabled, symbolically, to meet psychological needs and therefore are ofen reluctant to have them move toward true independent functioning.

Both for the sake of the disabled themselves, and in the interest of their families and the larger society, it is essential that disabled persons be enabled to become as independent as possible in terms of their social and recreational lives.

It is at this point that the interests of institutional or treatment centers, and community-based recreational and social agencies coincide. Both must be dedicated to returning disabled persons to the community with skills and attitudes that will permit them to function as happily and effectively as possible within a broad range of relationships and interpersonal spheres. Within the past decade, there have been major shifts in the organization of health and rehabilitation agencies that have focused on the need to integrate the disabled as fully as possible in community life.

This has led to the fundamental concept that therapeutic recreation cannot be viewed as a set of isolated services provided without overall direction, but must be organized along a continuum in which all elements are effectively coordinated. In order to meet the needs of disabled persons at various levels of illness and re-

covery, it is necessary to develop a logical and orderly progression of services.

Therapeutic Recreation as a Continuum

This concept may be illustrated in three ways: (a) a description of the *sequence of settings* for therapeutic recreation; (b) an analysis of the principles of *progressive patient care;* and (c) a presentation of *levels of involvement* by patients, with respect to voluntary choice of activity, and personal motivation.

Sequential Settings for Therapeutic Recreation

This may best be demonstrated with respect to psychiatric care. Today, every effort is made to prevent hospitalization in the first place, through the dispersal of community mental health centers which can lead to early diagnosis of illness, and the provision of special clinic services that can assist in keeping the patient functioning in the community. However, if this approach does not work, and if the patient must be hospitalized because of an acute condition, the following sequence of settings for therapeutic recreation may be developed.

1. *Full hospitalization.* While undergoing treatment on an in-patient basis, every effort is made to maintain contact with family and community groups through recreation programs. Outside organizations may provide parties, entertainments and similar programs. Patients themselves may move into the community on special trips and visits. At the same time, a process of recreation counseling (see page 208) is developed which helps the patient become aware of the role of recreation and leisure in his own life, and to develop a positive attitude—as well as knowledge and recreative skills—with respect to future participation.

---

[25] Nancy Hicks: "Life of Disabled is Tied to Family." *New York Times,* September 14, 1969, p. 73.

2. *Partial hospitalization.* Increasingly, instead of discharging patients directly from a custodial setting into complete freedom, the practice is developing of having them visit their homes for weekends, or work during the day and return to the hospital at night. An important ingredient in this process is to have patients who are undergoing this process of gradual resocialization take part in community-based recreation activities and social programs. Hospital personnel, working closely with community leaders, may refer patients directly, assist them with transportation, brief the receiving agency about them and continue to assist them in a variety of ways.

3. *Post-discharge arrangements.* In a number of communities, "halfway houses" or special social clubs have been provided for discharged mental patients, or for those who are undergoing day-clinic treatment. In addition to other services, such as educational, counseling or vocational training, such programs may offer a variety of recreational activities to ease the transition of the former patient back into community life.

Similar sequences may be found in other types of disability groupings. Mentally retarded adolescents or young adults may move from a special school or home, to a sheltered workshop or residence in the community, to full social independence. At each stage along the way, therapeutic recreation may be designed to meet current needs for constructive leisure activity, and to contribute to the process of education and growing capability for community living.

Principles of Progressive Patient Care

This concept is fundamental to every aspect of medical treatment or rehabilitation. It implies that, at each stage of the patient's illness and recovery, all aspects of treatment are geared to providing max-

imum benefit and moving him along constructively to the next stage. For example, in an early description of therapeutic recreation service in a military hospital for physically injured or orthopedic patients, service was carried on in the following way. Recognizing that day-by-day consultation with doctors, medical social workers and recreation specialists would not be possible for each patient, the basic responsibility for determining activity needs at each recovery level was assigned to the recreation specialist, after a general briefing on the medical limitations and individual or group problems of the patients.

1. *Post-operative and post-traumatic phase.* Here, the emphasis is placed on medical care, and on helping the patient make a healthy initial adjustment to the fact of his injury and the period of hospitalization that he must face. At this stage, the recreation specialist makes an early contact with the patient, and identifies interests that may be developed in the following stages.

2. *Traction Phase.* Here, the patient is confined to bed, and obviously limited in mobility, although not under intensive medical care. The emphasis is on providing individual attention to the patient, and helping him occupy his time creatively, by use of such activities as games, arts and crafts, and other pursuits that may be carried on individually, with limited mobility.

3. *Ambulatory Phase.* In this stage, the patient is able to move around the hospital, and to take part in varied activities of an individual interest, small-group, or mass nature. The effort here should be on reinforcing old interests and developing new ones that may be appropriate to the residual handicap left by the injury suffered—building on the strengths of the patient, and opening up new areas of recreational involvement for him.

4. *Disposition Phase.* Here, the emphasis is placed on providing experiences that will strengthen the patient's ability to meet his own recreation needs independently, and to develop associations and community involvements that will carry over effectively, following discharge from the hospital. It is at this

stage that the recreation counseling process described earlier is most important.[26]

Although this analysis deals with the physically impaired, a similar approach would obviously apply to psychiatric patients—the distinction being that their process of recovery would not be as likely to fit into such easily categorized phases.

Levels of Patient Involvement

Initially, it is often difficult for patients to make appropriate leisure choices; they may lack skills and interests, which compel others to make choices for them.

When a patient is *required* to do something, it may not have the desired elements of free choice, self-discovery and pleasure that true recreation can provide. It is the subjective experience of the patient that is most important. As Haun points out, a ball game is not necessarily recreation, but the absorbed involvement of the patient is. Prescribing calisthenics, softball or dancing may simply result in the patient undergoing exercise, but not receiving the values to be derived from true recreation.

Yet, it often is not possible to rely on the patient's self-motivation to bring him into activity. Both psychiatric and physically disabled persons frequently tend to resist involvement. Streeter writes:

It is terribly hard for seriously damaged people to reconcile themselves to their disabilities. Some of them spend months or years evading the issue by trying vainly to live as they did before their accident or illness. Families, struggling with their own feelings about a disabled patient, may drift away while he is in hospital. Permanent disability and long-term hospitalization often make for apathy and despair . . . . The complex pathology of the severely disabled, deeply troubled patient makes it specially urgent for him to take initiative

and decide for himself what he wants to do.[27]

What solution is there for this dilemma? Obviously, recreation may be offered on different levels in institutional settings:

Recreation can be offered as an informal, completely voluntary form of activity in the hospital program, often on a mass or large-group basis, without any close relationship to other adjunctive therapies or medical guidance and direction. In such situations, it clearly should not be designated as therapeutic. On the other hand, when it is medically oriented, guided, and approved, related to pathology, modified or adapted to meet individual patients' needs, interests, and capabilities, and when it has certain specific goals of rehabilitation in mind, it deserves the title.

What is important is that, even when it is "prescribed" for a given patient, the activity should not be approached in a compulsory fashion. A patient may be introduced to the activity, encouraged to participate, and given help—but cannot be forced to take part—or it is no longer recreation. Thus, the recreation worker will need to be ingenious in his effort to motivate patients and (particularly with psychiatric patients, who often are extremely withdrawn and reluctant to take part in recreation) fairly strong in his efforts to persuade. In the final analysis, however, unless the patient comes to the point of selecting activities for participation voluntarily . . . the approach will not have been successful.[28]

This varied approach to "prescribed" versus "voluntary" participation is illustrated in the breakdown of recreation program activities found in Veterans Administration hospitals. There, three major phases of recreation have traditionally been provided:

1. *General:* both active and passive services throughout the hospital, in the audi-

---

[26] Staff of Oliver General Hospital: "We Prescribe Recreation." *Journal of Health, Physical Education and Recreation,* November, 1951, pp. 12–13.

[27] George Streeter: *In* "Art Studio: Therapy in an Institutional Setting." *Information Center, Recreation for the Handicapped, Newsletter,* July-August, 1971, p. 1.
[28] Richard Kraus: *Recreation Today: Program Planning and Leadership.* New York: Appleton-Century-Crofts, 1966, p. 307.

torium, recreation lounge, outdoor areas, dayrooms and on wards. Only a general clearance for these activities is required, usually obtained from the Chief of Staff and the chiefs of clinical services.

2. *Specialized:* activities designed to meet needs based on specific disabilities, particularly of long-term patients in groups. This phase of the program is developed by the cooperative efforts of the medical and recreation staff, usually with recreation workers being assigned to specific services and developing programs for them.

3. *Prescribed:* individualized services which may be provided for individual patients at the specific request of the patient's physician, based on his needs, progress, and past participation in recreation.[29]

Seen more abstractly, patient participation should be helped to move along a continuum which extends from outer-directed involvement toward self-motivated, voluntary activity. Ball has developed a model of this continuum:

in which he wishes to participate, within the hospital setting.

Finally, on the *fourth* level, the individual is free to engage in whatever activity he wishes in his unobligated time; this is simply viewed as recreation, and is the ultimate goal of the entire process.[30]

Similarly, Frye and Peters have presented a sequence of stages showing how participants move from a situation in the clinical setting, in which the therapeutic recreation specialist exerts primary authority, to involvement in the community in which they are free to select and carry on their own choice of activity. This model involves five stages:

1. Recreator administers highly structured program under medical orders.
2. Recreator "sells" program to patient, motivates patient to participate.
3. Recreator and patient construct program together.
4. Recreator advises patient and community.

EXPERIENCE	TYPE OF TIME	MAJOR MOTIVATION
1. Activity for sake of activity	Obligated time	Drive is outer directed
2. Recreation education	Obligated time	Drive is outer directed
3. Therapeutic recreation	Unobligated time	Motivation is inner directed but choice of experiences is limited
4. Recreation	Unobligated time	Motivation is inner directed

On the *first* level, the patient engages in any activity, such as music, games or art, without conscious goals or purpose other than to provide reality orientation or diversion. Activity is carried on in time scheduled for recreation, with choice determined by the therapeutic recreation specialist.

On the *second* level, the individual is specifically counseled into activities which are based on an assessment of his needs and interests; the purpose of this phase is to help him develop constructive attitudes, knowledge and skills with respect to recreation and leisure.

On the *third* level, the patient begins to select therapeutically oriented activities

5. Patient free to participate in any activity available to him.[31]

Obviously, in some situations, such as the planning of programs for physically disabled persons living in the community, it may be possible to by-pass the early stages of this continuum. In other situations, such as nursing home settings, with a number of severely regressed residents who have suffered organic brain deterioration, it may not be possible for participants to exercise meaningful choices; it may be necessary for the recreation leader to select and direct all activities.

[29] Orientation Manual, *Physical Medicine and Rehabilitation.* Washington, D.C., Veterans Administration Department of Medicine and Surgery, March, 1966.

[30] Edith L. Ball: "The Meaning of Therapeutic Recreation." *Therapeutic Recreation Journal,* November, 1970, pp. 17–18.

[31] Virginia Frye and Martha Peters: *Therapeutic Recreation: Its Theory, Philosophy, and Practice.* Harrisburg, Pennsylvania, Stackpole Books, 1972, p. 43.

The Selection of Appropriate Activity

A final area of concern, with respect to the development of effective therapeutic recreation programs, has to do with the selection and provision of organized programs of activity. On what basis should activities be chosen? Obviously, they must be appropriate, in terms of meeting the overall goals of rehabilitation and therapeutic recreation service. However, to what extent are they to be geared to meeting the needs of patients in specific diagnostic categories?

This problem is related to the issue, described earlier, of whether recreation is to be regarded as a specific therapy. Essentially, this question has two subelements: (a) whether recreation is *comparable* to other therapies, and (b) whether placing emphasis on it as a therapy does not actually *diminish its value* for patients.

Paul Haun has taken the position that when recreation is conceived of and presented as a therapy, it may lose some of its key benefits, and, further, that it is *not* comparable to other medical techniques. He writes:

> The hospital recreation worker performs many services essential, in my opinion, to the welfare of the patient. I cannot, however, regard any of them as therapeutic, first because I have never been convinced that recreation in any of its forms is a specific instrument for the modification of a disease process comparable say to penicillin in the treatment of syphilis; second, because I am so fully persuaded of the psychiatric patient's need for recreation *as recreation* that I grudge any dilution of its potency through adulteration with alternative purposes. . . . It is because I believe that recreation is an essential human need that I want it for my patients.[32]

On the other hand, the equally distinguished physician, Howard Rusk, has stated: "I firmly believe that both indi-vidual and group recreation for patients have a direct relationship upon their recovery—these, in my opinion, are definitely adjunctive therapy."[33]

Therapy has been defined as a "planned conscious intervention intended to produce a change." Such an intervention must involve techniques that are not passive, accidental or happenstance, but ones that are known, understood and demonstrable. It may be reasonably argued that a variety of therapeutic techniques are widely used that *do not have* predictable and measurable effects. For example, psychotherapy itself is applied in many forms, and with varied degrees of success. Certainly, no psychiatrist or psychoanalyst is able to predict that a given patient will progress at a certain rate, or that a particular approach will ensure recovery.

It is less important to argue about the semantic meaning of the terms "therapy" or "therapeutic" than to analyze how and why recreation does operate in this way, and how it may be most effectively applied in rehabilitative settings. Obviously, it is most effective as therapy when it is carried on by skilled practitioners, working in close collaboration with medical authorities.

Rosen writes knowledgeably of the needs of psychiatric patients, and the ways in which recreation may be used as a specific tool in their treatment. She makes clear that the characteristics of psychiatric patients are such that it is not possible to present activities to them as "normal" people might visualize recreation:

> Certainly anyone who has worked with paranoid patients or with guilt-ridden, self-destructive personalities knows that even the most common events of everyday life, eating and sleeping, are frequently connected with fearful and anxiety-provoking fantasies. Objects themselves can take on symbolic significance to be feared or cherished far beyond their realistic meaning. The peculiar defensive systems erected

[32] Paul Haun: "Hospital Recreation—A Medical Viewpoint." *In Recreation for the Mentally Ill.* Washington, D.C., American Association for Health, Physical Education and Recreation, 1958, pp. 57–58.

[33] Howard Rusk: *Basic Concepts of Hospital Recreation.* Washington, D.C., American Recreation Society, 1953, p. 7.

by psychotic patients shut out and distort the environment and the people in it so that ordinary channels for communication and social interaction are obstructed. Psychiatric treatment is first and foremost concerned with breaking down these barriers, with whatever means are available. It attempts to enable the patient to function within the framework of the social community. Recreative experiences can be utilized to serve this purpose only when they are adapted to the particular needs of the individual patient. Finding the areas of accessibility to psychotic and emotionally disturbed patients may involve a great deal of experimentation in a variety of media. Resourcefulness and imagination in the adaptation of techniques are required . . . .[34]

While it is possible to make such generalized statements as, "strenuous physical activities or certain arts and crafts activities are useful for the release of aggression and hostility," or "group social activities are indicated for withdrawn or isolated patients," these *are* just generalizations. Often, the need to develop a convincing statement of the purpose of a field may lead to precise "laundry lists" of needs and recommended activities, which are superficial and misleading. Rosen points out that many of the personal elements intrinsic to the recreative experience are intangible and variable, and therefore defy a systematized method of cataloguing.

She comments that it is hazardous to ascribe to a particular activity a specific therapeutic effect:

> The practice of listing categories of activities into which patients with specific types of psychopathology can be neatly fitted is little more than a convenience devised by efficient management. In the hands of untrained personnel, the fallacies of such "systems" of selection are obvious.[35]

The treatment of the patient must be directed by the psychiatrist who makes the diagnosis, charts the various techniques or modalities that are to be used with him and evaluates his progress. The recreation specialist must work as part of the treatment team, using the tools of his profession with sensitivity to psychological needs. He plans a sequence of recreation experiences, appraising the patient's reactions and behavior, modifying his approach to use those activities which evoke the most constructive behavior and abandoning those which are unsuccessful.

It is necessary, in programming, to identify the specific therapeutic objectives for each patient, and to analyze the structure and characteristics of each activity. Rosen writes:

> It is important to know what physical skills and what degree of emotional maturity each activity might require to ensure satisfying participation. Some activities allow for a wide range of abilities, and their organization, materials and methods of presentation can be altered to accommodate many different individual needs. Other activities have a definite structural form and pre-requisite skills which limit their potential accessibility.[36]

It is necessary, in selecting activities for patient involvement, not to rely on classical diagnostic categories as much as on specific observable symptoms, such as disturbances in communication, social control, reality testing and interpersonal relationships. Throughout, recreation specialists must be patient, must seek to establish contact, must stress success and encouragement and, with severely regressed patients, must rely on sensory-motor activities which do not depend heavily on verbal communication.

Within community settings for non-hospitalized persons, there is a serious question as to whether many forms of recreation *should* be regarded as therapy.

For example, in a day camping program provided for retarded children by Camp Spindrift, a project of the Recreation Center for the Handicapped in San Francisco, the following objectives are cited:

---

[34] Elizabeth R. Rosen: "The Selection of Activities for Therapeutic Use." *Recreation in Treatment Centers,* September, 1962, p. 30.
[35] *Ibid.*

[36] *Ibid.,* p. 31.

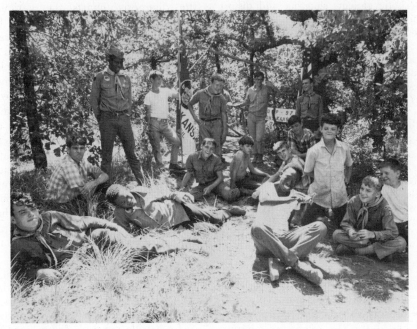

Boy Scout troop from Parsons State Hospital in Winfield, Kansas enjoys country outing.

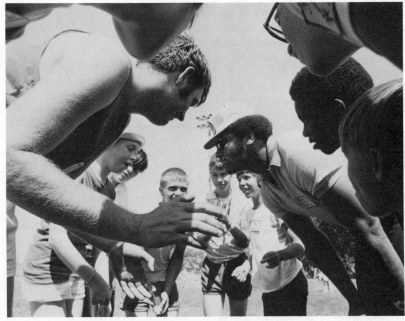

Youthful athletes at Parsons State receive special coaching from Buck Buchanan, pro football great . . .

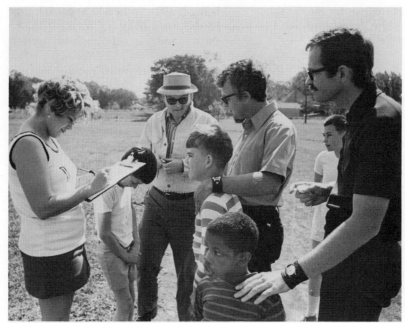

. . . while others sign up for competition in local Special Olympics.

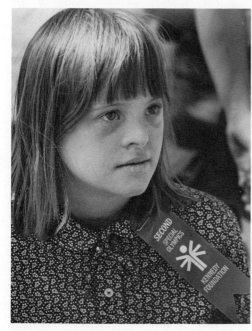

This young lady is proud of her second-place ribbon!

1. To provide fun in the out-of-doors.
2. To offer satisfying contacts with nature, so that the camper may acquire a sense of being at home in the out-of-doors.
3. To provide opportunities for group and individual experiences in a natural environment; to join in and contribute to a plan of living for a day, a week, or more.
4. To foster the growth of independence and self-direction in each camper.
5. To acquire new skills, hobbies, and interests that have long-time values.
6. To arouse a sense of curiosity, stimulate spontaneous expression, provide enjoyment, and accelerate the learning process.
7. To provide opportunities for new experiences, for emotional satisfaction, and for spiritual growth.
8. To foster better mental and physical health, courage, and confidence and to exercise mind and body in healthful activity.
9. To offer a range of experiences that will help to prepare the campers for resident camping.

10. To provide opportunities for the development of initiative, leadership, and a sense of responsibility.[37]

It is apparent that these goals are identical to those that might be cited for *any* day camp program. In no sense do they constitute "therapy" as such. However, in order to achieve them, and to make the program meaningful in terms of the special needs of retarded children, it is necessary to provide a higher degree of skilled leadership, a better ratio of leaders to children, a modification of program activities and a much more individualized approach to supervision than in normal programs. For retarded children, these program goals are particularly vital, and may contribute significantly to the socialization, growing maturity and improving self-concept of the campers.

Concluding Statement of Purposes

Summing up the rationale presented in this chapter, the following important goals of therapeutic recreation service may be listed. It is obvious that they vary widely, depending upon the group being served, the nature and degree of disability and the setting in which the service is provided.

General Objectives of Therapeutic Recreation Service

1. To provide constructive, enjoyable and creative leisure activities, seen as a general need for persons of all ages and backgrounds.
2. To improve morale, and a sense of well-being and interest in life, as opposed to depression and disinterest or withdrawal.
3. To help individuals come to grips with their disabilities, and build positively on their existing strengths and capabilities.
4. To help individuals gain security in

being with others, and develop healthy and outgoing social relationships and a feeling of group acceptance.
5. To emphasize positive self-concepts, and feelings of individual worth, through successful participation in activity.
6. To help individuals gain both skills and attitudes which will assist them in using their leisure in positive and constructive, as opposed to negative or pathological, ways.
7. For hospitalized patients, to help them build bridges for the successful return to community life.
8. To contribute to a sense of community in the hospital or in group life, and to promote an atmosphere in which it becomes possible to make progress toward recovery.
9. To give experience in mastering simple tasks and reality situations that may be of prevocational value.

Specific Objectives of Therapeutic Recreation Service

1. For disabled persons living in the community, to provide activities that they can share constructively with their families, or that they can carry on independently, thus minimizing their dependence on their families.
2. For psychiatric patients, to provide a positive means of releasing aggression or hostility harmlessly, relating to others constructively, coming to grips with reality and gaining leisure interests that will contribute to mental health.
3. For the mentally retarded, to promote both physical, social and intellectual functioning, to assist in developing social independence and to promote confidence and the ability to function in community settings.
4. For the physically disabled, to provide new skills and interests that compensate for lost functions or abilities, to provide practice in self-care skills and to assist in re-integration in community recreation programs.

[37] Report on Camp Spindrift, Annual Report of Recreation Center for the Handicapped. San Francisco, California, Summer, 1968, p. 22.

5. For the socially maladjusted, to assist in learning to develop effective social relations with others, to use leisure constructively, to learn to accept the values and rules of the larger society and to teach qualities of good sportsmanship and fair play.

6. For aging persons, to provide continuing social involvement, creative satisfactions and the opportunity to be of community service.

Guidelines for the Provision of Therapeutic Recreation Service

Finally, a number of guidelines for the provision of therapeutic recreation service are provided here:

1. Whenever possible, self-choice rather than compulsion should be stressed in the selection of activities.

2. Individuals should be encouraged to develop their own philosophy of leisure involvement, as true expressions of their own personality.

3. Activities should be provided that can be carried over independently in the community, after the process of rehabilitation is completed.

4. Emphasis should be placed on activities that contribute to the participant's feeling of competence and accomplishment.

5. Whenever possible, programs should be planned with the full involvement of those who are to be served.

6. The disabled should be integrated with the nondisabled, whenever possible, in carrying on recreational activities.

Other guidelines dealing with the actual planning and organization of therapeutic recreation programs are presented in later chapters of this text.

Suggested Topics for Class Discussion, Examinations or Student Papers

1. Outline the ways in which recreation serves as a component of healthy living for all persons; relate these to the process of rehabilitation for ill and disabled persons.

2. Present the arguments for and against considering recreation as a specific form of therapy, and take a position on this issue.

3. Show how therapeutic recreation service operates as a continuum in both institutional and community-based settings.

Chapter 3

Professional Development in Therapeutic Recreation Service

This chapter examines therapeutic recreation service as a career field today. It outlines its background and origins and describes the settings in which therapeutic recreation personnel are employed, as well as their job functions. It presents the past and present role of professional organizations in the therapeutic recreation field and explains the nature of other adjunctive therapists with whom recreation personnel have close working relationships.

Early Development of Employment in Therapeutic Recreation

The development of professional specialization in therapeutic recreation followed the overall pattern of recreation leadership in community and voluntary agencies. The field did not suddenly spring into being as an independent area of service. Instead, it gradually developed in a variety of settings, often with personnel with training in other fields assuming responsibility for it.

There were four major stages in the development of therapeutic recreation service:

1. *General responsibility.* During the early decades of the century, responsibility for supervising or providing recreation tended to be seen as a general responsibility, shared by such practitioners as adapted or corrective physical educators, occupational therapists, physical therapists, nurses, attendants and other ward personnel.

2. *Beginning specialization.* Beginning in the 1930s, but more pronouncedly after World War II, individuals began to be employed on a wide scale who had a *special* responsibility for recreation, and were known as "hospital recreation workers," "medical recreation workers," "recreation specialists for the ill and handicapped" or similar nomenclature. They were employed chiefly in large federal and state hospitals, particularly those concerned with mental illness and long-term care. In some settings, they had the title of "recreation therapist."

3. *Recognition of the field.* By the 1950s and 1960s, there began to be a much wider use of recreation specialists in institutions serving special populations. These included homes and training schools for retarded or emotionally disturbed children and adolescents, centers for physical rehabilitation, nursing homes and, to a lesser degree, penal institutions. At the same time, the term "therapeutic recreation" be-

came widely accepted. College and university training in this field was established.

4. *Extension to the community.* In the middle and late 1960s, therapeutic recreation service was extended to varied community settings. This trend was based on three factors: (a) the recognition that hospitals could only do their job properly if they were able to help discharged patients make successful transitions into community life, which compelled a concern with such settings; (b) the fact that an increasing number of city and county recreation and park departments began to establish special programs for, and in some cases, hire specialists to serve the disabled populations within their jurisdictions; and (c) the role of voluntary agencies serving such handicapped groups as the blind, deaf or cerebral palsied, in providing expanded social services, including recreation, social activities and camping.

As a consequence of these developments, the image of the therapeutic recreation worker became more sharply defined, and increasing numbers were employed in treatment centers and community agencies around the country. While there has been no definitive survey of the number of specialists in recreation service for the ill and disabled, there have been a number of studies of recreation within a particular region or type of service.

For example, Phillips reported in 1958 on a study conducted by the National Recreation Association in psychiatric hospitals throughout the United States.[1] Organized recreation programs were found in 456 hospitals providing psychiatric services; approximately 2780 full-time personnel were employed to conduct recreation in these institutions. It was found also that, in smaller institutions,

the ratio of patients to therapeutic recreation specialists was much more favorable than in the larger ones. In hospitals with under 300 beds, for example, there was one therapist for each 41 patients. In hospitals with between 700 and 3000 beds, the ratio was one to 220.

A more extensive study of recreation personnel in hospitals was carried out by Silson, Cohen and Hill in 1959.[2] It was found that, in the 1486 hospitals of all types that had organized recreation programs throughout the nation, there were 5236 full-time recreation workers. However, there were sharply contrasting patterns of employment among different types of hospitals, and a considerable number that had no full-time recreation specialists. For example, while almost all Veterans Administration and state hospitals had full-time employees with recreation titles, only a small percentage of municipal, county and voluntary hospitals had such employees. It was found that 30.8 per cent of the hospitals had *no* full-time recreation personnel, and 20.6 per cent had only one such employee on a full-time basis. In many hospitals, other personnel, such as occupational therapists, physical therapists, social workers, librarians and vocational rehabilitation specialists, had recreation responsibilities.

A number of studies carried on in the 1960s indicated a severe shortage of trained therapeutic recreation specialists. Berryman, in 1964, summed up reports from such states as Illinois, Indiana, Pennsylvania, California and Minnesota, showing that they had more than 500 recreation staff vacancies in state hospitals alone.[3] With the growth of municipal and voluntary hospitals, nursing homes, homes for the aged and community-based agencies and departments providing therapeutic recreation services, and with

---

[1] B. E. Phillips: *Recreation for the Mentally Ill.* Washington, D.C., Conference Report, American Association for Health, Physical Education and Recreation, 1958, p. 1.

[2] John E. Silson, Elliott M. Cohen, and Beatrice H. Hill: *Recreation in Hospitals: Report of a Study of Organized Recreation Programs in Hospitals and the Personnel Conducting Them.* New York, National Recreation Association, 1959, pp. 35–39.

[3] Doris Berryman: "Manpower for Therapeutic Recreation Service." *Recreation in Treatment Centers,* September, 1964, pp. 24–27.

a limited number of students graduating from colleges with specializations in therapeutic recreation, Berryman concluded that only a handful of persons existed to fill thousands of existing and expected vacancies.

It was estimated in 1968 by the National Center for Health Statistics of the Public Health Service of the United States that there were approximately 4000 recreation therapists in hospitals and other treatment centers throughout the country.[4] This statistic was undoubtedly conservative, in that it did not include many individuals working in community agencies, and did not cover those persons trained in other disciplines, with a major responsibility for providing recreation programs.

Emerging Functions of Therapeutic Recreation Specialists

Gradually, the functional role of therapeutic recreation specialists has become more clearly defined. In the late 1950s, Fred Chapman, professor of recreation at the University of Minnesota, carried out an analysis of the responsibilities of recreation workers in state, military, Veterans Administration and private hospitals.[5] The functions were grouped in three categories: *essential* duties, *highly desirable* duties and *desirable* duties:

Essential Duties

1. Organizes, directs, and supervises a recreation program for rehabilitation of patients.
2. Provides supervision for recreation staff (staff meetings, recruitment, recommendations, and evaluation).
3. Confers with medical staff or a physician in developing a recreational therapy program for patients.

4. Cooperates with other medical team members in the coordination of a program of activities for patients.
5. Directs and participates in an in-service training program for recreation staff.
6. Surveys program and makes recommendations for improvement.

Highly Desirable Duties

7. Prepares reports on progress of recreational program for staff meetings and other personnel.
8. Interprets recreation program to staff, volunteers, and the public.
9. Observes, interprets, and reports progress in the recreational therapy program.
10. Makes, reviews, and authorizes budget requests and expenditures within recreation department.
11. Addresses student nurses, other staff members, and interested community organizations on recreational therapy.
12. Orders and maintains necessary recreation supplies and equipment.
13. Interviews referred patients and plans recreation program modified for patients' limitations and needs.
14. Attends professional meetings away from the hospital.
15. Directs volunteers' activities, enlists their support and coordinates their efforts.
16. Keeps clinical notes, records, and reports on patients in recreation program.
17. Directs special holiday program for patients.
18. Assists in training of students from educational institutions.
19. Leads a planned recreation program for an intensive treatment unit of patients ("total push," selected groups, etc.)
20. Instructs individual patients in recreation (encourages participation, arranges schedules, and leads activities).
21. Arranges special entertainments for patients (circuses, plays, etc.)

The *desirable* duties identified in the study consisted chiefly of leading specific recreation activities for patients in the following areas: sports and games; social and folk dancing; nature and outing; motion pictures; music; parties; dramatics; hospital radio station, newspaper, or clubs; arts and crafts; assigning patients to activities and working with

[4] *Health Resource Statistics, 1968.* Washington, D.C., Public Health Service, U.S. Department of Health, Education and Welfare, 1968, p. 183.
[5] Fred Chapman: Findings summarized in B. E. Phillips: "Recreational Therapy: Duties of Hospital Recreation Personnel." *Journal of Health, Physical Education and Recreation,* April, 1957, p. 60.

relatives of discharged patients. It is worth noting that Chapman's analysis found that administrative and supervisory responsibilities of recreation therapists (and even such duties as preparing reports, addressing student nurses, ordering supplies or attending professional meetings) were seen as *more* important than providing direct leadership for patient activity programs.

In 1961, an influential statement was issued on the changing functions and roles of therapeutic recreation specialists. This statement was developed by the National Curriculum Conference on Therapeutic Recreation, and had important implications for the education of professional personnel in therapeutic recreation.[6] The expanding role of practitioners was seen as including the following elements:

1. Providing activities which serve therapeutic purposes.
2. Supervising and administering recreation services in a variety of settings, including institutions, the home and the community.
3. Training aides and volunteers.
4. Counseling the ill and disabled, to assist them in meeting their needs through recreative experiences.
5. Providing consultation service to communities and institutions planning programs for the ill or disabled, and helping them to implement such programs.
6. Interpreting therapeutic recreation to the community and particularly to the medical and professional personnel in allied disciplines.
7. Providing a continuity of recreation experience as the patient moves from the hospital or institutional setting through the rehabilitation process and into the community.
8. Expanding community recreation services to handicapped people of all ages who are not under direct medical supervision and who live in the community.

In contrast to such statements, there was the growing point of view that therapeutic recreation specialists, along with other hospital personnel, had to learn to use themselves in uniquely therapeutic ways. This concept, as developed by the Group for the Advancement of Psychiatry, became influential in many hospitals in the 1950s and 1960s. It is based on the view that the patient is forced to enter the psychiatric hospital chiefly because he has experienced severe difficulties in living in the outside world, particularly in terms of his relationship with others.

It becomes essential, therefore, that the hospital provide him with a new, non-threatening and highly supportive environment, a smaller, safer world in which living with others is not threatening, and in which he can overcome his tendency to withdraw from anxiety-provoking relationships. It is necessary that he find new personal relationships that help to gratify his needs, ease his communication with others and encourage his social participation. Within this context, the idea of the "open hospital" and the "therapeutic community" developed, with an underscored need for patient activities and experiences that would include meaningful relationships with people on every level in the hospital. Emphasis shifted away from providing activities for their own sake, to the psychodynamics of the personal relationship they were able to facilitate.

Simon described the concept of "therapeutic use of self" in the following passage:

> . . . the hospital must offer a controlled milieu in which the transferences of the patient may be expressed. Psychodynamics teaches us that these transferences are repetitions of relationships which existed in the early life of the individual. It would seem, therefore, that the hospital should present a model of the outside world in which the transference could take place and corrective emotional experiences come about— that the essential difference between the mental hospital and the community should be the presence of personnel trained to understand the patient's reactions and to use themselves therapeutically. In this atmosphere there should exist replicas of all the activities normally experienced by the patient in his community. Whatever the size

[6] *Report of Therapeutic Recreation Development Conference.* Sponsored by National Recreation Association's Consulting Service on Recreation for the Ill and Disabled. New York, Comeback, Inc., 1961.

or structure of the hospital, it should offer the equivalent, in as nearly a similar form as possible, of home and community. This . . . involves basic functions of living, eating and sleeping. . . . Everything is oriented, ultimately, toward re-establishment in the external world.[7]

This developing approach had considerable influence on *how* recreation personnel functioned, particularly in psychiatric institutions. In general, however, formal statements of the responsibilities of therapeutic recreation specialists have not attempted to encompass this approach. Instead, they tend to describe the more clearly identifiable functions. This is particularly true of job descriptions. As an example, a 1968 recruitment brochure published by the Veterans Administration describes the role of recreation therapists under the following two headings:

Patient Care and Treatment Program:

1. Teaching patients how to manage their leisure time.
2. Planning and conducting rehabilitative recreation on a voluntary, guided, or prescribed basis.
3. Programming of adapted sports; arts, crafts, and hobbies; motion pictures; music; radio-TV; dramatics and social activities.
4. Conferences with physicians and other hospital personnel concerned with the patients' problems and rehabilitation potential.

Administrative Responsibilities:

1. Planning and organizing a department of Recreation Therapy for the ill and handicapped.
2. Supervision of personnel who are administering the therapy program.
3. Responsibility for proper operation and care of modern facilities and equipment and requisitioning supplies.
4. Interviewing and orienting new employees.
5. Preparation of budgets.[8]

In a conference of recreation administrators, supervisors, counselors and other personnel, in February, 1971, at the Arkansas Rehabilitation Research and Training Center, the following areas of professional functioning were identified:

1. *Meeting Client Needs.* Need to develop differentiated programs to meet varied client needs; to structure some activities to have stronger therapeutic content; to coordinate recreation and other rehabilitation personnel more effectively; to promote better integration of discharged patients in the community, and to improve community opportunities for discharged or disabled persons.
2. *Staff Training Needs.* Need to be able to evaluate activity programs more effectively; to serve as therapeutic agents; to communicate with those in other rehabilitation disciplines; to develop effective and innovative programs; to help the profession become community-oriented as well as clinically-oriented.
3. *Meeting Research Needs.* Need to develop effective programs of research to measure outcomes and effects of recreation; need to develop experimental and demonstration projects, particularly in areas related to welfare programs, public offenders, alcoholics and drug abuse; need to develop better dissemination of research between researchers and practitioners, and among the various rehabilitation disciplines.
4. *Improving Communication with other Disciplines.* Need to develop more effective team approaches to providing services; to have recreation publications made available to therapists in other disciplines; to promote therapeutic recreation as a section of the National Rehabilitation Association.[9]

Professional and Service Organizations in Therapeutic Recreation

An integral part of the growing professionalization of therapeutic recreation has been the contribution made by professional and service organizations in pro-

[7] Benjamin Simon: "The New Trends in Rehabilitation." *Recreation's Contribution to the Patient,* North Carolina Recreation Commission, September, 1963, p. 11.

[8] *Recreation Therapists in V.A. Hospitals and Clinics.* Washington, D.C., V.A. Pamphlet No. 10-68, March, 1968, p. 1.

[9] Thomas W. Collingwood: "Report on Training Conference on Therapeutic Recreation within Rehabilitation." *Therapeutic Recreation Journal,* 2nd Quarter, 1971, pp. 88–91.

moting public awareness of this field, strengthening practices, improving curricula in higher education and developing standards for the selection of personnel. Among the major organizations to have contributed in this field are the American Recreation Society, the American Association for Health, Physical Education and Recreation, the National Recreation Association and the National Association of Recreational Therapists. Their contributions are briefly detailed in the section that follows.

HOSPITAL SECTION, AMERICAN RECREATION SOCIETY. This organization was formed in Omaha, Nebraska, in 1948. It promoted hospital recreation programs in a variety of ways by: (a) sponsoring special meetings on therapeutic recreation at the annual National Recreation Congress; (b) pressing for improved standards of training and selection, through its Standards and Training Committee; (c) advocating or sponsoring special national or regional conferences on hospital recreation, either independently or in cooperation with other organizations; and (d) developing effective relationships with other organizations in the fields of rehabilitation or recreation.

Initially through a newsletter and through articles in the American Recreation Society quarterly publication, *The Bulletin,* and later through articles and columns in the *American Recreation Journal,* the Hospital Section did much to promote interest in this field on the part of community recreation personnel.

RECREATIONAL THERAPY SECTION, AMERICAN ASSOCIATION FOR HEALTH, PHYSICAL EDUCATION AND RECREATION. This section of the overall organization serving health, physical education and recreation education, was formed in Los Angeles, California, in 1952. The Recreation Division of the American Association for Health, Physical Education and Recreation (a department of the National Education Association) had included three sections: *public recreation, voluntary and youth-serving agencies* and *institutional and industrial recreation.* The latter one divided, in April, 1952, into two autonomous sections: *industrial recreation,* and

recreational therapy. The interests of members of the latter section tended to be more heavily in special schools, or in adapted physical education programs, than in hospital-based recreational therapy. However, the section cooperated closely with other professional groups and, because of its natural linkage with colleges and universities that prepared recreation majors, made an important contribution to the field.

Through its monthly column, "Recreational Therapy," in the *Journal of Health, Physical Education and Recreation,* the Recreational Therapy section promoted awareness of this growing field. Also, it was active in developing conferences, stimulating research and attempting to improve professional standards.

NATIONAL ASSOCIATION OF RECREATIONAL THERAPISTS. This organization was founded at Bolivar, Tennessee, in February, 1953. Its initial membership consisted primarily of recreation therapists employed in state hospitals and schools, particularly in the southern and midwestern states. Although many were members of the American Recreation Society, they wished to develop a stronger professional focus on the role of the recreation therapist than was possible in this organization. This group worked closely with other organizations in promoting conferences, research and other action related to therapeutic recreation service. It published a quarterly journal, *Recreation for the Ill and Handicapped.*

CONSULTING SERVICE ON RECREATION FOR THE ILL AND HANDICAPPED, NATIONAL RECREATION ASSOCIATION. Although the National Recreation Association did not have a separate section or branch concerned with therapeutic recreation, it employed consultants who provided service in this field, working with hospitals and other agencies, beginning in 1953. The National Recreation Association's monthly magazine, *Recreation,* regularly contained a column, "Hospital Capsules," and the organization itself was represented in many professional meetings and conferences.

COUNCIL FOR THE ADVANCEMENT OF HOSPITAL RECREATION. The membership of these four organizations realized that there was a strong need for more effective evaluation of hospital recreation programs and an upgrading of personnel standards, as well as a system of registration or certification that might enforce such standards. To meet this need, they formed the structure that became known as the Council for the Advancement of Hospital Recreation, in November, 1953. This body was to serve as a vehicle for registration of qualified practitioners, to develop standards for training and clinical practice experience and to serve as a means for promoting communication among the other organizations in this field.

In 1956, the Council officially adopted personnel standards for Hospital Recreation Director, Leader, and Aide, and set out to promote a registration system for identifying those in the field who met these requirements. It also attempted to upgrade and improve the overall field of therapeutic recreation, and to develop a merger of the existing organizations in this field.

Mrs. Beatrice Hill, formerly a consultant with the National Recreation Association, formed an organization titled Comeback, Inc., which was designed to promote professional therapeutic recreation service. She also made a sustained effort to unify the field of therapeutic recreation service. However, this was not to be accomplished until the separate organizations representing the field agreed to merge in late 1965, forming the National Recreation and Park Association. This organization established a number of separate branches as substructures to represent the varied interests of its members. One of these, the National Therapeutic Recreation Society, absorbed the existing organizations concerned with recreation for the ill and disabled, and has functioned effectively in this area since that time.

NATIONAL THERAPEUTIC RECREATION SOCIETY. One of the key functions of this organization is to promote professional development by sponsoring or cosponsoring conferences, and by developing programs and special institutes for the annual National Recreation Congress.

For example, it cooperated in the sponsorship of a professional advisory conference on activity therapy in September, 1971, in cooperation with the Joint Commission on Accreditation of Hospitals, the Accreditation Council for Psychiatric Facilities, and other organizations representing occupational, musical, dance and art therapy, and mental health centers and psychiatric services for children. At the 1971 Recreation Congress in Houston, Texas, it provided an extensive pre-Congress Institute, with meetings devoted to such themes as:

"Programs and Standards for Nursing Homes"
"Psychodrama in Activities Programs"
"Comprehensive Programming for Emotionally Disturbed Children"
"Federal Supports for Therapeutic Recreation"
"Recreation Counseling for the Ill and Disabled"
"Therapeutic Recreation in Correctional Institutions"
"Planning Community Facilities for the Ill and Disabled"
"Recreation Services for Drug Abusers"

The National Therapeutic Recreation Society has appointed official delegates to represent the views of its members at important national meetings, such as the 1971 White House Conference on Aging. It has conducted district workshops to develop guidelines for the recruitment, training and employment of disabled individuals in the recreation and park field, and has sponsored research efforts with the financial assistance of federal agencies. In addition, it has published the quarterly journal, *Therapeutic Recreation Journal,* which today acts as a single spokesman for this united field.

The National Therapeutic Recreation Society maintains a voluntary registration program which defines standards for various levels of professional functioning. One problem has been that the registration standards have included the need for a specific number of years of experience working in the field under the direct supervision of a qualified supervisor. Since so many persons were employed in the past without appropriate qualifications, and have been upgraded to supervisory job levels, this created a problem for many otherwise qualified individuals. Since 1970, this requirement has been waived, and the registration standard now consists chiefly of academic education and professional experience (see page 227).

Despite these efforts, the National Therapeutic Recreation Society has not been able, thus far, to promote a more effective system of registration or certification that would ensure that only well-qualified individuals are employed in the field. In part, this is because there is such a diversity of employment agencies that it would be almost impossible to devise a system of certification that would apply to all positions and be readily enforceable. It also reflects the situation of the overall recreation field, in which certification has been approved in only a few states, and in which Civil Service hiring requirements are generally quite flexible.

A final important function of the National Therapeutic Recreation Society has been to influence government policy and to promote improved public awareness of the field. It has done this by vigorously presenting its views before government officials and committees, and by pressing for financial support of special projects serving the ill and disabled. The work of the National Therapeutic Recreation Society is also being carried on by sections of state recreation and park societies that have been formed in recent years.

OTHER ORGANIZATIONS. A variety of other organizations have promoted the overall rehabilitation movement, and, through joint projects, have cooperated with therapeutic recreation specialists. Among these organizations have been: the American National Red Cross; American Occupational Therapy Association; American Physical Therapy Association; Association for Physical and Mental Rehabilitation; National Association for Music Therapy; American Association of Rehabilitation Therapists; American Art Therapy Association; American Dance Therapy Association and the National Association of State Activity Therapy and Rehabilitation Program Directors.

Professional Education in Therapeutic Recreation Service

The development of special curricula in therapeutic recreation did not get fully under way until after World War II. In August, 1953, the Standards and Training Committee of the Hospital Recreation Section of the American Recreation Society reported that, of the 44 colleges and universities which offered degrees in recreation, only six had graduate or undergraduate degrees in "hospital" recreation. These were: Teachers College, Columbia University; New York University; Springfield College; the University of Minnesota; Purdue University and Sacramento State College.

However, a number of other colleges offered special courses in this field, or sponsored workshops and institutes that contributed significantly to professional practice. For example, the University of North Carolina hosted a series of Regional Conferences on Hospital Recreation, beginning in the mid-1950s, that brought together representatives of Veterans Administration, state, county and private and municipal hospitals, to discuss theory and present innovative practices in therapeutic recreation. Other colleges have sponsored or cosponsored similar programs.

An important step in developing special curricula was the conference on graduate curricula in therapeutic recreation sponsored by the National Recreation Association's Consulting Service on Recreation for the Ill and Handicapped, held in New York in 1961.[10] This meeting brought together leading recreation educators and practitioners, and sought to identify the changing competencies required of professional specialists in therapeutic recreation and to suggest curriculum models based on these competencies.

It made a number of recommendations, chiefly to the effect that professional practitioners required graduate education in a specially designed program that followed an undergraduate major in general recreation. On the graduate level, it recommended that emphasis be placed on

---

[10] *Report of Therapeutic Recreation Development Conference. op. cit.,* pp. 2–3.

mastery of medical and pyschiatric nomenclature, ability to adapt activities for the ill and disabled, and competence to meet new demands that went beyond the traditional function of providing activities, such as training of personnel, providing consultation services, interpreting the field to the community and to other disciplines and developing strong links to community agencies.

It recommended that such programs include a strong component of clinical experience (including observation, involvement in programs, record-keeping and evaluation). The graduate program should not be fragmented into such areas as psychiatric, orthopedic or general medical options, and should include a common core of information related to medical understandings and knowledge of other therapeutic disciplines.

Those attending the conference made recommendations for specific standards that all institutions in this field should meet, including: (a) having certain graduate courses available in other departments; (b) accessibility to medical centers; (c) sufficient financial resources to support curriculum needs; (d) a full-time qualified faculty member to teach in and direct the curriculum; (e) adequate facilities, including a specialized library; (f) appropriate standards of administration, including procedures related to admission, supervision, records and ratio of students to faculty; and (g) standardized degree requirements.

During the 1960s, as the rapid growth in therapeutic recreation programs created a shortage of qualified personnel, and as interest grew in this field as a specialized concern, the number of colleges and universities offering curricula in therapeutic recreation grew steadily.

In 1969, the Society of Park and Recreation Educators carried out a study of recreation curricula in the United States which revealed that, of 114 institutions identified as having a recreation or recreation and park program, 35 offered a major in therapeutic recreation service.[11]

It was found that the largest number of such curricula were in the Great Lakes and Southwest Pacific regions of the country. They tended to be located in departments or schools of health, physical education and recreation rather than in departments that placed emphasis on the management of physical resources or parks administration—logically so because of the emphasis on physiology, kinesiology, physical activities, psychology and special education in such schools or departments. No therapeutic recreation majors were found in curricula housed in colleges or schools of agriculture, forestry or natural resources.

Undergraduate curricula were offered in 28 colleges, while 26 offered graduate degrees. Despite this growth, however, the study found that there were only 531 students enrolled in all degree programs in therapeutic recreation (381 on the baccalaureate level, 135 on the master's, and 15 enrolled for the doctorate).

A similar situation has prevailed in Canada, where there has been a lack of specialized programs in recreation generally, until fairly recently. Many Canadian therapeutic recreation specialists received their training at such institutions as the University of Illinois or the University of Indiana. Within the past several years, however, a number of Canadian colleges have initiated recreation and park administration curricula; several of these are also providing specialized courses in therapeutic recreation service.

Courses Offered in Therapeutic Recreation Curricula

In 1970, Donald Lindley reported on a study revealing the types of courses offered in therapeutic recreation curricula, and their relative importance, as rated by college educators and practitioners in the field.[12] In an initial study of 30 colleges and universities offering therapeutic recreation curricula, he found that

[11] Thomas A. Stein: "Therapeutic Recreation Education: 1969 Survey." *Therapeutic Recreation Journal,* 2nd Quarter, 1970, pp. 4–7.

[12] Donald Lindley: "Relative Importance of College Courses in Therapeutic Recreation." *Therapeutic Recreation Journal,* 2nd Quarter, 1970, pp. 8–12.

courses tended to be grouped in nine major areas: (a) communication arts-public relations; (b) community institutions and organizations; (c) social science and psychology; (d) medical and psychiatric information; (e) recreation philosophy; (f) recreation administration; (g) recreation programs; (h) evaluation and research and (i) clinical experience.

On the *undergraduate* level, the most valuable courses were rated as follows, in order of importance: field work, introduction to therapeutic recreation, philosophy of recreation, social psychology, community organization in recreation, small group dynamics, foundations of recreation, internship, programming in therapeutic recreation and methods of recreation leadership. Courses dealing with other rehabilitation services, psychiatric or medical information, or program elements for specific disabilities fell far below the first ten.

On the *graduate* level, the most valuable courses, in rank order of importance, were: research methods, readings in therapeutic recreation, psychological aspects of disability, readings in recreation, research seminars, professional seminars, psychiatric and medical information and administration in therapeutic recreation. Realistically, while curricula consisting of such courses are likely to provide an excellent experience for students who have already had an undergraduate major in recreation, they tend to be more advanced than they should be for students who have only had a brief orientation to recreation as a professional discipline—or for students who have had no formal academic training in the field at all. This continues, then, to be a major problem for college and university educators who are concerned with preparing professional therapeutic recreation specialists.

COMMUNITY COLLEGE CURRICULA. In direct contrast to the trend toward specializing in therapeutic recreation on the graduate level, has been the growth of two-year community college curricula in this field. This has stemmed from two basic sources: (a) an awareness of the shortage of trained personnel in the field

to carry out the functions of direct leadership in hospitals and other settings; and (b) the general expansion of community college programs around the country to meet the academic and vocational needs of young people who are not motivated sufficiently, or otherwise unable to enter four-year colleges. Hutchinson described the rationale for such programs:

> Those students entering junior (community) colleges who seek a terminal education at the end of two years should be given the opportunity to prepare themselves as assistants in therapeutic recreation settings. A two-year course could develop some to become valuable technicians who, under professional supervision, could contribute much to the recreation program. The functional roles which seem appropriate for them are: movie projector operators and visual aids experts; radio operators, and/or television repairmen; games rooms operators; designers of posters, notices, and other visual materials; organizers of outings, picnics and camp trips; storeroom and equipment attendants; and program assistants.[13]

The programs developed in such two-year community college curricula have tended to cover the broad range of courses in community recreation, recreation history and philosophy, programming and leadership, methods of supervision and organization, special programs for the disabled and recreation skills. Despite the original conception of community college programs as terminal, two trends have developed among many community college graduates:

1. Those who found employment tended to move into actual leadership or supervisory roles rather than be restricted to the kinds of limited tasks described by Hutchinson. Thus, they represented a threat to those already in the profession, who felt that opening up job levels that had formerly required a bachelor's degree to community college graduates represented a lowering of professional standards.

[13] John L. Hutchinson: "Therapeutic Recreation Education: Programs and Proposals for Sub-Professionals." *Recreation in Treatment Centers,* September, 1964, p. 29.

2. The great number of positions expected to materialize for two-year graduates did not appear, and promotional opportunities were sharply limited. Thus, the bulk of community college students sought to transfer, following graduation, to four-year colleges, where they might complete their bachelor's degrees and become fully eligible for Civil Service and other professional positions.

Hutchinson also urged that—in order to relieve the shortage of therapeutic recreation personnel—intensive three-month training institutes be given to prepare recreation aides, including retired persons, to work in hospitals and other treatment settings. Such institutes have not generally been developed, with the exception of short courses which have been used to prepare recreation aides for nursing homes (an area of extreme shortage of personnel, in which the salaries have not been attractive enough to justify employing full-time, professionally-trained individuals). In some cases, specially-funded federal grants have been given to train minority-group persons from disadvantaged backgrounds in therapeutic recreation leadership. In general, however, only a limited number of positions have been created to employ such persons.

PERSONNEL-SHARING PLANS. Other attempts to meet the personnel shortage have included an experimental approach to having several institutions share the costs of employing a professional recreation director who would supervise the work of subprofessionals and volunteers in each of the agencies.[14]

Gehan describes a cooperative venture in Peoria, Illinois, in which six participating agencies (three general hospitals, a county nursing home, a private home for the aged and the Peoria Institute for Physical Medicine and Rehabilitation) joined together to establish a jointly operated activity therapy program. The program was modeled after pilot projects in nursing homes which were carried on by the National Recreation Association's Consulting Service on Recreation for the Ill and Handicapped. It consisted of employing a professionally qualified director of services, who surveyed and evaluated the needs, resources and existing programs in each of the cooperating institutions. He then developed plans for having persons in the community with skills in art, music or dramatics serve as part-time consultants to patients, staff personnel and volunteers in the participating institutions, in helping them develop programs.

It was also the director's responsibility to promote community interest in supporting the program, both financially and by providing volunteers who might work with patients and other employees. Public meetings were held, and an orientation course provided, to train those who would be working in each of the institutions. Gehan recommended that such programs be initially begun with the aid of foundation funds or other special grants, and that it then become the ultimate responsibility of the community to support them financially.

Another approach that has been used in many nursing homes to overcome the personnel shortage has been to have several institutions employ a consultant on therapeutic recreation, who then visits each of them regularly, supervising aides, nurses and other part-time or nonprofessional personnel in conducting actual program activities. In most cases, such arrangements do not constitute an actual cooperative plan on the part of the nursing homes. Instead, they simply represent a convenient means of hiring part of the time of a professional consultant to assist in program development, and of meeting state-imposed requirements for activity programs in nursing homes.

USE OF VOLUNTEERS. A final means of dealing with the personnel shortage is using volunteers to carry on actual programs. Clark sums up the values to be gained by the use of volunteers in a Veterans Administration hospital:

We believe that volunteers under medical staff leadership and guidance can make a valuable contribution to the care and treatment of patients. We believe the volunteer's contribution is made in two basic types of supplemental service to the patients; first, direct service in which the volunteers par-

---

[14] John Gehan: "Bridging the Gap." *Recreation,* May, 1961, pp. 261–262, 274.

ticipate in hospital-approved programs with and for the patients; secondly, direct service in which the volunteers provide equally valuable assistance as public relations ambassadors to the community, informing friends and neighbors about the care and treatment programs and the role of the community in assisting in these programs.[15]

In addition to these values, volunteers are able to relieve professional staff members of many time-consuming tasks that do not require a high level of training. They may provide specialized leadership skills lacking in the regular staff, thus extending the program and offering more highly individualized activities. The fact that they are offering their time without payment, because they *care,* is undoubtedly an important morale "booster" for patients. However, volunteers may constitute a serious adminstrative problem if they are not properly guided and supervised. Clark suggests a set of guidelines for this process:

1. *Organization.* It is necessary to have one individual who will coordinate and direct the volunteer program, acting as a liaison with community organizations which are the source of volunteers, and assuming this entire responsibility.
2. *Climate.* It is necessary, as a first step, to establish a climate for the constructive use of volunteers within the total scope and philosophy of the agency. Staff members—who may feel threatened by the use of volunteers who work for nothing and may have highly developed skills—should be helped to accept volunteers, and assured that they do not represent a danger to professional, paid personnel.
3. *Establish Need.* Before any volunteers are recruited or accepted, the agency should carry out a survey of its need for volunteers. After these have been established, "job" descriptions might be written for each possible volunteer assignment.
4. *Recruitment.* Generally this is carried on most effectively if there is an advisory council for voluntary services in the community. If not, contact must be made with service organizations that provide volunteers, and all forms of communication (radio, television, announcements, newspapers, and personal contact) should be used to reach potential volunteers.
5. *Screening and Selection.* The potential volunteer should fill out appropriate background forms and be interviewed by the member of the staff responsible for coordinating volunteer services. Such qualities as sincere interest, the ability to work with people and to accept the policies of the agency, dependability, and personal stability should be assessed in this meeting. Then the volunteer should be interviewed by the member of the staff responsible for the program to which he would be assigned.
6. *Orientation and Training.* All volunteers who are accepted should be given a thorough introduction to the agency, in which they are helped to understand its objectives and philosophy, and learn about its structure and operation. Such a process helps to develop an effective rapport between staff members and volunteers. There should also be a preliminary period of instruction of specific skills or methods of carrying out the assignment.
7. *Supervision.* This is a key element in the use of volunteers. A properly qualified, capable supervisor should observe the work of the volunteer, meet with him regularly, offer assistance when needed, help him recognize and solve his problems—and, if necessary, make recommendations for re-assigning or terminating the employment of the volunteer.
8. *Recognition.* Most volunteers do contribute an important service, which should be recognized. This may be done regularly through the year, by praise and recognition of achievements at staff meetings. Providing identification cards or other formal symbols of volunteer roles may be helpful. In addition, it is desirable to give volunteers scrolls or other concrete statements of appreciation, or to hold volunteer dinners or other formal ceremonies in which they are publicly recognized.

---

[15] Thomas J. Clark: "The Administration of Voluntary Services in a Recreation Program." *Recreation in Treatment Centers,* September, 1962, pp. 13–17.

A final important consideration in this chapter is the relation of therapeutic recreation specialists with other treatment modalities. In many hospitals and treatment centers, recreation has become incorporated in total rehabilitation departments, in which recreation specialists must work in close cooperation with occupational therapists, physical therapists and similar personnel. The following section provides concise descriptions of the different disciplines found in the hospital setting which may be provided as part of the rehabilitation process.

Activity and Adjunctive Therapies

Before it is possible to meaningfully consider the role of the activity therapies, or adjunctive therapies as they are sometimes called, it is essential to examine their relationship to the physician and the role he plays. This may be done with respect to two major types of medical settings: *physical medicine and rehabilitation,* and *psychiatric care.* Both are part of the broad process of rehabilitation, which involves the "cooperative efforts of various medical specialists and their associates in other health fields to improve the physical, mental, social and vocational aptitudes of persons who are handicapped, with the objective of preserving their ability to live happily and productively on the same level and with the same opportunities as their neighbors."[16]

The physician's responsibility today goes far beyond diagnosing, providing necessary surgical or drug treatment and then dismissing his patient. Instead, he must concern himself not only with the physical disability but also with the psychological, social and vocational problems of his patient. Pinner writes:

The need is not, in my opinion, diagnosis and specific treatment of so-called psycho-somatic diseases, but the recognition—which is not new, but so frequently forgotten and ignored—that every disease is psycho-somatic, that is, that it affects both body and soul.[17]

How is this whole person to be treated in the field of physical medicine? Krusen writes that rehabilitation, as practiced in modern treatment centers, is a multidisciplinary service directed by the specialist in physical medicine and rehabilitation, assisted by other specialists in internal medicine, pediatrics, orthopedic surgery, neurology, neurosurgery and plastic surgery. These physicians in turn are assisted by a team of associates in the allied health professions, which might include various types of therapists, as well as social workers, clinical psychologists and vocational counselors.[18]

Within the field of psychiatric treatment, occupational and recreational therapy have, since the 1930s, been operating under a model of prescribing individualized activities designed to meet patients' specific psychodynamic needs during the recovery process. This approach was popularized at the Menninger Clinic, and involved instructing members of the staff in precisely how to deal with specific patients. Activities themselves became a means of making psychodynamic diagnoses, and the adjunctive therapist developed elaborate schemes for prescribing specific activities for patients. Pattison comments that this model persists as a dominant model for the adjunctive therapies in psychiatric institutions for two reasons:

For one, it adheres closely to the traditional model of psychodynamic psychotherapy which focuses solely on the one-to-one therapeutic relationship. The adjunctive therapist in his occupational or recreational therapy represents an extension of the one-to-one model of therapy. The activities of the adjunctive therapist are intended to indeed be "therapy"; and the adjunctive therapist becomes a junior psychiatrist of sorts. Thus the work of the adjunctive therapist is determined and controlled by the psychiatrist who is the ultimate authority

[16] Frank H. Krusen, Frederick J. Kottke, and Paul M. Ellwood, (eds.): *Handbook of Physical Medicine and Rehabilitation,* Philadelphia, W. B. Saunders Co., 1971, p. 1.

[17] Max Pinner; *In* Krusen et al.: *op. cit.,* p. 4.

[18] *Ibid.,* p. 2.

on the diagnosis and psychodynamic treatment of the patient . . . .[19]

The second reason, in Pattison's view, for this model's continued use is that it supports the professionalization of the various adjunctive therapies. Typically, adjunctive therapists look to the psychiatrist to achieve identity and gain social and professional status. Thus, adjunctive therapists are urged to become educated in psychiatric diagnosis and in psychotherapeutic techniques. However, it is no longer taken for granted that the major value of the adjunctive therapies lies in their specific psychodynamic meanings. Instead, in many institutions, their contribution is seen chiefly as being in the area of creating a therapeutic environment.

The concept of "milieu" therapy implies that treatment consists chiefly of providing, guiding and maintaining activities which are therapeutic, and thus promoting healthy patterns of social interaction. Specifically, then, the adjunctive therapies should *not* be regarded as therapy in a literal sense, but rather as elements of the total treatment process which contribute to varied aspects of the patient's growth and recovery.

With this background, the following section describes a number of activities or adjunctive therapies which are prominent in the field of rehabilitation today.

Occupational Therapy

The field of occupational therapy has been broadly defined by the American Occupational Therapy Association as "any activity, mental or physical, prescribed by a physician as a valuable adjunct in contributing to and hastening recovery. Physically, its function is to increase muscle strength and joint motion as well as to improve the general bodily health; mentally, its function is to supply as nearly as possible normal activity through avocational projects and prevocational studies and training."[20] More recently, the U.S. Public Health Service described occupational therapy in these terms:

Occupational therapy (is) the use of purposeful activity in the rehabilitation of persons with physical or emotional disability. The occupational therapist, as a vital member of the rehabilitation team, determines the objectives of the treatment program according to the individual needs of each patient. This may include decreasing disability during the patient's initial phases of recovery following injury or illness, increasing the individual's capability for independence and improving his physical, emotional, and social well-being and developing his total function to a maximum level through early evaluation and experimentation for future job training and employment.[21]

Occupational therapy may be prescribed to accomplish any of the following objectives:

1. Specific treatment for psychiatric patients—to structure opportunities for the development of more satisfying relationships, to assist in releasing or sublimating emotional drives, to aid as a diagnostic tool.
2. Specific treatment for restoration of physical function—to increase joint motion, muscle strength, and coordination.
3. To teach self-help activities—those of daily living such as eating, dressing, writing, the use of adapted equipment, and prostheses.
4. To help the disabled homemaker readjust to home routines with advice and instruction as to the adaptation of household equipment and work simplification.
5. To develop work tolerance and maintenance of special skills as required by the patient's job.
6. To provide prevocational exploration— to determine the patient's physical and mental capacities, social adjustment, interests, work habits, skills, and potential employability.

[19] E. Mansell Pattison: "The Relationship of the Adjunctive and Therapeutic Recreation Services to Community Mental Health Programs." *Therapeutic Recreation Journal,* 1st Quarter, 1969, p. 17.

[20] John Eisele Davis: *Principles and Practices of Rehabilitation.* New York, A. S. Barnes and Co., Inc., 1943, p. 169.

[21] *Health Resource Statistics, 1968: op. cit.,* p. 145.

7. A supportive measure—help the patient to accept and utilize constructively a prolonged period of hospitalization and convalescence.
8. Redirection of recreational and avocational interests.[22]

It is apparent that a number of these goals are very similar to those of therapeutic recreation service. This is supported by the actual content of occupational therapy, which includes many clearly recreational activities.

However, a clear distinction must be made between therapeutic recreation and occupational therapy, in terms of professional preparation. Occupational therapists must graduate from a college or university accredited by the Council on Medical Education of the American Medical Association, in collaboration with the American Occupational Therapy Association. Such programs may have as a minimum requirement a four-year bachelor's degree, or a one-year certification program following the bachelor's degree, or a two-year Master's degree program. Normally, they include considerable work in the biological sciences, particularly human anatomy and physiology, behavioral sciences and physical and psychosocial dysfunction, as well as courses in occupational therapy principles and skills.

As indicated, most occupational therapy programs place a heavy emphasis on the use of manual activities, such as crafts or industrial skills, to help patients recover function with respect to writing, reading, self-care, homemaking and the use of prosthetic equipment, in order to increase mobility and the ability to function in various spheres of living.

The Veterans Administration stresses the arts and crafts aspect of the occupational therapist's work, emphasizing such activities as woodworking, leathercraft, ceramics, textilecraft and other creative projects:

The therapist provides planned treatment for motivation, functional restorations, work exploration and measurement of physical capacity. The program frequently requires adapting or devising equipment, splints and other self-help items to assist the patient in achieving a great degree of independence.[23]

Physical Therapy

Physical therapy is concerned with the restoration of function and prevention of disability following disease, injury or loss of a bodily part. It seeks to aid the normal progression of the healing process by serving to relieve symptoms and speed recovery.

Among the types of patients served by physical therapy are those suffering from chronic arthritis, rheumatism, forms of paralysis, organic and functional affections of the nervous system, digestive disturbances and various other severe trauma. Generally, physical therapy employs the following types of treatment:

1. Thermotherapy: radiant heat; artifically induced fever.
2. Light therapy: heliotherapy; artificial ultraviolet radiation.
3. Electrotherapy: Galvanic current; low-frequency currents (electrodiagnosis); high-frequency currents (long-and-short wave diathermy); static electricity.
4. Hydrotherapy: hot and cold, medicated, electric baths; douches and showers; whirlpool bath, therapeutic pool; colonic irrigation.
5. Mechanotherapy: massage; general and special exercise; occupational therapy.[24]

In addition, physical therapy includes the process of instruction, in that it is often necessary to teach patients and/or their families about the use of prosthetic and orthopedic appliances, the use of continuing therapeutic exercises and other home treatment procedures. Physical

[23] *Orientation Manual, Physical Medicine and Rehabilitation.* Washington, D.C., Veterans Administration Department of Medicine and Surgery, March, 1966, p. 20.
[24] Richard Kovacs: *A Manual of Physical Therapy.* 4th Ed. Philadelphia: Lea and Febiger, 1949, pp. 13–14.

[22] Helen S. Willard and Clare S. Speckman: *Occupational Therapy.* Philadelphia, J. B. Lippincott Co., 1971, p. 2.

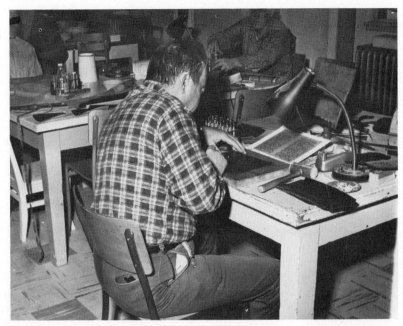

The Saskatchewan Hospital at Weyburn, Canada offers such creative activities as leather-carving . . .

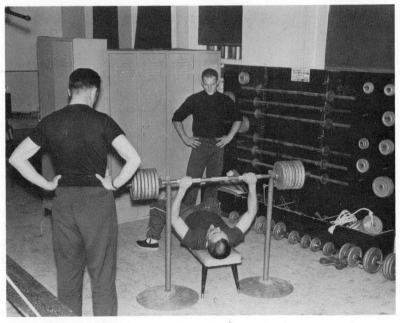

. . . and body-building activities.

therapy generally is regarded as having three major phases or applications:

1. *Prevention:* to prevent deformity or disability, instruction and practice may be given in corrective posture and movement techniques, muscle reeducation or progressive relaxation, as well as preoperative exercises given before surgical procedures.
2. *Diagnosis and treatment:* use of physical therapy as a form of testing, to assist the physician in establishing the diagnosis of certain conditions and in determining prognosis and the treatment required; treatment by medically prescribed physical therapy procedures and techniques.
3. *Rehabilitation:* this should begin the day the patient enters a hospital or rehabilitation center, and continue until maximum functional or organic recovery is achieved. It includes instruction in functional training, ambulation and self-care activities leading to maximum social and vocational independence.

Physical therapy is based on medical guidance and precisely-stated objectives. It is normally applied on a one-to-one basis, in which the patient is, for the most part, in a passive or recipient role; it has comparatively little effect on his social or emotional development. As in the case of occupational therapy, this field normally requires graduation from an approved school or department of physical therapy, and the passing of a state board examination.

Corrective Therapy

Corrective therapy is the treatment of patients by medically prescribed physical exercises and activities designed to strengthen and coordinate functions and to prevent muscular decline resulting from lengthy convalescence or inactivity due to illness.[25] It places emphasis on functional training and practice in the more ad-

vanced stages of rehabilitation, and makes use of various types of exercises and modified sports activities. In addition, it may provide instruction in the use of orthopedic and prosthetic appliances.

The Veterans Administration employs the largest number of personnel specifically identified as corrective therapists. Generally, corrective therapy in the V.A. hospitals includes the following types of treatment activities:

1. Conditioning exercises to develop strength, endurance, neuromuscular coordination and agility; reconditioning exercise to prevent both physical and psychological deconditioning.
2. Exercises and resocialization activities for psychiatric patients, specifically oriented toward the accomplishment of psychiatric objectives.
3. Teaching self-care activities, including personal hygiene.
4. Teaching of functional ambulation and elevation techniques, including the use of all types of prosthetic devices.
5. Therapeutic swimming (hydrogymnastic) programs.
6. Corrective and postural exercises prescribed and administered for specific conditions.
7. Conditioning, reconditioning, self-care and motivation activities for aged and infirm patients.
8. Special activities in the reorientation of the blind.
9. Training in the operation of manually controlled motor vehicles, where appropriate.

Corrective therapy may be provided in ward or clinic situations or in outdoor exercise or games areas. Normally, prescription for corrective therapy is given on an individual basis, although the program of activity itself may be carried on in a group setting.

The title "corrective therapist" is normally given to persons who work in this field in hospitals, nursing homes and rehabilitation centers. The minimum educational requirement is a baccalaureate in physical education from an accredited school, which should include a strong component of courses in anatomy, kinesiology and related courses, followed by a

---

[25] *Orientation Manual. op. cit.,* p. 183.

period of clinical training involving 400 to 600 hours in an affiliated hospital approved by the American Corrective Therapy Association.

Adapted Physical Education

A field that is closely related to corrective therapy is *adapted physical education.* This term is normally applied to programs of modified physical activity provided in educational settings to meet the needs of atypical students with physical or psychological disability. In some settings, the term "corrective physical education" is used.

In adapted or corrective physical education, the activities of students should be highly individualized, with the choice and modification of activity based on medical diagnosis, prescription and supervision. Its application should mean that all students in a school setting are able to engage in some form of physical education:

> Adapted physical education is for every student who cannot safely or successfully participate in the regular program. Adapted physical education should not be limited to students with postural, orthopedic, and organic conditions. The program should include students with visual handicaps and hearing impairment, as well as those with intellectual limitations, behavior problems, perceptual-motor difficulties, and (other) physical impairments. In addition to students with chronic conditions, adapted programs should provide for those recuperating from injuries and accidents and those convalescing from long or short term illnesses.[26]

Adapted physical educators are not as fully trained in this field, and do not deal with individuals who are as severely disabled as those served by corrective therapists in hospital settings. In general, corrective therapy and adapted physical education tend to share similar objectives and to employ the same types of activities.

---

[26] See *Journal of Health, Physical Education and Recreation,* May, 1969, p. 45.

Adapted physical educators make greater use of modified games and sports, while corrective therapists rely more heavily on various types of individualized exercises and functional training activities.

Other Activity Therapies

Although occupational, physical and corrective therapy are the best known forms of activity or adjunctive therapies, a number of other therapies are used in various rehabilitation settings.

Educational Therapy

Educational therapy is the utilization of instruction in academic areas of education, consciously used to develop the mental and physical capabilities of hospitalized patients. Instruction given at various levels may be accredited by recognized educational authorities. It may be restricted to classwork in such subjects as English, mathematics or the physical or social sciences—all carefully geared to the capabilities of those taking part, and with teaching methods designed to meet individual needs.

In addition, in some programs of educational therapy, discussion groups serve to promote motivation and social involvement. Such sessions may include current events discussions, travelogues, seminars on problems of aging, human relations or similar topics. Educational programs of this type are becoming increasingly important in treatment plans for chronic, long-term geriatric patients, and in some cases have been blended with "sensitivity training" or "encounter group" methods to promote interaction, awareness and involvement on the part of aging patients. One approach to using discussion groups in this way has been titled "remotivation therapy."

Educational therapists are normally people who hold a college degree with a major in education, combined with several months of training in a clinical setting.

Manual Arts Therapy

Manual arts therapy is the use of industrial arts activities of vocational value in programs of actual or simulated work situations that help patients prepare for return to community life and successful vocational adjustment.

In part, such therapy is used to appraise patients' reactions, functional ability, emotional status and aptitudes, in order to help them in planning realistic rehabilitation goals relating to post-hospital employment or involvement in a sheltered workshop. In addition, manual arts therapy may have the same goals as occupational therapy, in terms of direct stimulation and improvement of the patient's physical and mental functioning. Typically, seven broad categories of manual arts therapy are: metalworking, woodworking, electrical work, graphic and applied arts, agriculture and hospital industries. Within these categories, the demands of many types of job operations can be duplicated, and the patient's level of performance evaluated.

The normal preparation of a manual arts therapist consists of a college degree with a major in industrial arts, agriculture or some other related field, followed by a period of between two and seven months training at an approved hospital or rehabilitation center.

Music Therapy

The use of music for therapeutic purposes is found more widely in psychiatric treatment programs than in physical rehabilitation settings. Emphasis is placed on the use of music as a means of promoting group dynamics, nonverbal communication and individual expression. Both improvisation and instruction in technical skills are stressed, with the emphasis usually on instrumental music.

Music is generally viewed as a medium through which disturbed patients may be reached and involved, and in which they may find not only emotional expression and release but also a growing sense of self-worth. It is regarded as a supportive therapy that facilitates other treatment methods. A number of colleges offer degree programs in music therapy today. To meet the standards of the National Association for Music Therapy, qualified music therapists must complete a six-month internship in approved psychiatric hospitals affiliated with their institution.

Industrial Therapy

This field consists of the therapeutic use of activities related to the operation of the hospital. Formerly it was known as "hospital industry"; it involves the patient working in such capacities as: laborer, carpenter, kitchen worker, electrician, plumber, clerk-typist, laboratory technician, psychiatric aide or nursing aide. In some settings, such assignments of patients (e.g., unskilled labor, laundry help, grounds maintenance and the like) have represented little more than a form of cheap labor that helps to keep the hospital going. However, when properly supervised, industrial therapy has real value for patients. A Veterans Administration statement to this effect holds that:

> The motivation provided, the acceptance engendered, the socialization encouraged, the psychodynamics observed provide definite therapeutic benefits for the patient which far outweigh the benefits the hospital may receive from the patient's efforts.[27]

The distinction between industrial arts and manual arts therapy is that the former generally involves performing a real work function which is significant in the operation of the hospital, while the latter is basically a form of modified instruction and treatment within a clinic or workshop setting. Industrial therapy is not normally carried on under the guidance of specially-trained therapists, but is most valuable when selective placement techniques are used and patients are carefully observed and evaluated.

There is a growing body of opinion that work in itself is an important form of therapeutic experience and makes a significant contribution to the patient's feeling of self-worth and importance, as well

---

[27] *Orientation Manual. op. cit.,* p. 27.

as to his growing readiness for discharge to the community and ultimate vocational adjustment. This view is based in part on the high value that modern society places on work as a human endeavor. It also is based on the nature of work which relates patients to reality-based situations, providing a structure to their lives, and a sense of concrete accomplishment.

Art Therapy

Like the field of music therapy, art therapy is generally regarded as a form of treatment which provides the opportunity for healthy self-expression and growth, self-awareness, communication and relation to society. Art has been widely used in the past as a means of understanding the dynamic elements in a patient's illness (it is chiefly used in psychiatric therapy), and helping him express himself and recognize the source of some of his own difficulties through non-verbal forms of expression.

In recent years, there has been a growing recognition of the value of creative expression in healthy personality development and integration. Art therapy generally focuses on the freer forms of artistic expression, such as drawing, painting, modeling and sculpture. It is commonly seen as a highly flexible, individualized experience, in which patients select their own project and proceed at their own pace, with the encouragement and help of the art therapist. In some settings, an art studio is simply made available for the voluntary use of patients, unlike other forms of therapy which may be prescribed and carefully structured for them. The brochure of one psychiatric institution simply states:

> There is paper and paint and people and music and pencil and chalk and ideas and ink and wood and canvas and coffee and book and clay and you—if you choose.[28]

Art therapy may also be used for specific hospital projects, such as the design of Christmas cards and the provision of posters or other art work for departments of public information, recreation or volunteers. A number of colleges or special schools have initiated special training programs for art therapists which include course work in psychology, psychopathology, rehabilitation and therapeutic methods, as well as art techniques.

Bibliotherapy

This field consists of the guided use of reading to promote patient recovery. Normally, it is carried on by hospital librarians who become specialists in understanding patient needs, and who help them in selecting books, magazines or stories that will meet their interests and promote specific aspects of reintegration. Generally, it does not constitute a separate professional field with its own area of training, but represents the work of librarians who become knowledgeable in the area of psychodynamics, and who work closely with medical personnel in understanding and guiding patients in their reading programs.

Play Therapy

This form of therapy is generally carried on with younger children in hospital or psychiatric treatment settings. In the hospital, it may be used with both general medical and psychiatric patients. In one general hospital setting, it has been described as having the following goals:

1. To offer diversional activity to the child while undergoing medical treatment, thus continuing as much normal play as possible.
2. To help alleviate tension or feeling of homesickness, thus aiding orientation by establishing a better rapport with hospital personnel and other children.
3. To promote normal development, in spite of physical, mental or emotional disability.
4. To promote staff and parental understanding of the purpose, use and selection of play experiences and equipment.[29]

---

[28] "Art Studio: Therapy in an Institutional Setting." *Information Center Recreation for the Handicapped, Newsletter,* July–August, 1971, p. 1.

[29] Eloise C. Parker: "Play Therapy." *American Journal of Occupational Therapy,* September–October, 1952.

When used as a form of treatment with disturbed children, play therapy is normally carried on by specially trained therapists with a strong background in guidance and psychotherapeutic principles and techniques. Usually, it is unstructured; children are encouraged to use a variety of media—toys, play equipment, clay, finger-painting, construction materials, dolls, clothing and similar free-expression materials—in a completely free way. They play either individually or in small groups, with a therapist who encourages them, helps them resolve difficulties and talks with them about what they are doing and why, but does *not* instruct or guide them in any formal way. Play therapy is used as a means of understanding disturbed children and diagnosing the bases of their illness, and also of helping them express themselves in nonverbal ways. For severely disturbed children, play may represent the only way to encourage self-expression and communication, and may represent the first step in the process of communicating with a therapist and beginning the treatment process.

Dance Therapy

Like art and music therapy, dance therapy is based on the view that expressed feeling, meaningfully shared, can aid in the integration of the personality and growth in the ability to relate to others. It is particularly useful in work with individuals for whom words are difficult or impossible.

Dance therapy utilizes the tools of basic dance movement and rhythmic action as a means toward nonverbal communication. In many hospitals, both psychiatric and physically disabled patients may be involved in social forms of dance, such as folk, square and social dancing, as part of the overall recreation program. When it is applied as dance therapy, it consists of a simplified and unstructured form of modern or creative dance, permitting highly individualized, free personal movement. The dance therapist aids individuals or groups of patients in discovering

their own capabilities for expressive movement, using simple music, drum rhythms, or even vocalization and other improvised sounds, as accompaniment.

At its most effective, dance therapy is carried on in close consultation with psychiatrist and other hospital personnel, and with close attention being paid to the psychodynamic needs and recovery process of individual participants. There has been an increasing amount of research and special training in this field, encouraged by the American Dance Therapy Association.

Homemaking Therapy

The specialist in this field is customarily referred to as the "homemaking rehabilitation consultant." Such individuals are usually college graduates with a degree in home economics or occupational therapy, followed by in-service or graduate training in work with the physically or mentally disabled. Degrees or work experience in such fields as dietetics, nutrition or home economics, or practical experience in homemaking and child care are also valuable attributes.

The homemaking rehabilitation consultant adapts knowledge of home management, family finance, nutrition and similar subjects to meet the needs of disabled persons who have housekeeping responsibilities to which they will return, on discharge. The specialist may either provide direct retraining experiences in these areas to patients, or may, as a resource specialist, counsel other persons on the rehabilitation team. His goals should be to strengthen the skills of patients in these areas, and to help restore their confidence in being able to handle family problems, at which they may have failed in the past.

Status and Role of the Therapeutic Recreation Specialist

This chapter has thus far examined the early development, patterns of employment, functions of and professional education in therapeutic recreation service. It should be understood that in many institutional settings, therapeutic recreation does not function as a separate department but instead is a service division within a total department of rehabilitation, or part of a department of activity or adjunctive therapies.

In conclusion, the question should be asked: what is the present status and degree of acceptance of therapeutic recreation service as a specialized field of rehabilitation or community service?

PRESENT DEGREE OF RECOGNITION. As the early sections of this text have indicated, there has been a steady growth in therapeutic recreation service, at first in hospitals and other treatment centers, and more recently in community-based programs. This growth testifies to increased recognition given to this field by the public at large, by community recreation and park officials and by hospital administrators and doctors in general.

However, this recognition is still on a somewhat tenuous basis. Community recreators, for the most part, see their function with respect to therapeutic recreation service as limited to sponsoring Senior Citizens clubs or providing an occasional special program for the mentally retarded or physically disabled. Few have fully accepted the view that this area of service represents a major responsibility of the municipal recreation and park departments. Fewer still have developed meaningful links with institutions in order to facilitate after-discharge programming for disabled persons.

In many hospitals, the view of recreation is that it is chiefly a diversional activity, and thus deserves lower priority than other services that are more closely related to treatment goals. In part, this attitude stems from the fact that, unlike occupational therapy and physical therapy, both of which are certified fields requiring clinical training under medical supervision, the field of therapeutic recreation does *not* require such training. In many institutions, those working in recreation have come from other disciplines, and have little specialized preparation for their work.

This problem is made more complex

by the fact that many therapeutic recreation specialists today work in settings where medically-oriented training is *not* essential. The recreation leader who works in a Senior Center, a home or school for the retarded, a correctional institution or similar setting, may require varied kinds of information related to that disability and its treatment goals and procedures—but it is not basically medical information.

Thus, it is essential that fuller attention be given to the nature of professional education in therapeutic recreation service today, as well as to the kinds of selection, accreditation, registration or certification procedures that might be used to insure a higher standard of professionalism among workers in this field.

Professional Education and the Work of Professional Organizations

As indicated earler, a 1969 survey revealed that 35 colleges and universities offered degree programs in therapeutic recreation service. This number is increasing steadily. In addition, many other departments with recreation and park programs offer one or more special courses in therapeutic recreation service—although these do not constitute degree options.

Many of these programs are minimal in terms of staffing, courses offered and, particularly, clinical affiliations. While the most desirable method of upgrading therapeutic recreation curricula would be to develop accreditation procedures that would enforce adequate program standards, the attempt made to develop such a process—the National Recreation Education Project—has not yet achieved success.

It is a high-priority function of the National Therapeutic Recreation Society, in coordination with the Society for Park and Recreation Educators, to develop recommended curricula in this field, as well as standards relating to clinical placement, admissions, faculty and similar matters. Whether or not such standards can be enforced depends upon the capability of the professional organizations involved. Such efforts often prove to be divisive in the long run. However, it is apparent that they constitute the most promising means of upgrading professional education, producing more highly qualified practitioners and thus ultimately improving the status of workers in this field.

Need to Clarify Roles, Functions and Accomplishments

Just as in the overall field of recreation, the roles and functions of therapeutic recreation specialists are extremely complex and varied. Unlike the physical therapist, who has a clearly defined set of objectives and techniques, the recreation worker may have goals and methods that vary widely, according to the setting in which he is employed and the patients he is serving.

Therefore, it is necessary to define more sharply each of these specialized areas of service, as to the needs of those served and the unique responsibilities or functions of the therapeutic recreation specialist in each of them. It is quite apparent that this varies widely, from institution to institution—even within a particular area of service, such as psychiatric care. It is clear also that the other fields of professional service described earlier also impinge on recreation. Occupational therapists frequently assume major responsibility for recreation in their institutions. Corrective therapists frequently conduct modified games and sports activities. Music, art and dance therapists often provide services that might be regarded as recreational.

This confusion of role is made more complex by the fact that in an increasing number of departments of activity therapies, especially those committed to the "milieu therapy" approach, the functions of *all* practitioners have become blurred.

Again, it should be the responsibility of college and university educators in this field, and of those in professional organizations, to carry on systematic research to clarify roles and functions. Following this, it would be appropriate for them to make recommendations regarding the assignment of responsibilities that might be helpful to those responsible for organizing services in institutions, communities or in federal or statewide systems of rehabilitation. Closely attached to this is the need to conduct more effective research related to effective methodology in therapeutic recreation service, and to the legitimate outcomes of such programs.

Suggested Topics for Class Discussion, Examinations or Student Papers

1. Identify and describe several of the major functions carried out by therapeutic recreation specialists in hospital settings today. In what significant ways do these extend beyond the provision of an activity program?
2. What are the key ways in which the National Therapeutic Recreation Society serves to promote professional service in this field?
3. Contrast the work of specialists in other fields of activity therapy (such as occupational or physical therapy) with that of therapeutic recreation specialists. How do these fields differ? How do they overlap?

Chapter 4

Recreation and Mental Illness

Mental illness is a complex form of human disorder. Medical authorities have at best only limited knowledge of the causes and symptomatology of functional mental illness. Indeed, there are no clear-cut criteria for defining this disorder, or for characterizing a person as mentally ill. Despite these facts, it is clear that mental illness constitutes a major social problem today. It is said to affect one out of every ten persons in the United States, with psychiatric patients occupying almost half of all hospital beds at an economic cost of about three billion dollars a year.

Concepts of Mental Illness

In modern psychiatry, there are two conflicting approaches to characterizing mental illness.

The older approach, which might be characterized as the *disease model,* suggests that the psychotic behavior of a disturbed individual unfolds inevitably from a defective psychological or neurological system that is essentially contained within the person. Symptoms of mental disorder are not caused by the social system in which the individual exists; mental illness is considered in the same manner as a virus infection or other physical illness might be.

The more recent approach, which might be described as the *maladaptive model,* takes into account the social en-

vironment—including the family, neighborhood and larger community—of those persons who are described as mentally ill. The mentally ill, according to this viewpoint, should not be thought of or treated as diseased persons, but rather as individuals with severe problems of adjustment. Thus, disturbed behavior is simply seen as maladaptive, and often caused by stresses of the social environment and the inability of the individual to meet these stresses—rather than by pathology as such.

There is no clear line of distinction between so-called normal and abnormal behavior. Unlike physical illness, in which the norm is the structural or functional integrity of the body and in which medical science has little difficulty in identifying "illness," it is difficult to identify, along the range of possible actions, the point at which human behavior shifts from a normal to an abnormal form of expression.

Medical science has, however, suggested certain criteria for identifying the mental health of individuals. These critieria are rather broadly stated as: personal adjustment, personality integration, personal maturity and growth and social or group involvement. The actions of persons, in terms of whether or not they are able to function effectively in terms of family, vocational responsibility or other interpersonal relationships, are used to determine whether they are mentally healthy.

Physicians have established two major divisions in the classification of the mentally ill: disorders associated with organic brain disturbance, and disorders of psychogenic origin.

Chronic brain disorders, which result from severe, lasting damage to cerebral tissue, may effect impairment of judgment, memory or orientation. Epilepsy is an example of a brain disorder usually caused by physical injury to a tiny but critical part of the brain. Temporary injury to brain tissue may result in acute behavioral malfunction, from which the patient recovers. These two examples fall within the realm of organic brain disturbance.

In contrast, disorders of psychogenic origin have no apparent physical cause. Temporary personality disorders may be triggered by acute stress and tend to involve previously normal individuals who have a good potential for recovery. Another form of disorder is the presence of neurosis or psychoneurosis which is related to acute anxiety and partial inability to function effectively; this normally does not require hospitalization, although psychotherapeutic treatment may be helpful. Frequently, psychosomatic illnesses, such as migraine headaches or hypertension, may be connected to such neuroses. Other forms of character disorders may result in various symptoms, such as alcoholism, drug addiction or severely antisocial behavior.

Functional psychosis is the most severe and disabling psychogenic disorder, and it is to this category that the term mental illness is most frequently applied.

Functional psychosis usually involves a severe degree of personality disorganization and a progressive loss of contact with reality. It is customarily classified today under one of four headings: *schizophrenia, manic depression, involutional states* and *senility*. These represent the major disabilities of patients in mental hospitals today.

Schizophrenia

Schizophrenics are characterized by a striking withdrawal from society and from emotional ties with other persons. This may be caused by the general social alienation of the person, or loss of the ability to think in meaningful and logical terms. Five common characteristics of schizophrenics are: (a) withdrawal from reality; (b) autism; (c) emotional distortion; (d) delusions and hallucinations; and (e) abnormal or bizarre behavior.

Persons suffering from schizophrenia often have a history of social inadequacy. They tend to be disorganized persons who have never developed adequate roles or self-concepts. In the face of emotional difficulties or disappointments, they tend to withdraw into a fantasy world. They no longer communicate meaningfully with others, and their thought processes become disorganized and unreal. As a consequence, schizophrenics are unable to relate to or understand others, take meaningful social roles or function meaningfully in their families or in society at large.

Schizophrenic disturbance can be further categorized into the following groups.

SIMPLE SCHIZOPHRENIA. Persons suffering from this disorder are not always confined to mental hospitals, but may simply lead undemanding, socially withdrawn lives. Simple schizophrenics are generally isolated, with few friends and with jobs requiring only superficial contact with others; they often have peculiar habits of dress or speech.

HEBEPHRENIC SCHIZOPHRENIA. This frequently emerges at puberty, a time of physical change and emotional stress. The individual's thoughts become confused and his language unintelligible; he may be prone to hysteria, or uncontrollable laughter or rage. Hebephrenic schizophrenics often report hearing voices or other forms of hallucinations. They may ritualize their lives in great detail, apparently as a means of controlling their environment and avoiding ambiguous or threatening situations.

PARANOID SCHIZOPHRENIA. This common disorder often involves patients having a strong sense of persecution. They may feel that their entire environment is hostile and threatening, that people are plotting against them, and even that they are inhabited by, or controlled by, other persons. Paranoid schizophrenics tend to be suspicious of others and to resist social communication or emotional contact.

Manic Depression

Many persons experience mild depressions. These deepen markedly in the psychotic form of this disorder. The patient feels sad and lonely; his thought processes and behavior slow down. He refuses to respond to others, and the entire functioning of his mind, memory and thought processes is retarded. Depressive persons may become suspicious and irritable, and have frightening hallucinations, although, most commonly, they become slow and drowsy, sitting or lying in one spot for hours on end. Ultimately, the patient may become suicidal as a result of his feelings of hopelessness and lack of worth.

It is the nature of the manic-depressive patient to swing violently in emotional mood from extreme elation to severe depressive states. In the manic, or "high" state, he may have feelings of great optimism and become extremely energetic and overexcited, talking incessantly. He may develop unreal, grandiose images of himself. His judgment becomes faulty, he is easily distracted and may readily fly into sudden rages. When exhausted, he may then swing into a state of severe depression.

Involutional Psychosis

This disorder is similar to the extreme state of depression found in those with manic-depressive psychoses. It tends to occur for the first time in later middle age, along with general physical and intellectual decline. Patients complain of insomnia, excessive anxiety, restlessness and concern about unimportant matters; often they fall into spontaneous periods of weeping. Suicidal impulses and delusions of hypochondria are also frequently seen in involutional states. Those with involutional psychosis tend to remain in the depressive state, and not to recover spontaneously, as sometimes occurs with manic-depressive individuals.

Senility

In senile patients, progressive mental deterioration occurs as a result of the degenerative brain changes and arteriosclerosis that affect many older persons. Withdrawal from social contacts, a narrowing of interests and a general lessening of alertness and awareness of the environment are typical of senile patients. Often they become extremely confused, with severe memory impairment, even of recent events.

Causes of Mental Illness

In attempting to identify the causes of mental illness, it is first necessary to recognize that this term has never been precisely defined. Even today, the exact nature of mental illness in terms of personal behavior or psychological state has not been given a universally acceptable description, and diagnostic categories like those just presented are frequently modified or changed in the literature.

In past centuries, physicians tended to accept the view that all mental illness resulted from anatomical lesions of the brain or nervous system. This view, which dominated the practice of neurology and psychiatry in the United States until the turn of the 20th century, held that only the body could become diseased; the mind could not. As a result, only those who had suffered organic brain damage were regarded as legitimately mentally ill. All other disturbed persons were held to blame for their actions, and often prosecuted as willful criminals.

Sigmund Freud was responsible for the view that mental illness should be regarded as a functional maladjustment, without discernible anatomical basis. He conceived of the role of the psychiatrist or psychoanalyst as a practitioner of the science of the mind rather than of the brain and nervous system. According to Freud, all persons—even those who are considered mentally healthy—tend to adjust to life's problems by creating subtle delusions of reality and employing defence mechanisms to deal with stress and problems of human relationships.

Freud sought to eliminate the sharp differentiation between neurotics and so-called normal people. It was his view that abnormal psychology merely represented an exaggerated picture of processes that were at work among all human beings; the mentally ill were seen as caricatures of their more smoothly functioning brethren, and the state of the disturbed constituted a mirror held up to human nature in general.[1]

Despite the influence of Freudian theory in discouraging the doctrines of 19th century pathology, the view that mental illness is the result of biochemical inbalance or disturbance has been repeatedly presented during the present century. Pavlov, the Russian physiologist, drew a connection between schizophrenia and physiology in the overdevelopment of the process of cortical-based inhibitions which resulted in the individual's withdrawing from the outside world.

Recent scientific research has indeed demonstrated that biochemical and electrochemical disturbances accompany certain clinical manifestations of mental illness. Scientists have found that the brain encompasses a complicated system of nerve connections between arousal structures in the brain stems and the many areas of the cerebral cortex. Specific chemicals are employed in these connections to transmit impulses. They either arouse or retard the operation of brain processes, and their proper functioning is the basis of balanced behavior, including the generation of moods, appetites, desires and drives. Other pathways in the brain are concerned with countering such arousal activities by diminishing or inhibiting their effects.

In clinical cases of severe psychosis, it has been shown that the excitatory pathways and their chemicals have sharply increased their activities. This results in an increased state of arousal, which becomes difficult to handle. The patient becomes distracted and confused, and often overwhelmed by hallucinations, rages and other disorders of mental functions. In contrast, in depressed states, the patient does not appear to be properly aroused, with the likelihood that the arousal pathways in his brain are not sufficiently stimulated. In short, it is hypothesized today that both the explosive thought processes and behavior of the manic patient and the extreme withdrawal of the severely depressed individual are caused by physiological malfunctions.

It has still not been determined whether biochemical malfunctions of this type are the *cause* or the *result* of functional mental disturbance. Certainly, there is a strong body of professional medical opinion that holds that the primary cause of mental illness lies in environmental and social factors, and that psychosis results not from a chemical malfunction, but from inability to handle the stresses of daily living.

Those who take this position stress that mental illness is, in fact, a problem that all persons have to some degree. It is not seen as a disease in the classical sense, but rather as the result of the inability to cope with life in the fashion that social norms accept as mentally healthy. Since all persons deviate occasionally from what is considered normal behavior, some authorities have argued that it is wrong to classify such deviation as mental illness. Meyer writes:

> We are all in fact, at times mentally ill. Most, however, are never so far down on the continuum, or for long enough periods of time as to require professional assistance. The number requiring professional assistance varies by definition. If you define mental illness as needing 24-hour-a-day residential care, the number is indeed small. If you define mental illness as a condition which interferes with maximum performance and a reduction in happiness and self-fulfillment, you are talking about a massive number of people, perhaps 50 to 75 per cent of our total population.[2]

---

[1] Donald Fleming: "The Meaning of Mental Illness." *The Atlantic Monthly,* July, 1964, p. 73.

[2] Martin W. Meyer: "Recreation and Mental Health." *Dialogues with Doctors.* Raleigh, North Carolina, North Carolina Recreation Commission, Bulletin No. 41, April, 1968, p. 18.

Some authorities, critical of current psychiatric treatment processes, hold, in fact, that there is no such thing as mental illness in a medical sense.

Thomas Szasz, for example, characterizes mental illness as the impersonation of society's stereotype of madness by individuals whose real impairment concerns a problem in living. Mental illness, unlike a physical disease or defect, is perceived as a strategy of the individual to help himself cope with a psychological crisis or to get help from others. Since the behavior norm upon which the diagnosis of mental illness is based is a psychosocial and ethical standard, Szasz argues that it is illogical to attempt to "cure" it by medical means.

Carrying the argument further, Szasz argues that mental illness is a false concept that serves to hide and disguise, behind the facade of the term "mental illness," certain real problems in human needs, aspirations and values.

Therefore it is his position that it is wrong to diagnose cases of "mental illness" as forms of disease that should be treated. He argues vigorously against the present system of treatment by forced custodial care in mental hospitals. Szasz holds that if an individual has violated certain ethical, political or social norms, he should be permitted to do so—provided that he has not broken the law—in which case he should be sent to prison. Otherwise, he regards mentally ill persons as those who have broken out of their normal social role classifications and tried to define their own identities; and he sees the normal process of psychiatric treatment as forced repression by an organized society of individuals who are socially deviant.[3]

Other authors have presented similar points of view. Thomas Scheff, for example, suggests that most chronic mental illness represents a form of role playing in response to stereotypes that are established by society. He points out that at times of stress, severe depression or so-called psychological "crisis" states, many persons tend to be unsure of their own feelings and to behave in ways that deviate from normal behavior. They tend to be in a highly suggestible state, and are vulnerable to the suggestion by others that something is wrong with them, that they are "sick" or "going mad."

To support this argument, Scheff points out that the images of insanity in our society are continually reaffirmed and stereotyped, through childhood games, mass media imagery and ordinary social interaction. The disturbed person gradually adopts this stereotyped role; this is why so many mental patients seem to have the same "symptoms." The process of becoming a confirmed deviant, of being "mentally ill," is completed when the traditional imagery of insanity becomes part of the disturbed person's own orientation, and he accepts it as a basis for guiding his own behavior.

Scheff suggests that the assumption of the role of being "crazy" is used as a means of adjustment by the patient, because he is just as confused about his own behavior as are the observers. He prefers the role of insanity as a replacement for his normal self image, which has broken down under stress; the label of "I'm going mad" is preferable to the feelings of nothingness that the severely depressed person feels. He concludes that the mentally ill person has in a sense become a forcibly type-cast actor, forced into this role by society's reaction to his personal crisis. Ultimately, he cannot control his behavior; chronic mental illness is on the border between the volitional and the nonvolitional.[4]

The arguments made by Szasz and Scheff have been strongly supported by other authorities. Erving Goffman, for example, writes:

> . . . I want to stress that perception of losing one's mind is based on culturally derived and socially engrained stereotypes as to the significance of symptoms such as hearing voices, losing temporal and spatial orientation, and sensing that one is being followed, and that many of the most spectacular and convincing of these symptoms

[3] See Thomas S. Szasz: *Law Liberty, and Psychiatry: An Inquiry into the Social Uses of Mental Health Practices.* New York, The Macmillan Co., 1963.

[4] Thomas Scheff: *Being Mentally Ill—A sociological Theory.* Chicago, Aldine Publishing Co., 1966.

in some instances psychiatrically signify merely a temporary emotional upset in a stressful situation, however terrifying to the person at the time. Similarly, the anxiety consequent upon this perception of oneself, and the strategies devised to reduce this anxiety, are not a product of abnormal psychology, but would be exhibited by any person socialized into our culture who came to conceive of himself as someone losing his mind.[5]

A final eloquent spokesman for this point of view has been R. D. Laing, who has gone the furthest in criticizing the disease model of mental illness, and has implied that there is nothing really wrong with the person described as "mentally ill." Instead, Laing holds, it is the environment that has somehow gone wrong.

He argues that madness is not a disease to be cured, but results from the conflict between an outer "false" self and an inner "true" self. He suggests that this split is begun in childhood, when children have certain needs and feelings which they wish to express, but which they are taught by parents to suppress or change in order to be socially acceptable. By sheer social force, Laing argues, this inner self is compelled to become isolated from the false outer state that arises in compliance with society, and gradually becomes alienated from relatedness to the outside world.

In what is frequently referred to as a "nervous breakdown," the individual experiences the sudden removal of the veil of the false self, which served to maintain an appearance of outer normality but did not reflect the true feelings of the inner self.

In Laing's view, getting a person to behave in a conforming way, acting adaptively to the norms of society, is not a "cure" for what is disturbing him. He suggests that the traditional mental hospital approach attempts merely to restore the split between the true, inner, and the false, outer self. While it produces an outward compliance in the individual, and an ap-

parent "cure," it has merely denied the validity of the inner self.

In response to this, Laing developed a radical new approach that was carried out in an institution in England called Kingsley Hall. This involved an experiment in communal living, in which residents, all of whom had come from traditional mental institutions, were permitted to make up their own rules of operation instead of accepting old ones. The purpose of the Kingsley Hall experiment was to see what would happen if disturbed people were allowed to completely abandon their outer selves and let their "inner selves," which emerge during psychosis, take over. They were urged to follow their impulses completely rather than attempt to curb them, so that they could live and grow through their own "madness." No attempts at all were made to urge them to return to "normality," and no restrictions were placed on the behavior of members.

Kingsley Hall yielded some remarkable results. Many of its members, who had not been "cured" by years of treatment in traditional programs of psychiatric therapy, and who had been locked up for sustained periods in mental wards, were able to leave therapy and lead emotionally happy lives.[6]

While there is a growing body of agreement with Szasz, Scheff and Laing, the predominant opinion today is that there *is* such a phenomenon as mental illness—and that it is a disorder that prevents or inhibits happy and effective living in society. While treatment approaches vary considerably, an increasing number of therapists today are moving toward a "behaviorist" view of mental illness.

The Behavioral Psychology Viewpoint

The behaviorist holds that all human behavior is the result of learned associations of stimulus and response that the individual has been conditioned to adopt. Behavior generally is seen as coming about as a response to external pressures rather

[5] Erving Goffman: *Asylums: Essays on the Social Situation of Mental Patients and Other Inmates.* New York, Doubleday and Co., Inc., 1961, p. 132.

[6] See R. D. Laing: *The Politics of Experience.* New York, Ballantine Books, Inc., 1967.

than coming from within, as a coherent unfolding of the personality.

In this approach, human behavior is seen as adaptive; the actions of even the "strangest" individual are perceived as the long-term result of social influences to which he has learned to adapt. Therefore, his behavior is neither normal nor abnormal, right nor wrong; it is simply how the individual has *learned to* act. The goal of behavior therapy today is to get the mentally ill person to re-adapt to society's norms, by learning to act in ways that are considered normal. Only the part of the person's self which comes into contact with the outside world is important for the behaviorist. The so-called inner self is nonobservable, and therefore meaningless.

The behavioral therapist rules out any introspective report by the patient on his own mental processes, and instead is concerned solely with his observable external behavior. It is the behaviorist view that if the symptoms of abnormality can be arrested, then the person has been cured. Neurotic or even psychotic behavior is seen as the product of defective learning, and can be unlearned by intensive reconditioning and reeducation processes. Typically, alcoholism has been treated by "aversion therapy"—consisting of putting emetics in the patient's drink so that alcohol becomes distasteful rather than pleasurable.

Freudian psychotherapists see this approach as dealing superficially with the surface manifestations of underlying neurosis. They argue that if the therapy succeeds in removing or repressing a specific symptom, it will be replaced by another symptom, until the neurosis itself is uncovered and dealt with. Freudians see behavior therapy as a form of symptomatic relief which removes the outward evidences of disturbance without attacking the essential disturbance in personality or giving the patient any real insight into his own needs.

Trends in Psychiatric Care

Humanitarian attempts to care for and heal the mentally ill began about 150 years ago. Prior to that time, mental illness had been considered to be a result of witchcraft or possession by spirits, and its treatment had been carried on by such primitive measures as flagellation, confinement in dark cells and severe contrivances for mechanical restraint, shock treatments, and purging the sick person through emetics or bleeding.

The first half of the 19th century saw a new philosophy of treatment titled "moral therapy." This method emphasized kinder treatment of the insane, as well as the view that they should become involved in occupational and recreational activity.

Moral therapy also emphasized the need to keep institutions small, so that personal contact between the patients and the supervisor could be maintained. During this period, high rates of curability, often as high as 90 per cent, were reported for hospitals that had adopted this approach.

By the 1870s, a new approach replaced the moral therapy method. Mental institutions became largely custodial in nature. Recoveries and discharge rates declined to below ten per cent in many hospitals during the first two decades of the 20th century. Many psychiatrists believed that less than five per cent of schizophrenics could be expected to recover. Tourney attributes the growing therapeutic nihilism—as this period has been termed—to "personnel problems, budgetary difficulties, hospital overcrowding, the large proportion of chronic cases, and a dogmatic depersonalized theoretic approach to insanity."[7]

However, during this period a number of the basic principles underlying modern care for the mentally ill were first developed. Individual patient treatment, open-door policies, patient freedom, voluntary admissions, home and after-care services and sheltered or specially arranged employment for patients were all experimented with during this period.

Before the end of the 19th century, owing chiefly to the efforts of Sigmund

---

[7] Garfield Tourney: "Psychiatric Therapies: 1880–1968." *In:* Theodore Rothman, (ed.): *Changing Patterns in Psychiatric Care.* New York, Crown Publishers, Inc., 1970, p. 12.

Freud, attention was given to the effectiveness of the new method of psychotherapy in treating the mentally ill. This approach gave emphasis to the direct relationship between the physician and the patient rather than reliance on medical or surgical procedures. Techniques of dream analysis, exploration of the unconscious, free association and the use of transference were developed, based on a growing body of theory of psychoneurosis as the cause of mental illness. Psychotherapy tended to be offered chiefly in clinics and private practice, and to devote itself to the treatment of psychoneurosis, while its success with psychotic patients in mental hospitals was limited.

During the 1930s, new approaches in the field of somatic therapies were employed, including the use of insulin coma, convulsive therapy and lobotomy. Tourney writes:

> Two broad schools of psychiatry emerged, the organic-physical treatment oriented, and the psychodynamic-psychotherapeutic group. The former focused on psychotic patients, and the latter largely on the psychoneurotic and characteriologic problems.[8]

Somatic therapy as developed in the 1930s survives today in the use of electroconvulsive therapy for the treatment of depression. However, it aroused interest in the use of physical therapies and drugs in the treatment of psychotic patients; this paved the way for the two most recent and promising developments in psychiatry, *psychopharmacotherapy* and *community psychiatry*.

Psychopharmacotherapy

The recent revolution in drug-based psychotherapy began in 1951, when the French scientist Laborit synthesized chlorpromazine (Thorazine). This became widely used as a tranquilizer and accounts for the major portion of drug treatment today. Along with similar drugs, such as reserpine, chlorpromazine is used in such conditions as anxiety states, agitated depressions, manic states and schizophrenia. The effect of these drugs is to calm the overly aroused nerve systems in the brain.

The second phase of the psychopharmacological movement began in 1954, when iproniazid (Marsilid) was found useful with severely depressed patients. This drug and other "psychic energizers" which stimulate the arousal pathways in the mind began to replace convulsive therapies—particularly electroconvulsive treatment—in the care of depressive illness.

Since the mid-1950s the increase in the use of drugs in the treatment of the mentally ill has been tremendous. As an example, the total number of psychopharmaceutical tablets dispensed by the Boston State Hospital grew from 113,503 tablets in 1955 to 1,675,190 tablets in 1965—a more than tenfold increase. Similarly, the use of tablets in outpatient care has grown tremendously.

Many investigators regard psychopharmacology as palliative rather than curative. They claim that although drugs are useful in the reduction of symptoms, they do not hit at the basic causes of mental illness. The value of psychopharmacology appears to lie chiefly in its use with other therapeutic methods. It has made a great number of patients more accessible and amenable to treatment and has been used in combination with psychotherapy, milieu therapy and other specific treatments.

> An immediate and outstanding value is the control of tension and of disturbed behavior, reflected in the virtual elimination of restraint and seclusion in the department's institutions.[9]

The psychopharmacologic revolution has done much to change the nature of mental hospitals and of psychiatric care in general. In recent years, there has been a marked shift from large, impersonal mental hospitals devoted chiefly to custodial care, to smaller institutions based

---

[8] *Ibid.*, p. 35.

[9] *Treatment in the Modern Mental Hospital.* Albany, New York, New York State Department of Mental Hygiene, 1966, p. 1.

on the therapeutic community model, and, most recently, to the development of community mental health centers.

Within institutions, because it is no longer necessary to confine many patients, a new emphasis on activity and adjunctive therapy has been made possible. In general, there is a stronger push toward treating patients and getting them out of the hospital—or avoiding institutionalization in the first place. Fewer patients are neglected, and the total resources of the hospital may be used for therapeutic purposes. Emphasis is placed on helping patients return to community life by a combination of resocialization, living skills and work readiness experiences.

It should be made clear that medical opinion is still somewhat divided regarding drug therapy. Some psychiatrists regard psychopharmacotherapy as a "chemical strait jacket," in that it simply serves to make patients more docile, allowing overburdened hospital staffs to control them easily. In their view, doctors simply tend to do things *to* patients rather than work meaningfully *with* them. However, it is clear that one major benefit of this therapeutic innovation has been the sharp decrease in the number of patients confined on a long-term basis in large, isolated, custodial-type asylums, and the corresponding increase in the use of community mental health centers or small local hospitals or units in general hospitals. The purpose of the latter approach to treatment is to maintain disturbed persons in the community, or to reintegrate them as rapidly as possible.

Community Psychiatry

This represents the most important and promising recent trend in psychiatric care. Deriving its principles from the idea of social causation of mental illness, community psychiatry stresses the need to understand the familial, social and cultural milieu of each patient. The community psychiatry approach also defines mental illness broadly, and includes, as part of its concern, delinquency and crime, sex offenders, addicts and alcoholics, as well

as mentally retarded and isolated senile persons.

The chief emphasis in community psychiatry is to help patients move rapidly toward adjustment and constructive living in family and community settings. This works through decentralized mental health centers to prevent hospitalization or, when it is necessary, to get patients back into the community as rapidly as possible. Emphasis is placed on using a variety of groups or resources in the community, such as family, friends, employers, health and welfare agencies or sociorecreational organizations, to support and work with patients. Thus, the problem of isolation and resistance against treatment that often occurs when patients are taken a great distance from home and institutionalized may be minimized.

> Emphasis is placed . . . on treatment in the community, the utilization of clinic resources, day and night hospital units, crisis-oriented therapy, rehabilitation and aftercare, hospitalization in psychiatric units in general hospitals, earlier discharge, use of halfway houses, and the establishment of special programs for the mentally retarded, aged, alcoholics, and addicts. The education of the public regarding mental illness becomes paramount in helping change community attitudes toward the mentally ill.[10]

The community psychiatry movement was given a strong impetus by the Mental Retardation Facilities and Community Mental Health Centers Construction Act of 1963. This legislation stipulated that, in order to qualify for federal funds, a community mental health center must provide at least five essential services: (a) inpatient services; (b) outpatient services; (c) partial hospitalization services, including at least day-care; (d) emergency services provided 24 hours per day within at least one of these three categories; and (e) consultation and education services available to community agenices and professional personnel. In addition, adequate services were defined as including such other components as

---

[10] Garfield Tourney: *op. cit.,* p. 32.

diagnostic services, rehabilitation programs (including vocational and educational activities), pre-care and after-care services including foster home placements, training and research and evaluation.[11]

Many community mental health centers maintain some type of social group today to which patients can be referred, either by hospitals, psychiatrists, outpatient community clinics or other social agencies. In most cases, such clubs serve as an intermediary step for the patient to move from a treatment center to a more active social life. Another technique of helping patients in their return to community life is the halfway house. These are places where discharged persons can live, in the company of professional staff members and other former patients. It provides a means of helping them adjust to community life before attempting to live independently. Halfway houses offer alternatives to living alone in run-down hotels, or having to return to unsympathetic or overanxious relatives.

Within this entire context, the social life that becomes available to patients or former patients, and the degree to which they are able to become effectively reintegrated in community life, are of crucial concern.

Recreation in Psychiatric Treatment

Although it has not been possible to develop valid scientific evidence to show that recreation can either prevent or cure mental illness, it has been widely accepted that recreation makes an important contribution to psychological well-being. Meyer writes:

> Basically, recreation is an experience which leaves one refreshed, rejuvenated, fulfilled, happy, content and at peace with oneself and the world. It reinforces companionship, group belonging and esteem, mutual interests, concern for our fellow human beings. It is a happy, productive, creative and positive experience, fostering a feeling of well-being. It does not leave us isolated,

withdrawn, anxious, apprehensive, suspicious, hostile, fearful and totally sick inside. The outcomes of recreation, the very experience itself, are so closely related to positive mental health that one may consider them as almost synonymous.[12]

Individuals with poor mental health often have exaggerated feelings of worthlessness, inferiority, deficiency in body structure, athletic ability, intellectual performance or other personal characteristics. Commonly, such individuals have few friends and are not valued members of groups of their peers. Unable to achieve normal relationships, they frequently become supersensitive to social slights, apprehensive about failure and rejection and ultimately withdraw from social contacts.

Recreation has the capability for providing such individuals with the opportunity to be successful and to develop feelings of self-worth. It has other important functions as well, in terms of maintaining healthy emotional status. One of these is its potential for providing a release for the socially acceptable discharge of violent or hostile emotions. Recreation may be used to strengthen or develop such defense mechanisms as repression, displacement of affect, substitution, sublimation, and compensation. While it may be argued that these mechanisms do not deal with the fundamental neurotic problems that affect emotionally unstable persons, the fact is that they make it possible for many such individuals to live with themselves and others in a reasonably happy and constructive way.

Thus, recreation provides a means of dealing with one's antisocial or unhealthy impulses. Meyer writes:

> A classic example is the "substitution" of dangerous aggressive impulses, such as the desire to destroy or kill, to a more acceptable, but none-the-less aggressive activity. Kicking a ball, striking at a punching bag, chopping wood, throwing a rock at a target, can serve as initial substitutions. These

[11] Ardis Stevens: "Recreation in Community Mental Health." *Therapeutic Recreation Journal, 1st Quarter,* 1971, p. 16.

[12] Martin W. Meyer: "Recreation, A Positive Force for Mental Health." *American Recreation Journal,* September-October, 1964, p. 140.

impersonal and socially harmless acts can be further redirected or refined to more meaningful releases, with rules established as controls, such as in the organized sports of soccer, handball, archery, football and tennis. As aggressive impulses are brought under control or redirected . . . important defense mechanisms can thus be established which may serve as a safety valve when dangerous aggressive impulses are ready to explode . . . .[13]

Art, music, dance and similar activities may also serve as desirable forms of release or sublimation. The kinds of pathologic, high-risk, destructive play described earlier can be made less appealing by providing more constructive and self-enhancing activity.

Typically, recreation programs in psychiatric institutions have been designed to achieve the goals of helping to improve patient morale, provide constructive outlets, promote resocialization, redevelop capacities for creative self-expression and the enjoyable use of leisure and promote the patient's capability for independent community living, following discharge from the hospital.

Programs, as described earlier, have been designed on a variety of levels: for mass participation on a voluntary, non-prescribed basis; group or ward activities with specially designed components to meet the needs of patients in certain classifications of illness; or individually prescribed activities geared to meet the unique needs of each patient. Many hospitals have developed extensive schedules of activities throughout the week, with the opportunity for patients to engage in them on a varied basis, depending on their own capability and need.

During the 1930s, 1940s and 1950s, recreation departments tended to be separate units of hospital service, although they may have been administratively placed within departments of rehabilitation, social service or activity therapies. In general, the role of recreation therapists in mental hospitals was fairly sharply defined. However, the growing trend toward the activity therapy approach has made

a radical impact on the use of therapeutic recreation techniques in psychiatric settings.

Activity Therapy Approach

As described in Chapter Three, the activity therapy approach includes various types of rehabilitative therapies, such as occupational therapy, physical therapy, recreational therapy, educational therapy and work therapy. The basic premise underlying this method is that, by prescribing a diversified program of manual and creative activities, patients are given incentives, outlets and means of creative satisfactions. Pertinent data are provided to the psychiatric treatment team regarding the patients' reactions, aptitudes, interests and social adjustment.

Woloshin and Tamura point out that within the rehabilitative-adjustive model, support is given for productive behavior instead of inappropriate behavior. Essentially, the method is geared to the behavioral psychology viewpoint described earlier:

The message that should be clearly communicated is that staff respects the patient enough to expect something of him. He is expected to participate in his program and activities, to contribute to his community, and be productive rather than "crazy." . . . the rehabilitative-adjustive approach is based upon those things which are tangible and easily seen. . . . The staff and patient can chart progress more readily through tangible accomplishments . . . than through therapeutic gains in a one hour interview. If a person indeed can be productive and see the results of his productivity, it is an assumption that behavior modification takes place. Deep insight need not occur within this model for behavior modification to begin. An enhanced self-image and a greater belief in one's ability to be productive, to trust oneself and to trust others can result in further ego strengthening and social growth.[14]

[13] *Ibid.*

[14] Arthur Woloshin, and Robert Tamura: "Activities Therapy in a Community Mental Health Center." *Therapeutic Recreation Journal,* 1st Quarter, 1969, p. 31.

This approach has generally been accepted throughout the country. As an example, in 1964, the Joint Information Service of the American Psychiatric Association and National Association for Mental Health, in conjunction with the Division of Community Psychiatry of Columbia University and the Department of Mental Health of the American Medical Association, published a survey titled "The Community Mental Health Center—An Analysis of Existing Models." Ten mental health centers in the United States and one in Saskatchewan, Canada, were studied in depth. All of these centers were reported as putting a strong emphasis on occupational and recreational therapy, with considerable emphasis on the resocializing aspects of these programs. In addition to the use of formally trained recreation therapists, these centers made use of other personnel, such as social workers, occupational therapists, rehabilitation counselors, nurses and volunteers, to assist in program development.

Within the activity therapy program, the primary thrust today is toward the maximum "push" in helping "rapid-recovery" patients move toward discharge. Because of the use of drugs, many patients are able to move freely around hospital grounds or even to go into the community on trips or work sessions—where this would not have been possible in the past. Almost every aspect of programs in many of the newer mental hospitals is geared directly toward developing competence for community living.

RECREATION COUNSELING. One unique aspect of recreation as a component of activity therapy is the extent to which it is placing emphasis on preparing psychiatric patients for return to the community. Many institutions have developed a new "recreation counseling" program, with the following objectives: (a) to help patients maintain and strengthen their existing affiliations with family, friends, churches, lodges and civic groups; (b) to help patients form new ties with individuals and groups; (c) to teach patients to make effective use of available community resources for recreation; and (d) to mobilize community resources for fostering mental health.

Recreation counseling, according to Humphrey, should include procedures designed to evaluate each hospital resident's recreational interests, and planned efforts to expand and enrich these interests and skills during the treatment process. It should also include a conscious effort to have patients engage in community recreation programs while institutionalized, and the involvement of community groups in recreation activities carried on within the hospital setting. Finally, it should provide not only guidance to help discharged patients find desirable leisure outlets in the community, but also follow-up assistance to help them function effectively in such settings.

Increasingly, the movement in this field has been away from emphasis on *treating* patients with recreation, toward *making use* of recreation as a social interaction medium. The major value of recreation with mental patients is seen not as the opportunity to provide individualized psychodynamic prescriptions of activity, but rather as the opportunity to play and create in a manner which allows the patient to recapture his own sense of individuality and meaningfulness.

Milieu Therapy

It has become widely accepted that psychiatric disorder is integrally related to the social milieu in which it has developed. As a consequence, the conviction has grown that the community in which he is *treated* must be a healthy and constructive one if the patient is to regain a positive relationship with his family and community. This viewpoint is the basis of "milieu therapy," which stresses the importance of the total physical and social climate in which the patient is treated. Stanton has written:

The onset, symptoms, and recovery rates of major psychiatric illness are decisively influenced by the environment within which the patient is observed and treated.

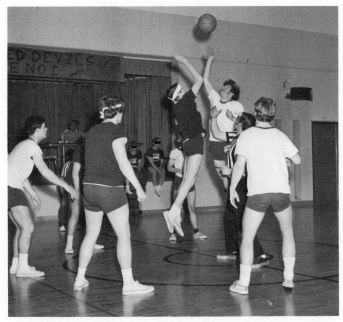

Program activities at the Traverse City, Michigan State Hospital include sports competition . . .

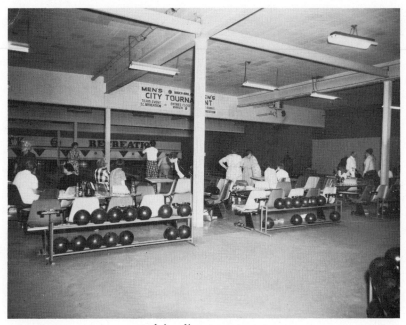

. . . and bowling tournaments.

. . . There is no patient "untreated" by his environment—only patients "treated," well or ill.[15]

Milieu therapy is concerned with *all* aspects of the hospital environment, including its physical structure, the opportunity for patients and staff to interact with each other in emotionally supportive ways, and the provision of a wide range of important experiences and activities that support meaningful change. In short, the total philosophy of the hospital must be therapeutic, and in every aspect of hospital life therapeutic agents must be at work:

> The concept of the therapeutic or curative community may be described as an arrangement in which all of a patient's time in the hospital—not just the time he spends in therapy—is thought of as treatment. The milieu in which he finds himself—i.e., the hospital, is seen as exerting a powerful influence upon his emotional life and behavior. Every contact, every casual conversation with a fellow patient, a nurse, even a kitchen helper, is regarded as potentially therapeutic. Milieu therapy . . . is an attempt to take into account what psychiatrists have called "the other 23 hours in the day"—to treat mental illness through a careful restructuring of the social environment.[16]

The therapeutic community concept represents a radical departure from the traditional view of a mental hospital as a custodial institution or "asylum." The asylum was deliberately located at a place far from the community—to afford the patient protection from the stress of daily life or the problems that had beset him, and probably also to "remove" him from the family as a source of grief or shame. Within such hospitals there was little sense of community life or interaction; patients were not expected to make decisions, exercise judgment or function responsibly.

[15] Alfred Stanton: *In* V. Cumming and E. Cumming: *Ego and Milieu.* New York, Atherton Press, 1969, p. v.
[16] Maggie Scarf: "In the Therapeutic Community Patients are Doctors." *New York Times Magazine,* May 25, 1969, p. 109.

The proponents of the milieu therapy approach claim that removing patients from social stress and meaningful community roles serves to make their return to society more difficult, because of the prolonged period of dependence they have experienced. Their social skills and ability to face the outside world may have atrophied during hospitalization, and they may understandably fear that there is no longer a place for them among family and friends, and in the vocational world.

Milieu therapy, therefore, is committed to making a patient's stay in the hospital a replica of the social interactions of ordinary life—in terms of social and recreational activities, work, civic or community responsibility, human relationships and other significant aspects of life. Within the therapeutic community, patients, while being treated for their illness, are encouraged to function as fully as possible in settings that are realistic and make real demands on them.

Typically, many mental hospitals maintain an open-door policy for large numbers of patients. Patients are encouraged to have frequent contacts with the outside community:

> The principle of the open door was established as a general policy for New York State hospitals, and patients responded by taking new interest in their surroundings, their personal appearance, and other members of the hospital community. This was the beginning of an overall liberalization program that permitted patients to move freely about the institution, that encouraged them to choose their companions, their activities, their clothes, to assume responsibilities for themselves and others—in short, *to function as normally as possible while being treated for illness. . . .*

A new flexibility in hospital management is also developing. Patients are encouraged to go home for brief visits, weekends and "vacations." In addition to the full time resident patient, there is now the "day patient," who lives at home and spends his days at the hospital participating in regular treatment programs, and the "night patient" who lives in the protected environment of the hospital but goes out to work during the day. As the average length of hospitalization decreases, families are urged to keep a place for the patient in the home and help him maintain his community ties.

The community itself, evincing a more understanding and accepting attitude, has made it possible for many more patients to leave the hospital and continue their treatment in the department's outpatient clinics. Treatment in the community has become more feasible because convalescent patients may be maintained on sustaining doses of the tranquilizing drugs.[17]

Current Trends in Therapeutic Recreation

What has been the total impact of the milieu therapy and decentralized mental health centers movements upon therapeutic recreation service? First, it should be made clear that theoretical statements of philosophy, or of idealized programs, do not always portray the reality of what goes on in institutions. The reality is that many institutions are badly overcrowded, and that many patients still exist in chronic wards, or "extended-care" facilities for older, highly regressed patients, while newer, smaller centers, situated in and around cities, represent the big push for patients with more hopeful prognoses.

The very notion of the therapeutic community, with the idea that every staff member, every aspect of living, every physical or social element of hospital life serves as a supportive therapeutic agent, belies the reality of crowded wards, overworked personnel who may be moonlighting because of poor salaries, and a lack of cooperation among disciplines, or the difficulty in developing meaningful relationships with community groups. Nonetheless, the new approaches are exciting ones. They have had a significant impact on therapeutic recreation service in the following ways.

SHIFTING OF EMPHASIS IN ACTIVITIES. In the traditional psychiatric hospital recreation program, in addition to numbers of special events or other mass activities, there were normally a variety of regularly

[17] *Treatment in the Modern Mental Hospital: op. cit.,* pp. 2–3.

scheduled sports and games, arts and crafts, music, dance or other social programs which patients were, in effect, assigned to, as part of regular ward or building unit schedules. Today, the emphasis has shifted away from this type of clearly recreational activity, frequently in the direction of activities which have an informal, less structured, social-learning kind of orientation.

Instead of learning dances, games or crafts, or playing sports or music—with the emphasis on the activity involvement—many departments are today providing activities in which patients become involved in self-discovery processes—which are heavily based on "encounter or sensitivity group" activities. As an example, one such program in a New York State Department of Mental Hygiene mental hospital schedules the following kinds of activities throughout the week:

grooming (male)	cooking
grooming (female)	small crafts
bowling	"psycho-
newspaper group	gymnastics"
coffee and	hootenanny
conversation	self-expression
psychodrama	exercise group
open shop	small groups
dance therapy	ward clean-up
drama and poetry	movies

Such activities are more personally involving, less demanding of skills and much freer in terms of permitting expressive behavior than more traditionally oriented recreational activities. They imply that the group leaders will play a therapeutic role and, presumably, that they have certain kinds of distinct skills in leading such activities. Whether they are more or less valuable in terms of the fundamental goals of therapeutic recreation than the traditional kinds of activities, is not easy to measure.

UNIFICATION AND THE BLURRING OF PROFESSIONAL ROLES. In some large psychiatric hospitals, a "unitization" scheme has gone into effect, under which patients are grouped according to their residence or "catchment" area. The purpose of this is to strengthen the element of community affiliation and, presumably, to facilitate planning for return to the community, recreation counseling and community-patient interaction. What it has meant in a practical sense is that patients with all degrees of illness or recovery stages, and of various ages and backgrounds, are lumped together in hospital units rather than housed according to age and type or severity of illness, as in the past. In this type of structure, staff members no longer serve their hospitals on a system-wide basis, planning overall hospital activities and acting as specialists within their areas of competence. Instead, they are attached solely to their units and assume roles that contribute generally to the therapeutic community process—but in which they do not specialize in their fields of particular training or skill.

In an increasing number of hospitals, staff members working in such programs are no longer identified according to their professional specialties but are simply titled activity therapists. The implication of this is that they no longer will be presenting specific areas of activity in which they are highly competent or gifted leaders, but instead will simply be promoting group process and the therapeutic interaction of patients and staff. Whether they are competent to do so, or are simply operating as somewhat unskilled therapists is a moot point. In any event, the notion of recreation *as* recreation appears to have suffered a decline in such settings. Instead, the group process and the experience of living, planning and sharing decision-making together appear to be the primary emphases.

DEVELOPMENT OF COMMUNITY-BASED FA-CILITIES. The community mental health movement has had a profound impact in breaking down the rigid walls that have separated psychiatric patients from community life in the past. Recreation has become an important part of special day-care and night-care programs. In many communities, it is now provided as part of day-center programs which, operating as satellites to a hospital structure, or existing independently in the community, meet the needs of discharged mental patients who require a protected setting or

are living at home and are receiving psychiatric clinical counseling for part of the day.

For example, in Rockland County, New York, the Elmwood Club for discharged mental patients serves over 100 members with 11 part-time workers on staff, aided by 35 volunteers and student leaders. The goals of this program are the following:

> . . . individual self-fulfillment; development of a sense of self-worth; creative use of self; emphasis on healthy aspects of personality, focusing on strengths, development of new skills and encouraging the emergence of old ones; belief in the ability to manipulate one's environment, to change undesirable parts of it; to participate fully in what life has to offer; and a positive approach to life based on day-to-day existence, but one with careful planning of activities over an extended period of time with concrete goals in mind.[18]

Many of the members of the club work either full-time or part-time while others attend a local community college or work in a sheltered workshop. The club meets for parts of three days or evenings each week, and engages in social recreation activities, home crafts, discussion groups, grooming activities, community service programs (dramatics, dancing and singing), parties, trips, cooking, exercise and games and similar activities.

In addition to such activities, the members of the staff work closely with social workers and other staff members at nearby state or veterans hospitals and with social workers from the Rockland County Department of Social Services. Volunteer workers include both college students on field-work placement assignments and local high school students. Many other community mental health centers have begun to sponsor such services.

Mental Hospital Programs

This chapter concludes by providing descriptions of the activity therapy or recreation programs in a number of hos-

---

[18] *Annual Report, Elmwood Club.* Rockland County Mental Health Association, 1970.

pitals in the United States and Canada. Obviously, it is not possible to give full details of such programs. In each case, some of the more interesting aspects of the program are provided, along with examples of rating or evaluation forms, personnel assignments and program schedules.

Athens Mental Health Center, Athens, Ohio

This center provides both inpatient and outpatient services, assisting persons in a 15-county area of southeastern Ohio who have a "major" mental illness, and assisting less severely ill persons in a five-county area. Multidisciplinary teams of mental health workers operate through four major treatment units: (a) Community Services, for outpatients and acutely disturbed inpatients; (b) Adolescent, for inpatients up to 18 years of age; (c) Geriatric, for inpatients 65 years of age and

older and (d) Continued Care, for patients requiring long-term hospitalization.

The history of this hospital reflects changing trends in psychiatric care throughout the United States. Founded in 1874 as the "Athens Lunatic Asylum," its name changed to the "Athens Asylum for the Insane," the "Athens State Hospital," and finally the "Athens Mental Health Center." Its treatment procedures also shifted through the years, from a primary emphasis in the 1950s to work on the farms and hydrotherapy, to a heavy use of lobotomies, and finally to the use of psychiatric drugs coupled with a strong emphasis on the activity therapies and the therapeutic community approach. The inpatient population has been reduced from 1800 to about 600; in addition, several hundred outpatients are treated monthly.

The treatment staff is organized into several departments (see chart). Of these the Activity Therapy Department includes the following services: Volunteer Services,

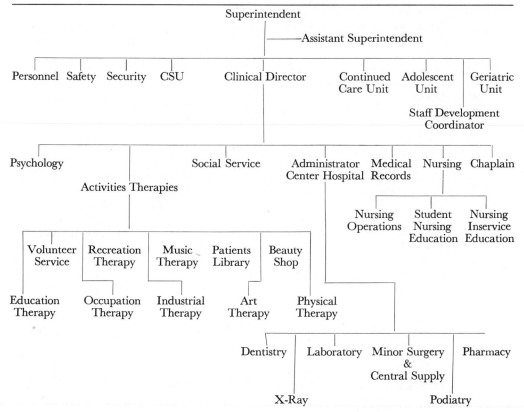

Administrative structure of Athens Mental Health Center.

Patients' Library, Beauty Shop, Recreation Therapy, Music Therapy, Physical Therapy, Education Therapy, Industrial Therapy, Arts Therapy and Occupational Therapy (including Arts and Crafts shop, and Home Management). The emphasis within this overall department is on providing real-life situations that are educative or reeducative, that will reequip patients to adjust to the demands that will be made on them by society after discharge.

A key element in this program is provided by an evaluation committee which is responsible for appraising patients (based on past history, medical record admission information and personal interview), determining the needs and interests of clients and assigning them to appropriate placement groups or patients. This committee also is responsible for reporting periodically on each patient's progress and for recommending changes in assignments. The goals of all elements of the Activity Therapy Program are clearly outlined. For example, the Vocational and Work Training Center seeks to meet the following goals:

1. Develop ego, strength, and self-worth.
2. Provide maximum reality contact through work.
3. Learn to establish standards and techniques.
4. Learn to follow a routine by use of verbal or written instruction.
5. Learn to use already established methods and procedures.
6. Learn to recognize limits set by a given task.
7. Use those work structures that are good in serving the client's dependency needs.
8. Permit client some control of his situation by the use of structure and control implicit in jobs.
9. Encourage decision making and planning.
10. Teach responsibility through care of equipment and tools. . . .[19]

This department provides work assignments in several categories: maintenance

department (power house, pulling ashes, shoveling coal and cleaning), dietary department, farm, store room and sewing room, laundry, commissary and paint shop. Similarly, each service within the Activity Therapy Department has clearly outlined goals and procedures.

Recreation is offered in conjunction with other creative activities, such as art, music and drama therapy. Activities are divided into two classes, based on the nature of participation required:

1. Passive participation
   (a) Movies
   (b) Theatre
   (c) Church services
   (d) Art exhibit
   (e) Bus rides
   (f) Concerts
   (g) Trips to Columbus Zoo
   (h) Spectator sports
2. Active participation
   (a) Club activities (press club, garden club, cooking club, literary club, drama and radio club)
   (b) Adapted sports (softball, basketball, shuffleboard, horseshoes, touch football, bowling)
   (c) Glee club and choir activities
   (d) Individual music lessons (voice, piano, organ, guitar and brass instruments)
   (e) Music appreciation groups
   (f) Art therapy groups
   (g) Social recreation (dances, parties, teas, picnics)
   (h) Tournaments (pool, checkers, bowling, ping-pong, table shuffleboard, cards and horseshoes)
   (i) Camping (overnight and day camping)
   (j) Library (regular lending services, literary and current events groups, for both leisure time and educational purposes.

The facilities used include an extensive variety of shops, studios and other recreation areas at the hospital itself, as well as other resources in the community, such as schools and colleges, hobby groups, service clubs, fraternal organizations, families and friends.

---

[19] *Activity Therapy Manual.* Athens Mental Health Center, Athens, Ohio, 1971.

Mt. Sinai Hospital, New York, New York

The psychiatric unit within Mt. Sinai Hospital in New York City provides a useful example of activity therapists employed in a significant role as fully integrated members of the psychiatric treatment team. The rationale for this role is stated thus:

The Activity Therapist is responsible for full-time in-patient psychiatric care. The patients involved are not confined to bed; yet they must remain within the hospital for an average stay of 35 days. The patient generally spends only one-and-a-half hours a week with his resident psychiatrist; if he has a private psychiatrist, he will usually spend five hours a week with him at best. The balance of the patient's time, a considerable part of the day and the entire evening and weekend time, the patient's treatment plan is implemented by his Activity Therapist. There is considerable need for this care; in psychiatric illness, the constructive use of this time is of the utmost importance toward the patient's recovery. An Activity Therapist must be professionally trained for this responsibility. His activities must facilitate the patient's recovery, and bring him back to healthy functioning, by restoring an interest in life and constructive action; and guiding the patient to an awareness of his unhealthy mental habits, pointing the way to a positive change toward healthful balanced attitudes. This must be done with the cooperation of the nursing staff, regarding medication and medical problems; and the programs must complement the doctor's long-range treatment goals for the patient.[20]

The time of Activity Therapists at Mt. Sinai is about equally divided between servicing an inpatient unit and working on the ninth floor of the hospital, where activities and programs are provided on an all-hospital basis. They have the following specific responsibilities for their own units:

1. Supervision of patient government-type meetings.
2. Leading of activity planning sessions for events that will take place on weekends or evenings when Activity Therapists are not present.
3. Attendance and participation in daily morning group meeting with patients and staff, and follow-up discussion meetings with medical and nursing staff.
4. Attendance and participation in twice- or thrice-weekly unit conferences with medical, nursing and social work personnel, where new admissions are interviewed and discussed.
5. Staff meetings with medical, nursing and social work personnel, to bring out and discuss inter-staff problems.
6. Meetings between the chief resident and Activity Therapists, and the unit chief and Activity Therapists, to keep each of these individuals aware of patients' progress.
7. Meetings with nursing staffs of individual units, to exchange information regarding patients.

In addition, Activity Therapists attend weekly staff meetings of their own group, in which they deal with the mechanics of running the program, such as scheduling, planning of special events, problems relating to equipment, supplies and similar matters. They also meet in regular in-service seminars concerned with evolving new types of programs designed to best serve psychiatric patients today. Essentially, Activity Therapists are responsible for three types of group experiences: leisure-time groups, prevocational groups and rehabilitative groups. In each situation, they must serve as resource persons (with emphasis on skills involved in the activity) and as facilitators of group process. The team approach to the use of the Activity Therapist is illustrated in the listing of meetings to which he is committed, as well as in the following statement:

Since his function is that of a professional within the Department of Psychiatry, it is necessary for the Activity Therapist to have a working double professional vocabulary: one relating to activities, and one involving psychodynamics, psychopathology, and psychopharmacology. The foregoing knowl-

[20] *Departmental Manual.* Mt. Sinai Hospital, New York, 1971.

edge is essential when writing in nursing report books on the individual units, and in filling out evaluation sheets on patients in . . . ninth-floor activity groups, and in verbally sharing information on patients with the medical staff. . . .[21]

Each form of activity in which patients engage is seen as providing a particular kind of challenge and a special opportunity to observe and evaluate patient skill and response. As an example, within the area of arts and crafts, two activities may be cited as described in the department manual: *group collage* and *drawing*. These illustrate the kinds of elements that Activity Therapists must be aware of, and the ways in which they use activity to examine and encourage patient growth.

Group Collage

Response to many and varied stimuli—ability to organize stimuli—make choices—inhibit response to others.

Assess alternatives—plan and organize.

Translate ideas into images.

Reality testing: realism of idea in relation to materials.

Adaptation: ability to compromise, alter ideas or materials to achieve a result, accept limitations of external reality, such as time or materials.

Nature and degree of creativity and originality.

Eye-hand coordination—field ground discrimination.

Collaborative-independent relationship skills.

---

[21] *Ibid.*

Ability to engage in mutual problem solving.

Interpersonal roles: initiator, clarifier, organizer, helper, doer, director, encourager, etc.

Ability to listen to and respond to ideas of others.

Handle conflict—mediate—deal with conflict between our needs and those of others.

Tolerance for conflict—opposing opinion.

Drawing

Ability to organize—when expectations and external limits and controls are not evident or are ambiguous.

Ability to be goal-directed in face of anxiety, ambiguity.

Ability to develop ideas and imagery.

Capacity for tolerating and dealing with the unknown, untried.

Ability to depict ideas—move from ideation to image.

Ability to exercise volition.

Nature of emotional-impulse control.

Ability to abstract, generalize.

Comfort with feelings, thoughts.

Reality orientation.

In general, the emphasis is on open-ended, creative kinds of activities or projects, and on experiences that are rooted in feeling and fluid group relationships, and which provide self-discovery opportunities. Various forms are used in evaluating patient performance and making recommendations for activity. Here is an example of such a form used in the Mt. Sinai psychiatric treatment program:

Performance Evaluation Summary and Program Recommendations

Patient's name: _____   Date: _____

Unit: _____

I. Evaluation summary: Performance deficits and strengths related to:
    (A) Self-concept and identity
    (B) Need-drive adaptation
    (C) Interpersonal and social relations
    (D) Cognition and problem solving
    (E) Perceptual—Motor functions
    (F) Life tasks skills and vocational adjustment

II. Program focus and recommendations:
   (A) Program focus
      1. Remedial:
         (a) deficits in performance skills around which program is to be structured
         (b) essential characteristics of remedial activities
      2. Supportive:
         (a) existing skills, capacities and interest which should be sustained and/or protected
         (b) essential characteristics of supportive activities
      3. Life tasks skills and vocational adjustment
         (a) areas and level of daily life tasks skills and vocational adjustment needs toward which rehabilitation program should be directed.
         (b) activity and/or task assignment recommendations
         Staff: _____

Various inventories, forms or rating scales are used as part of the evaluation and counseling process in Activity Therapy at Mt. Sinai. For example, this department has patients fill out (if they are not able to do so independently, they are assisted) a comprehensive background profile. Here are excerpts from this form:

Educational, Vocational and Interest Profile

   I. Identification: Name _____ Address _____
      Age _____ Family Members _____
  II. Education (includes dates, diplomas or degrees, type of program, courses most enjoyed and most disliked, etc.)
 III. Avocational experiences:
      Hobbies: What activities or hobbies do you enjoy doing during your leisure time? Please list. How did you become interested in each?

      Check your special skills, talents or outstanding abilities and state whether skillful or average in each case:

Singing _____

Debating _____

Dancing _____

Photography _____

Sewing _____

Arts and crafts _____

Playing instrument _____

Needlework _____

Woodworking _____

Painting _____

Sports
   Teams: Baseball _____
      Volleyball _____
   Individual: Tennis _____
      Skiing _____
      Swimming _____

 IV. Family occupational inventory: (includes questions about age, educational background, major area of work or occupation, interests and hobbies of father, mother, sisters, brothers, spouses or other close relatives)
      (The profile also asks specific questions regarding:)
      Hobbies, work or other activities as part of early background of patient or shared with family.
      Total vocational experience record. Attitudes toward various jobs, qualities of employer, special vocational skills and work experience.
      Personal ambitions and self-perceived abilities, strong points, weaknesses and interpersonal relationships.

A final example of program development taken from the Mt. Sinai program is a sample schedule for a period of several weeks in February and March, 1972, listing activities and the times they are offered, the location and the criteria for admission to the group. The schedule is prepared for the entire week; however, only a portion of it is presented here.

Department of Psychiatry, Therapeutic Activities Division
February-March Activity Schedule
Patient Activities on the 9th Floor KCC; Monday, February 21—Sunday, March 26

MONDAY

TIME	GROUP	ROOM	CRITERIA FOR ADMISSION TO GROUP
Morning			
10:15–11:15 A.M.	Painting group	Room 3 OT area	By referral only
10:15–11:15 A.M.	Sewing workshop	Room 1 OT area	By referral only
Afternoon			
1:30–2:00 P.M.	Body awareness		
2:00–3:30 P.M.	Current events Discussion group	Music room gym area	Voluntary
2:00–4:00 P.M.	Clay workshop	Room 4 OT area	By referral only
2:30–3:30 P.M.	Gym for pediatrics	Gym	Pediatrics only
5:00–6:00 P.M.	Planning for leisure time	Room 2 OT area	By referral only
Evening			
7:00–8:00 P.M.	Gym for child psychiatry	Gym	Child psychiatry only

TUESDAY

TIME	GROUP	ROOM	CRITERIA FOR ADMISSION TO GROUP
Morning			
10:15–11:30 A.M.	Crafts workshop	Room 3 OT area	By referral only
10:15–11:30 A.M.	Food a la carte		By referral only
10:15–11:30 A.M.	Production lines	Room 4 OT area	Two separate groups—tie dye workshop and candle making workshop. By referral only
Afternoon			
2:00–3:30 P.M.	Painting group	Room 3 OT area	By referral only
Evening			
6:00–7:00 P.M.	Gym-free time	Gym	Voluntary
7:00–8:00 P.M.	Gym for child psychiatry	Gym	Child psychiatry only
8:00–9:00 P.M.	Gym—volleyball, basketball, table tennis	Gym	Voluntary

WEDNESDAY

TIME	GROUP	ROOM	CRITERIA FOR ADMISSION TO GROUP
Morning			
10:00–10:45 A.M.	Social dance instruction	Gym	By referral only
10:15–11:30 A.M.	Crafts workshop	Room 3 OT area	By referral only
10:15–11:15 A.M.	Food nutrition group	Room 5 OT Area	By referral only
10:15–11:30 A.M.	Production lines	Room 4 OT area	By referral only
Afternoon			
2:00–4:00 P.M.	Sewing workshop	Room 1 OT area	By referral only
2:30–3:30 P.M.	Gym for pediatrics	Gym	Pediatrics only
Evening			
5:30–6:00 P.M.	Coed body movement and exercise group	Gym	Voluntary
6:00–7:00 P.M.	Volleyball instruction	Gym	Voluntary
7:00–8:00 P.M.	Men's physical fitness group	Gym	By referral only
8:00–9:00 P.M.	Gym—volleyball, basketball, table tennis	Gym	Voluntary

Saskatchewan Hospital, Weyburn, Saskatchewan, Canada

For a period of years, this hospital represented one of the major institutions for psychiatric care in Western Canada, with a patient count in the late 1950s of well over 1500. As part of the shift to smaller, community-based institutions and more flexible treatment services, the patient load has now been reduced to 350, chiefly of extended-care patients. The following describes the recreation program of the hospital prior to its recent shift in focus.

STAFF. Two staff members, a recreation supervisor and an assistant, both of whom hold diplomas in psychiatric nursing and have completed three-year certification courses in recreation, are responsible for this program. They are assisted by nurses who encourage patients to take part in activity, while the recreation staff members act as providers, guiders and enablers.

FACILITIES. Compared to a municipal institution like Mt. Sinai, the Saskatchewan hospital has extensive facilities which, in turn, make possible an extremely varied program. These areas and buildings include: a curling and skating rink, poolroom, shuffleboard areas, music rooms, hobby rooms, game rooms, sports field, auditorium, gymnasium, picnic areas, miniature golf course, lawn bowling courts, croquet courts, horseshoe pits, library and other specialized facilities. In addition, the recreation department uses buses and camp rental procedures to provide vacations for both in- and outpatients. outpatients.

GOALS OF HOSPITAL. To facilitate the discharge of larger numbers of patients, the recreation department has placed emphasis on three major goals: (a) retraining in social and recreational skills; (b) fostering independence; and (c) exposing the patient to the community. It has structured its operation so that it is similar to the normal model of citizens living in the community. During the hours of 9 to 5, patients engage either in occupational therapy or in work assignments, either in a sheltered workshop manufacturing wood products or in hospital de-partments, such as the laundry, gardens or plumbing shop. Recreation is provided after 5 P.M. or, by prescription with special patients, between 9 and 5 P.M.

PROGRAM ORGANIZATION. This is carried out in the following ways:

1. By assigning several facilities and activities to each patient unit of the hospital.
2. Through the general function or core program, which is scheduled five nights a week for those patients who are able to attend them independently.
3. Providing equipment and activities for unit-building living rooms (day rooms) to serve patients who are too sick to leave this area.
4. Services for outpatients. The recreation staff of the hospital is also active in planning and setting up programs for youth, the physically disabled or elderly people in the adjacent community, by providing consultation, offering workshops and helping to establish youth coffeehouses and sports programs, nursing home activities and other events.

EVALUATION OF PATIENTS. Both in the assignment of patients to activities and in the evaluation of their continuing participation and progress, a five-point rating scale is used by staff. The patients are rated with respect to their attendance and participation in recreation and social activities, on the following scale:

5. Attends willingly and participates in activity as it would be expected of someone in a similar situation in the community._____
4. Attends willingly but is mostly a passive observer._____
3. Will attend, but only after protesting about it._____
2. Usually refuses to attend._____
1. Considered too ill to attend._____

Patients are rated each week on these points, and their status charted on an overall graph that extends over a period of several months, thus providing an overall picture of their progress as seen by recreation therapists and nurses.

In addition, two other devices are used to ascertain patient needs and interests and to evaluate systematically their participation in recreation activities. The first is a recreation interest questionnaire (see below), and the second an evaluation form for patient participation and interaction (page 89). The latter measures patient involvement in three types of activities: group activities, spontaneous activities and "voucher activities." The latter refers to activities which the patient attends, for which he pays with vouchers that have been paid him as a reward for work. The entire hospital operates with a system of such vouchers or "chits," through which the patients may purchase merchandise, candy, clothing and similar articles, or gain admission to special events at the hospital. The purpose of this device is to encourage appropriate spending within areas of personal responsibility. Patients are expected to spend a certain minimum amount each month in certain recreation activities, as evidence of social involvement.

Recreation Interest Questionnaire

Date:

Name ——————————————— Age ——— Occupation ———————————

Home Address ————————————— Town ————————— Rural —————————

In your community,

do you have:	*did you ever:*	*would you like to learn:*
——— a rink	——— curl	
——— a bowling alley	——— bowl	
——— a theatre	——— attend shows,	
——— a pool hall	dances, bingos	
——— a swimming pool	——— play pool	
——— a golf course	——— swim	
——— a community hall	——— golf	

Do you belong to any clubs such as:

——— a home makers club   did you ever ——— would you like to ———

——— a square dance club

——— a Legion society   Do you have any hobbies?

——— a church organization   What games or instruments have you enjoyed playing?

——— a craft club (What?)

What types of activities would you enjoy (Yes, No, Don't know):

Quiet Games	*Active Games*	*Social Activities*
——— playing cards	——— volley ball	——— community singing
———	——— darts	——— tours
———	——— shuffleboard	——— picnics
———	——— croquet	——— parties
——— table games	——— horseshoes	———
———	——— ring toss	———
———	———	
———	———	

Entertainment	*Hobbies and Clubs*
——— bands	——— drawing and painting
——— plays	——— leathercraft
——— slides	——— wood carving
——— variety shows	——— rug making
——— television	——— needlework
——— sports events	——— gardening
——— speakers	——— cooking and baking
——— discussion groups	——— reading

When you return to your home would you like help from anyone to join in any activities or clubs there may be in your town? ———

Comments:

Evaluation Form for Patient Interaction and Participation

NAME		ATTENDANCE			PARTICIPATION AND INTEREST						VERBAL INTERACTION DURING ACTIVITY				WARD——
Date	Group Act. (1) Spont. Act. (2) Voucher Act. (3) Activity	Refuses	With Persua- sion	Will- ingly	Does Not Partici- pate	Spec- tator (Shows In- terest)	Partici- pates with Persua- sion	Partici- pates Freely	Assists in Start- ing Activity	Assists Others	None	Some When Spoken to	Some Spon- taneous Inter- action	Inter- acts Freely	Comments

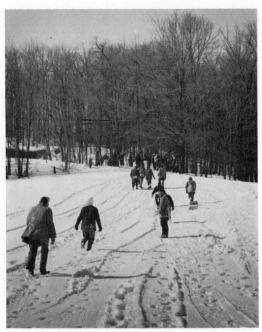

Many psychiatric hospitals provide varied out-door recreation programs. Here, at Traverse City Hospital, patients enjoy a wintry outing with tobagganing . . .

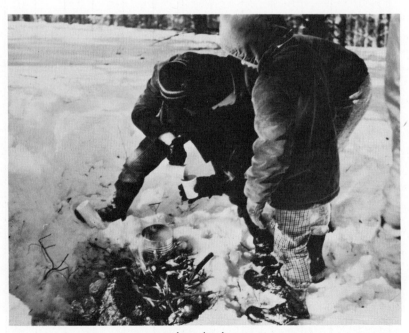

. . . a cookout in the snow. . .

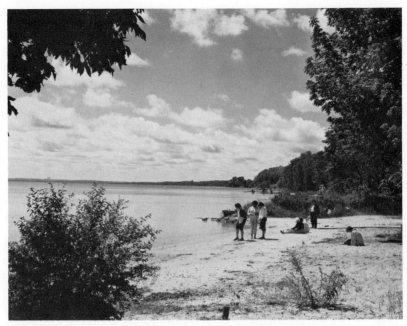

. . . *a picnic at a nearby lake.* . .

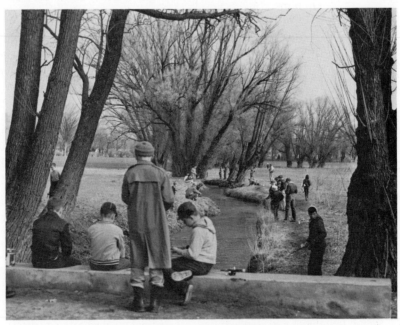

. . . *and a fishing expedition for younger patients.*

PROGRAM ACTIVITIES. This includes a substantial number of activities, both inside and outside of the hospital setting. In a recent year-end report, the following were listed (partial listing).

Social Activities

Coffee groups in
   city
Dances
White Cross socials
Seasonal parties
Whist tournaments
Scavenger hunts
Darts tournaments
Barbecues
Wiener roasts
Music listing
Bingo in hospital
   and city
Checker
   tournaments
Pool and pool
   tournaments
Picnics
Ping pong
   tournaments

*Education and
Cultural Activities*

Films
Art contests
Magazine
   subscriptions
Weekly newspaper
Library services
Craft sessions
Musical sessions
Talent shows
Cooking contests

   Physical Activities

Archery
Curling
Broomball

Shuffleboard
Miniature golf
Fishing
Ice fishing
Bowling in city
Gymnasium
   activities
Lawn bowling
Horseshoes
Croquet
Volleyball
Floor hockey and
   tournaments
Badminton
Soccer
Tobogganing and
   sleigh riding

*Audience
Activities*

Weekly movies
   (popular)
Weekly
   educational
   films
Curling matches
   in city
Band
   performances
Caroling
Hockey games in
   city
Television sports
   watching
Softball in city
Fair in city
Karate
   performances
Tours of city sites
   of interest

Substantial numbers of hospital patients also have been taken on one-week vacations, based on satisfactory performance in the industrial therapy (work program), satisfactory social behavior and payment of vouchers at an approved level. In addi-

tion, a selected group of outpatients have been taken on similar vacations. These consist basically of trips each day to scenic sites, parks, picnic areas and spectator events in various parts of southeastern Saskatchewan.

PATIENT COUNCIL. A final interesting aspect of the Saskatchewan Hospital has been its patient council, which functions in the following ways: (a) as a patient union in dealing with problems related to patient employment in the industrial therapy program; (b) helping to plan and critically evaluate the recreational services in the hospital; and (c) dealing with patient complaints regarding individual treatment programs or general ward affairs.

The officers of the patient council are elected from the general patient population every three months, or whenever a presiding officer is discharged or regarded as too ill to hold office. General meetings are held weekly and deal with a variety of problems, as well as hear reports from various patient committees set up to deal with aspects of hospital life. Once a month, 25 patient representatives of all the units in the hospital meet with the recreation staff to discuss and critically evaluate recreation activities. Their suggestions are implemented, unless they are regarded as detrimental to hospital or treatment goals. Reports are made regularly to the general meeting of the patient council.

As mentioned earlier, the Saskatchewan Hospital has been recently converted from an institution serving the general mentally ill population to a "level four" facility, designed to serve older patients (chiefly in the 45 to 70 age range) who have been the victims of long-term institutionalization and extreme decentralization. As described in the official guidelines:

> This level of care is for persons of all ages who do not require acute hospital care and treatment but do require regular and continuous medical attention, highly skilled technical nursing provided under appropriate supervision on a 24-hour basis, and, in addition, special techniques for the improvement or maintenance of function. Patients at this level require initial and continuing medical assessment involving investigation and diagnosis for which ap-

propriate facilities must be readily available. The aims of treatment are to control the disease process, to achieve maximum recovery of function, to prevent further disability, to retard deterioration, and to alleviate pain and distress.[22]

Realistically, these patients are regarded as poor-prognosis, long-term care patients, who have little or no prospect for recovery, and will probably spend the remainder of their days within the facility. It is believed that when such patients are permitted to become completely passive, they deteriorate sharply, both physically and mentally. However, "where there is a therapeutic environment in which there is motivation and stimulation for patients to be as independent as possible, even those with poor prognoses may improve."

This, then, represents a final concern

for therapeutic recreation specialists in the field of the mentally ill. While there has been a tremendous push toward serving those who are capable of quick recovery and discharge, and toward the development of the therapeutic community, and linkages to community life, as well as community-based programs serving the mentally ill in a variety of ways—it also is apparent that there is a substantial population of mentally ill patients who are *not* candidates for discharge. These individuals must be served, and the risk is that, in the pressure toward using intensified services to treat those with more favorable prognoses, the needs of the chronic or long-term patient will be ignored. It seems clear that in the years ahead, there will continue to be an important need for services for such patients, and that new techniques and approaches for serving them effectively in custodial situations will have to be developed.

---

[22] *Annual Report.* Saskatchewan Hospital, Weyburn, Saskatchewan, Canada, 1971.

Suggested Topics for Class Discussion, Examinations or Student Papers

1. Describe the effect of widespread reliance upon drug-based treatment in psychiatric institutions on therapeutic recreation service.
2. What special emphases should be given to therapeutic recreation service in institutions operating according to the "milieu therapy" and "therapeutic community" model?
3. Outline an imaginative and comprehensive recreation program for a modern psychiatric hospital or community-based aftercare or mental health center.

Chapter 5

Recreation for the Mentally Retarded

This chapter provides an understanding of the scope, causes and effects of mental retardation, and of the place of recreation in institutional or community programs designed to meet the needs of the mentally retarded. Emphasis is placed on the role of recreation in promoting social independence and job capability for the moderately or mildly retarded, and on recreation's function in minimizing disability and in enriching the lives of *all* retarded children, youth and adults.

The Nature of Mental Retardation

Although mental retardation has traditionally been defined as a function of intelligence (with an I.Q. of below 75 identifying the retardate) this is an unfortunately narrow view. A more sophisticated definition of the mentally retarded is likely to include the following elements:

1. It is generally agreed that mental retardation is a condition that *originates during the developmental period;* i.e., before the age of 18.
2. The key concept in many definitions is that of *mental subnormality.* In many cases, this concept has been used as the sole criterion of mental retardation.
3. A significant element in identifying

mental retardation has been *social inadequacy:* the inability of the retarded person to function effectively in a social setting.
4. The view has been widely shared that mental retardation must have an *organic cause,* such as an organic defect in the brain or some other significant pathology of the central nervous system.
5. A final concept is that mental retardation *cannot be cured.* This view is closely related to the belief in an organic cause; if a brain defect exists, it cannot be remedied.

None of these concepts can stand independently. It is obvious that some persons with I.Q.s of under 75 can function effectively in society and are *not* labeled as retardates, while others with I.Q.s of over 75 are so regarded. The notion of social inadequacy is a highly variable one, differing from culture to culture. It is possible to demonstrate pathology of the central nervous system in only 20 to 25 per cent of the mentally retarded—although this may be because of a lack of sufficiently refined instruments. Finally, it is obvious that mild forms of mental retardation *are* curable, at least in the sense that many individuals who have been classified on this level enter community life, hold jobs and live as responsible citizens.

Recognizing the difficulty of defining the term, the American Association on Mental Deficiency suggests the following:

> Mental retardation refers to subaverage intellectual functioning which originates during the developmental period, and is associated with impairment in adaptive behavior.[1]

If a person has a low I.Q. and is socially adequate, he is not to be regarded as mentally retarded. If a person lacks social competence but has a high I.Q., he is not, by definition, mentally retarded. Only when both elements are present is one considered mentally retarded.[2]

Numbers and Types of Mentally Retarded

There are believed to be approximately six million mentally retarded persons in the United States today; approximately three out of each hundred Americans are retarded to some degree. Half of these are children under the age of 20. The mildly retarded comprise 89 per cent of the total number. Moderate retardates are six per cent, severely retarded about three and one-half per cent, and profoundly retarded about one and one-half per cent of this population.

The life expectancy of the mildly retarded is about the same as that of normal persons. Although the development of antibiotic drugs which reduce fatal pulmonary illness in the severely and profoundly retarded has resulted in more of these individuals living to adulthood, their life expectancy is still shorter than that of the overall population.

Once he has lived to the age of five or six, the retarded child has a reasonable expectancy of living to adulthood. Following the school years, many mildly retarded individuals gain an adequate level of socially adaptive behavior and a degree of economic independence, and are able to blend into community life. Thus, a proportion of persons who were identified as mentally retarded in childhood are no longer classified in this way as adults.

Approximately 126,000 retarded persons are born each year. The causes of mental retardation are many. They include the following: (a) genetic or hereditary factors; (b) problems incurred during pregnancy or in childbirth; (c) illness, disease or accident; or (d) social or environmental deprivation.

Among the hereditary and genetic factors is chromosomal imbalance which causes Down's syndrome, commonly known as mongolism, which affects 1 out of 600 children. There are several other metabolic or chemical factors inherited from the mother which can cause retardation; a mixture of incompatible Rh factors may also be responsible.

There are some 200 diseases a woman can have during pregnancy which may lead to mental retardation in her child. Loss of oxygen during childbirth, the mother's diet or medication or accidents during pregnancy or childbirth may all result in brain injury causing retardation. Fortunately, modern science is developing preventive measures and mothers are being taught more effective approaches to pre- and postnatal care, so that retardation stemming from such causes can be minimized.

Other illnesses, such as meningitis, or injuries incurred in childhood, may lead to mental retardation. Lead poisoning and malnutrition are believed to be frequent causes of retardation among young children in poverty-stricken areas.

There is increased awareness of the role of the social environment in causing mental retardation. Lack of stimulation and cognitive input in the family setting means that a much higher proportion of children in extremely poor neighborhoods are classified as mentally deficient than those in middle- and upper-class families. This differentiation becomes increasingly marked during the elementary grades, as does the actual percentage of children classified as mentally retarded.

[1] Herbert J. Prehm: *In* Larry L. Neal: *Recreation's Role in the Rehabilitation of the Mentally Retarded.* University of Oregon, 1970, pp. 9–11.
[2] Rick Heber: *In* Larry L. Neal: "Recreation for the Mentally Retarded." *Therapeutic Recreation Journal,* 1st Quarter, 1968, p. 11.

CATEGORIES OF RETARDATION. There are a number of different systems under which the mentally retarded may be classified. Prehm points out that these include: (a) the *legal-administrative* system found in the laws of most states and cities, which judges which children, youths or adults are eligible for educational, residential or other forms of special social services; (b) the *educational* system, which customarily classifies the retarded into three groups— educable, trainable and custodial (totally dependent); and (c) the *psychiatric* classification system.[3]

In the past, the psychiatric system divided mental retardates into categories called *morons, imbeciles* and *idiots*. Today, these demeaning terms are seldom used.

Instead, the most common classification systems are those which relate to educational potential, and capability for independent living. Generally, these two factors appear to be highly correlated. In terms of potential for independent living, as a wage-earner, member of a family or resident in community life, adaptive capability is an extremely important factor. The following terms are widely used today to classify the retarded:[4]

RETARDED. Behavioral traits within each category of retardation have been classified (see Table 5–1, next page).[5]

Heber suggests that each retardate should be evaluated with respect to the following behavioral impairments:[6]

1. *Personal-Social Factors.*
   a. Impairment in cultural conformity, involving dependable or reliable social behavior, as opposed to behavior which is persistently anti-social or asocial.
   b. Impairment in interpersonal relations, implying inadequate ways for relating to peers and/or authority figures, or for recognizing the needs and feelings of other persons in interpersonal situations.
   c. Impairment in responsiveness and consistent motivation, involving typical inability to resist short-term gratification of needs, and to strive for long-range goals.
2. *Sensory-Motor Skill Impairment.*
   a. Motor skills, involving disability in large and fine motor movements.
   b. Speech skills—including such disabilities as stuttering, lisping, or other poor vocalization patterns.
   c. Auditory limitations, in understanding and responding to the speech of

LEVELS	DEGREE OF IMPAIRMENT	EDUCATIONAL	I.Q. RANGE	PERCENTAGE OF RETARDED POPULATION
I	Borderline or mild	Educable	52–67	89.0
II	Moderate	Trainable	36–51	6.0
III	Severe	Custodial	20–35	3.5
IV	Profound	Totally dependent	Under 20	1.5

Of these groups, it has been estimated that approximately 95 per cent, comprised chiefly of mild and moderate retardates, live in the community, primarily with their families. The five per cent who are classified as severely or profoundly retarded are heavily dependent on others for even the most basic forms of care (most cannot dress or feed themselves or attend to toilet needs without help), and are often institutionalized.

ADAPTIVE CHARACTERISTICS OF THE

others, beyond what might be expected on the basis of measured intelligence.
   d. Visual limitations, involving inadequate response to visual stimulation, beyond what might be expected on the basis of measured intelligence.[6]

Needs of the Mentally Retarded

Often, the retarded person is set aside from the rest of society and is heavily de-

[3] Herbert J. Prehm: *op. cit.,* p. 13.
[4] Adapted from Larry L. Neal: "Recreation for the Mentally Retarded." *op. cit.,* p. 4.

[5] *Ibid.,* p. 14–15.
[6] *Ibid.,* pp. 16–17.

Table 5–1. *Levels of Adaptive Behavior*

	PRE-SCHOOL AGE 0–5 MATURATION AND DEVELOPMENT	SCHOOL AGE 6–21 TRAINING AND EDUCATION	ADULT 21 SOCIAL AND VOCATIONAL ADEQUACY
Level I	Can develop social and communication skills; minimal retardation in sensori-motor areas; rarely distinguished from normal until later age.	Can learn academic skills to approximately 6th grade level by late teens. Cannot learn general high school subjects. Needs special education particularly at secondary school age levels.	Capable of social and vocational adequacy with proper education and training. Frequently needs supervision and guidance under serious social or economic stress.
Level II	Can talk or learn to communicate; poor social awareness; fair motor development; may profit from self-help; can be managed with moderate supervision.	Can learn functional academic skills to approximately 4th grade level by late teens if given special education.	Capable of self-maintenance in unskilled or semi-skilled occupations; needs supervision and guidance under serious social or economic stress.
Level III	Poor motor development; speech is minimal; generally unable to profit from training in self-help; little or no communication skills.	Can talk or learn to communicate; can be trained in elemental health habits; cannot learn functional academic skills, profits from systematic habit training.	Can contribute partially to self-support under complete supervision; can develop self-protection skills to a minimal useful level in controlled environment.
Level IV	Gross retardation; minimal capacity for functional in sensori-motor areas; needs nursing care.	Some motor development present; cannot profit from training in self-help; needs total care.	Some motor and speech development; totally incapable of self-maintenance; needs complete care and supervision.

pendent on his family. However, it is clear that with intensive training, care and attention, a high proportion of retarded persons can be integrated into the community, and can be enabled to function as useful citizens.

In the past, the mentally retarded were often confused with the mentally ill; even today, many individuals make no clear distinction between these two disabilities. They were cruelly treated by society, locked in attics, hidden away from the world, confined in prisons and madhouses or—too often—completely ignored. Even today, many parents of retarded children view them with a mixture of apathy and shame. Particularly among families in disadvantaged areas, the signs of retardation are ignored until it is too late to provide remedial services that might have minimized disability. Often, needed educational and community services are not provided.

However, over the past 15 or 20 years, there has been a growing realization of the scope of this problem, as well as of the fact that retardation is a disability stemming from identifiable causes and may be minimized and dealt with constructively.

It is now widely understood that the mentally retarded have the same basic needs as all other human beings. They have very strong human needs for love and understanding. They require food, shelter, work, if they are capable of it, and other interests and involvements that will provide their lives with meaningful activity and a sense of accomplishment.

Programs Serving the Retarded

For many years, the only programs serving the retarded were those of custodial institutions—either publicly operated homes and schools for the most severely impaired, or private homes or schools. In recent years, a number of public and voluntary organizations have been established to promote needed services for the mentally retarded. These include the following:

1. The National Association for Retarded Children, a private organization involved in a comprehensive program, including research, education, counseling, recreation and promoting public awareness of the needs of the retarded. This body operates both on a national level and through local or regional chapters.
2. The American Association for Mental Deficiency, a voluntary, nonprofit organization involved primarily in research concerning causes and effects of mental retardation.
3. The Federal Department of Health, Education and Welfare, which operates through a Mental Retardation Branch, promotes research and professional training in special education, and other services for the retarded, and provides financial assistance to special projects.
4. The Division of Mental Retardation of the Council for Exceptional Children, which promotes research, education and special community services for the retarded.
5. The Kennedy Foundation, a philanthropic organization which operates institutions for the retarded, supports research and demonstration projects and promotes innovation in the field of institutional care and community services.
6. The American Association for Health, Physical Education and Recreation, which has designed tests for the retarded and has promoted broad programs of physical education and recreation for this group.

In addition to these national bodies, there are many state and municipal organizations which have promoted a variety of services and programs, including education, vocational rehabilitation, sheltered workshops, recreation and legislation to serve the needs of the retarded. They have focused on research for the causes and prevention of mental retardation, on the development of new forms of rehabilitation that might succeed in helping retarded persons live independently in the community, and on providing programs of public relations that might improve public understanding of this problem.

Although many of these organizations have been operating for a considerably longer period, a major breakthrough was achieved in 1962, when the President's Panel on Mental Retardation, instituted by President John F. Kennedy, recommended a new, comprehensive program to serve the mentally retarded. This program made specific recommendations dealing with research, manpower, treatment, education, vocational preparation, legal protection and the development of federal, state and local programs for the mentally retarded. This was the first large-scale effort to come to grips nationally with the problem of mental retardation. It began a decade of development in which many of the goals which private organizations had been working for over a period of years were realized.

An example of legislation developed in this period was Title V, the Mental Retardation Amendment of 1967. This federal act provided $10 million over a period of three years to assist in the training of personnel and provide aid to programs already established. Another federal contribution was the Hospital Improvement Program, designed originally by the National Institutes for Mental Health and then shifted to the Office for Mental Retardation, which was designed to upgrade the care of the mentally retarded in state institutions.

Recreation in the Rehabilitation of the Mentally Retarded

One of the significant outcomes of the President's Panel on Mental Retardation was the recognition of the vital role played by recreation in working with the mentally retarded. It had already been recognized by many professionals that recreation served a variety of useful purposes with the retarded, but the Panel was the first influential national body to affirm this value:

> The retarded child, like other children, needs opportunity for healthy, growth-promoting play. The adolescent's vital need for successful social interaction and recreational experience is frequently intensified by isolation resulting from parental overprotection, the numerous failures he experiences in school and occupational pursuits, and by his exclusion by normal groups from everyday play group and social activities. For the retarded adult, opportunity and constructive use of leisure time may prove a major factor in maintaining community adjustment.[7]

The specific values of recreation for retardates lie in four major areas: (a) physical capacity and development; (b) social maturity and group adjustment; (c) contribution to vocational adjustment; and (d) constructive use of leisure time.

PHYSICAL DEVELOPMENT. The physical appearance, strength, stamina, motor skills and overall development of the mentally retarded are often inferior. Often the mentally retarded have not even mastered the basic skills of self-care. Since physical development is important not only for its own sake and because it contributes to the health of the individual but also because one's physical status is an important factor in having a positive self-concept, it is essential that retarded individuals be given full opportunity to gain physical skills and experience leisure pursuits.

Often these individuals are not involved in school-sponsored physical education programs, and they may be excluded from sports programs that serve children and youth in the community at large. An important contribution of recreation, therefore, is to provide games, sports, aquatics, conditioning programs and self-testing activities that help the mentally retarded reach their full potential of physical development. When such programs are pro-

vided, many retarded children and youth are able to compete with nonretarded youngsters on an equal basis in team and individual sports.

SOCIAL DEVELOPMENT. Many retardates are isolated from the mainstream of community life. Perceived by others as "different" because of their appearance and behavior, they are often excluded from peer groups and find it difficult to establish meaningful social relationships with others.

Often they are unmotivated in terms of social involvement and are overprotected by their families. Childish and immature behavior is frequently considered to be an inevitable part of their make-up, and they often are tremendously insecure in group settings—partly because of repeated failures and rejection by others. Carefully planned recreational activities, either in segregated or integrated group settings (in which they share social contact with the nondisabled), may do much to overcome these limitations.

VOCATIONAL ADJUSTMENT. Many retardates find it difficult to function well in a regular educational environment. They are often able to function more effectively in special vocational classes which are geared to their capabilities, and which equip them to hold jobs, either in regular industry or service trades, or in sheltered workshops in the community.

However, even when the retarded youth is successful in mastering the skills necessary to hold a job, he may fail to hold one down and function independently in the community. Francis Kelley, Superintendent of the Mansfield, Connecticut, State Training School and Hospital, states:

> It has been confirmed that many young retarded people have not been able to adjust in the community and have had to be placed in institutions because they have not been able to adjust during leisure, rather than because they failed to perform satisfactorily on the job, or . . . in the home. . . . As we provide for the education, vocational training, occupational and spiritual needs of the retarded, it is equally imperative that we do not overlook (their) recreational rehabilitation and social needs. . . . The presence of this "plus fac-

---

[7] President's Panel on Mental Retardation: *A Proposed Program for National Action to Combat Mental Retardation*. Washington, D.C. U.S. Government Printing Office, October, 1962.

tor" often makes the difference between a happy life in the community or commitment to an institution.[8]

CONSTRUCTIVE USE OF LEISURE. One of the major problems of the mentally retarded is the use of their leisure time which, for many, constitutes the entire day. Burghardt comments:

> We must realize the fact that in some instances the recreational skills mastered by the mentally retarded will constitute their major achievements and their most important assets. There is slim hope that their reading, writing, arithmetic and vocational aptitudes will assure them of acceptance by society. Thus, the skills they acquire as a result of the recreational program could mean more to them than they ever would to a normal person, insuring a reasonably successful social life.[9]

For many retardates, the empty hours in their day are characterized by lethargy, frustration and a feeling of uselessness. Too often, they spend their waking hours sitting alone or watching television endlessly. Higher-performing retardates in the adolescent age bracket may become involved in delinquent behavior because of a lack of other stimulation or interesting involvements. Thus, carefully planned recreation programs can do much to provide a useful and pleasurable existence for the retarded.

Finally, recreation may greatly help to promote the *mental development* of retarded children and youth. Broadly conceived, recreation may involve creative activities, hobbies, learning experiences, trips and similar experiences which broaden the range of knowledge and personal involvement of participants. Since retardates are so often deprived of the normal range of developmental experiences, it is essential to enrich their lives in this way.

Even programs of physical activity may do much to improve the mental performance of the mentally retarded. A British researcher, Dr. J. N. Oliver, reported dramatic results from a specially designed physical activity program for the retarded. All subjects improved significantly in physical ability, fitness and strength, and 25 per cent showed marked gains in intellectual performance.[10]

Goals of Recreation Programs for the Retarded

Summed up, then, the goals of recreation programs for the mentally retarded are the following:

1. To improve physical growth and development, enhance motor skills and lend confidence to participants by improving bodily build and physical fitness.
2. To minimize or prevent social isolation by helping the mentally retarded gain friends and adjust to social situations, minimizing atypical behavior and appearance and teaching social interaction skills.
3. To teach skills for the creative and constructive use of leisure, and to provide regular opportunity for hobbies, pastimes and other leisure involvements, either at home or in institutional or community settings.
4. To contribute to the retardate's ability to function independently in the community, and thus to hold down a job, where other ability levels permit this.
5. To improve language skills and develop other cognitive abilities, and to broaden the range of knowledge and environment contacts of the retarded.
6. To provide practice in self-care activities, thus enhancing the individual's capability for independent living.

---

[8] Francis P. Kelley: "Recreational Services for the Retarded—An Urgent Need." *Recreation in Treatment Centers*, September, 1964, pp. 12–13.

[9] Edward T. Burghardt: "Recreation for the Retarded: An Aid to Balanced Living." *Recreation in Treatment Centers*, September, 1964. p. 12.

[10] See Julian Stein: "The Mentally Retarded Need Recreation." *Parks and Recreation*, July, 1966, p. 574.

7. To improve the morale and quality of family living by helping to make the retardate less of a burden, and a more capable and autonomous individual.

Planning Services for Age and Functional Levels

Obviously, the kinds of recreational programs which may be provided for the mentally retarded must be geared closely to their capabilities. These, in turn, may be classified in two ways: (a) on the basis of chronological age; and (b) in terms of functional performance levels.

Planning on the Basis of Chronological Age

There is a temptation, in working with the retarded, to give excessive weight to demonstrated levels of social immaturity or limited mental development, and to treat ten or twelve-year-olds as if they were children of primary-grade age. However, as much as possible, it is desirable to carry on activities suitable for each age level, with whatever modifications may be necessary to make it possible for participants to be successful in them. In some classifications, the retarded are assigned to three major age levels: *pre-school age* (up to the age of five), *school-age* (six through 20), and *adult* (20 and over).

However, a more discriminating breakdown would be on the basis of the following divisions: pre-school, elementary school age, adolescence and early adulthood.

PRE-SCHOOL AGE. During this period of early childhood, it is essential that children who have been diagnosed as mentally retarded be given as wide a range as possible of those developmental play experiences which normal children receive. The emphasis should be on providing equipment, settings and structured leadership in games, environmental play, music, dance, drama and other creative experiences, simple arts and crafts, hobbies, group activities, neighborhood trips and

similar program elements. The emphasis is on providing activities that will build on the existing capabilities of the child and prevent further disability, and that will provide a healthy self-concept. Within many forms of early childhood play, beginning concepts related to the language arts, arithmetic and other forms of learning that contribute to academic capability may be introduced.

ELEMENTARY SCHOOL AGE. This is generally considered a key stage of growth, in helping the retarded child realize his full potential, and in developing a healthy and well-adjusted personality. Play programs should be designed that promote physical vigor and well-being, a range of leisure interests, satisfying and confidence-giving social adjustment, and that make the retarded child as independent as possible. All the activities that are normally provided for children in this age range may be offered, although many may be modified to permit successful accomplishment.

ADOLESCENCE. During this period of growth, it is essential that teen-age retardates be helped to adjust to the fact of their disability and to gain a realistic picture of their strengths and weaknesses. A considerable amount of emotional and practical support should be given to this age group, whose members face the problem affecting all teen-agers—making the transition from childhood to adulthood—complicated by their unique status in society. While they require adult guidance, adolescent retardates may assume a considerable degree of leadership in their own recreation and social activities.

EARLY ADULTHOOD. Recreation programs established for this age group in community settings should continue to offer skills instruction and general participation in activity, including remedial help in developing appropriate behavior and appearance, social adjustment and other elements of personal guidance. However, as much as possible the emphasis should be placed on informational and counseling services, which help young retarded adults develop their own leisure activities and social groups. Not infrequently, a community center will act as host to such a group, with an advisor provided by a local chapter of the voluntary association serving the mental retardation field.

In addition to chronological age, another useful way of developing program services is by assessing the degree of social independence of the children who are to be served. Avedon and Arje outline four descriptive categories which provide a basis for making such determinations. These are: *socially-independent, semi-independent, semi-dependent* and *dependent.*

For those in the first two classifications, it is essential to provide the kinds of counseling and community involvements that strengthen the retarded individual's capability for living and working in the community, thus preventing social isolation. Semi-dependent children, who generally are not able to hold positions, even in sheltered workshops, should be given the opportunity for community contacts through trips and other forms of recreational involvement. Dependent children, who usually are in institutions, should have a strong stress on physical development and self-care programs. On this level, although past practices have been almost completely custodial, it is important to provide intensive treatment services that may bring about improvement in functioning. In some situations, when even the most severely retarded children have become involved in intensive programs of physical recreation, they have progressed to the point that they were able to be reassigned to higher-functioning levels.[11]

Institutional Recreation Programs

In general, the most diversified programs of recreation tend to be found in state or privately operated schools or homes for the retarded. Several examples follow.

[11] Elliott M. Avedon, and Frances B. Arje: *Socio-Recreative Programing for the Retarded, a Handbook for Sponsoring Groups.* New York, Teachers College, Columbia, Bureau of Publications, 1964, pp. 15–18.

Plymouth State Home and Training School, Northville, Michigan

This state school for the retarded has a comprehensive program which operates 12 hours a day, six days a week, under a staff of ten activity therapy leaders, four of whom are specialists in skills areas. The goal of the Plymouth State School, as described in a descriptive manual of the Activity Therapy Department, is to:

> . . . provide a program of therapy that will facilitate the acquisition of physical and social skills by the resident that will make him an acceptable member of the community into which he may be placed or [in the institutional setting]. . . .[12]

A wide variety of physical, social and creative activities are designed to meet both the universal human needs and the specialized needs of the residents. Over 540 residents are served each day in the program and are grouped according to functional ability. Different groups (four levels are identified) are assigned priority on different kinds of activities. Each activity area (there are twelve) is designed to meet a specific set of rehabilitative goals. Based on participation and other information gained about residents, evaluation forms have been developed which determine the potential for community placement within the area of social living capability.

State Colony, Woodbine, New Jersey

In some institutions, programs have been developed for the severely and profoundly retarded. At the State Colony in Woodbine, New Jersey, a special program of activities was developed for ninety such residents, all highly hyperactive. Patients were carefully screened and placed in heterogeneous groups, according to levels of disability. The groups were conducted as carefully controlled learning sessions,

[12] *Activity Therapy Manual.* Plymouth State Home and Training School, Northville, Michigan, 1971.

making use of simple wooden games and puzzles, tools and other manipulative experiences. Emphasis was placed on developing routines with which the residents might become familiar, a relaxed atmosphere and repetition of simple actions.

Over a period of time, it was found that many of the residents gained in the ability to play constructively with toys, to follow rules and instructions and to play independently within the group structure.[13]

State Training School and Hospital, Mansfield, Connecticut

In this institution, considerable stress is placed on developing social training and recreational opportunity for all children, at whatever level of retardation. With the help of volunteer college students from the nearby University of Connecticut, teen-age girls are involved in a good grooming project which has a marked effect on their appearance and social behavior.

Physical activities, including softball, swimming, baseball, basketball and even football (played competitively with other high schools), serve to counteract the common obese and physically weak appearance of many retarded children. Other recreational activities at the Mansfield school include weekly dances for the residents every Saturday, birthday parties, picnics, field trips, a swimming and camping program and special seasonal activities to celebrate holidays like Christmas, Halloween and Easter. Children from both educable and trainable classifications are admitted to the school program at an early age, and are trained for eventual return to the community whenever possible.

Many other institutions have developed elaborate programs of recreation service, both for discharge-bound residents and for those whose prognosis is lifelong custodial care. However, it should be stressed that the majority of mentally retarded children and youth are not institutionalized, but live with their families. It has been estimated that, for each 1000 school-age children in the average community, there are approximately one totally dependent child, four trainable mentally retarded children and 25 educable retardates. Only the most severely retarded of these are institutionalized.

Of the others, Ramm writes:

> The retarded child living at home has little recreation opportunity. He may make friends with the children in his special class at school, but unlike the normal children who can play with their school chums in the neighborhood after school hours, retarded children are transported from their homes in different parts of town and have few friends in their own neighborhoods. A similar situation exists with mentally retarded adults who work in a centrally-located sheltered workshop, or who do not work at all. These people are victims of enforced leisure. They have a six-to-eight-hour time block each weekday and more on weekends or holidays during which little or no activity is available to them. Many just sit and watch television.[14]

As a consequence, a number of city and county recreation departments are now providing extensive recreation services for the mentally retarded. Their objective is not only to provide diversion but also to assist in the total development of the retarded.

Community-Based Programs

During the past several years, a pilot program has been organized in Washington, D.C., to provide services for the mentally retarded in the community.[15] Its goals have been two-fold: (a) to develop a comprehensive set of recreation opportunities for the retarded; and (b) to develop a set of principles and procedures as guidelines in the promotion of multi-agency cooperation in this field.

[13] *Report.* State Colony, Woodbine, New Jersey, 1971.

[14] Joan Ramm: "Challenge: Recreation and Fitness for the Mentally Retarded." Washington, D.C., American Association for Health, Physical Education and Recreation, 1966, p. 1.

[15] Helen Jo Mitchell: "A Community Recreation Program for the Mentally Retarded." *Therapeutic Recreation Journal,* 1st Quarter, 1971, pp. 3–8.

The city is divided into nine areas, each with a center where a variety of activities are provided for the retarded, such as arts and crafts, music, bowling, nature pastimes, golf, trips, self-help classes and aquatics. The program is staffed by 46 members of the city's recreation staff, who have received in-service training at the University of Maryland, and who are assisted by volunteers. Serving approximately 450 retardates, the program receives the cooperation of varied community agencies and parents' clubs, and departments of the federal government as well. The program is carefully monitored and assessed to determine its effectiveness, and has succeeded in arousing a high level of community concern about the needs of the retarded.

Another leading program which has been developed to serve the retarded in the community is the Recreation Center for the Handicapped in San Francisco. This nonprofit corporation has been influential in bringing happiness and companionship to mentally retarded and physically disabled children, youth and adults of varied races and creeds in the San Francisco, California, metropolitan area.

With assistance from both private and public agencies, and with appropriations from the city and special federal grants, the Recreation Center for the Handicapped operates both integrated and segregated services for the mentally retarded. It also operates a laboratory that assists in the training of college students and others in the field of therapeutic recreation. As an example of its work, in 1969, out of 500 children served, 225 had made sufficient progress to be accepted in city schools for the retarded, or in special classes in regular schools. The Center also provides educational talks, films and lecture series designed to educate the public on mental retardation.

One of its special projects is Camp Spindrift, a program sponsored with the assistance of the Kennedy Foundation and other community organizations. Operating in a wooded environment as a day camp, Camp Spindrift serves 181 campers with a program that places stress on developing living skills and social independence. Many of the campers who formerly had been extremely dependent on their families have now been able to take part in special overnight camping programs; others have shown remarkable progress in varied activities, and in being able to communicate effectively, take social responsibilities and make friends.

In some cases, camping programs for the retarded have been sponsored by school systems, or by state schools or hospitals for the retarded. For example, San Diego, California, has been one of the pioneers in school camping for elementary age children. For a number of years, it has included a special unit for retarded boys and girls in its program at Camp Cuyamaca. Within an integrated social structure, it was found that many of the anticipated problems did not exist, and retarded youngsters were able to function effectively in the camp setting.

Camping is of particular importance because it changes the environment of the retarded child radically and puts him in a living situation where he is much more dependent on his own efforts. Camp Confidence, a year-round camping operation for the retarded, operated in connection with Brainerd State Hospital in Northern Minnesota, stresses the need for young retardates to develop self-confidence, social adjustment and specific skills in the areas of camp living, nature and crafts, sports and conservation education. The keynote of the camp is "learning by doing." Endres writes:

> If our primary objective . . . is to develop social adjustment within the individual, the camp setting and outdoor education [offer] a natural laboratory. . . . The mentally retarded do not basically learn best by being "told" or "shown" what to do. They must physically experience a given situation to attain comprehension and understanding. Within the aesthetic setting of a camp, they are able to experience things first hand, through outdoor education classes. Such a relaxed atmosphere usually allows for better individual and group counseling. Nature has a way of relieving our tension and anxieties and as such we are better able to live with ourselves, as

well as being more considerate of our fellow man.[16]

Recognizing that recreation activities are not usually carried on with retarded persons as ends in themselves—but rather as means for bringing about therapeutic change in participants—at the same time, it is essential that activities be carefully geared to the capabilities of participants. The following section therefore describes a number of activity categories which are widely used with the mentally retarded, and shows how they are organized and modified where necessary.

In selecting activities, it is wise to bear the following principles in mind:

1. The mentally retarded have the same basic needs as other individuals for self-respect and a feeling of accomplishment.
2. Wherever possible, activities chosen should be appropriate for the chronological age level of retarded participants.
3. Retardates tend to have a short attention span; activities should therefore be diversified and should have a time limit determined by the behavior of the individuals taking part.
4. The mentally retarded also tend to have a low level of frustration. Therefore, games and other activities should be simplified, where necessary, and the teaching process should be done in stages.
5. The mentally retarded usually do not respond well to "talking about" an activity but learn better from direct participation.
6. Repetition is essential for retardates in learning most activities and skills.
7. Recreation can serve as an important stabilizing factor in the lives of the mentally retarded and should be organized in an orderly fashion, following a familiar schedule.
8. While the leader may have other social or educational goals in mind, activities must provide fun and a sense of enjoyment for participants.

Useful Activities for the Retarded

Recognizing these characteristics, those responsible for recreation programs for the mentally retarded have tended to emphasize the following areas of activity: (a) sports and physical fitness activity; (b) creative experiences: arts and crafts, music, dance and drama; (c) games; (d) social activities; (e) training in living skills; (f) special events and trips; and (g) camping.

Sports and Physical Fitness Activity

Some of the most successful programs for the retarded include such activities as bowling, skating, swimming, volleyball, track and field and similar activities. In addition to the physical benefits of sport, these activities provide the opportunity to engage in healthy competition, to strive toward a goal, to gain a sense of accomplishment and to feel that one is part of a group.

In general, when a given sport is presented to a group of retardates, it is necessary to teach the basic skills much more painstakingly and slowly than with other children of similar chronological age. It may be necessary to simplify the rules, and even modify the structure of the game, in order to ensure success and enjoyment for the participants. However, it is possible for the retarded to gain a high level of skill performance in sport; as indicated earlier, in some institutions they engage in team competition with other schools.

One of the sports programs which has received considerable attention in recent years has been the Special Olympics—a national competition which brings together teams of retarded children and youth from cities throughout the United States. They engage in various sports and fitness events and, ultimately, national champions are selected. Carried on with funding by the Kennedy Foundation and other public and private sources, the Special Olympics have been sponsored by

---

[16] For a description of Camp Confidence, see: Richard Endres: "Northern Minnesota Therapeutic Camp." *Journal of Health, Physical Education and Recreation,* May, 1971, p. 75.

major cities throughout the United States, such as Chicago, and have had thousands of retarded participants.

In some cases, major athletic programs have been promoted for the mentally retarded on a state-wide level. In Ohio, for example, the Ohio Athletic Association coordinates sports and physical activities in schools and institutions for the retarded. It arranges competitions and assists in providing transportation for visiting teams; it also provides modified rules and procedures for the more complicated sports in order to standardize practices throughout the state.

In many institutions, physical conditioning programs, such as stunts and tumbling, gymnastics or systematic exercise routines, have been developed for retarded residents. In general, there is widespread support for all forms of physical activity for the retarded, although some have warned of the dangers inherent in overemphasis on competitive sport. A report issued by the American Association for Health, Physical Education and Recreation commented:

> Undue emphasis is often placed upon participation in complex and complicated sports or athletic events in physical education and recreation programs for the mentally retarded. Frequently the retarded are placed in sports activities they don't understand, and in which their chances for success are minimized because of the intellectual function required by the activities themselves. An inadequate foundation of fundamental motor skills combined with too-early introduction to complicated sports skills also promotes failure for the retarded.[17]

Recognizing this, many institutions place stress only on the very informal and casual use of sports activities, usually for higher-functioning retardates. Many activities are approached in an exploratory, "fun" way, as well as other activities that involve the mastery of a single, fairly basic

skill. Typical of such activities are bowling, skating and swimming. To demonstrate how such activities are presented in an institution serving the retarded, the following descriptions of objectives of activity are excerpted from the leadership manual of the Plymouth State Home and Training School in Northville, Michigan. They deal with *bowling, roller skating* and *swimming.*[18]

BOWLING

Objectives. The objectives for this activity have two parts: those appropriate for non-physically handicapped residents, and those appropriate for residents with additional handicaps.

1. Non-handicapped residents should learn to bowl in turns and remain seated when they are not bowling. They should learn to hold onto the ball using thumb and middle two fingers (of either hand) and to swing either arm in a pendulum motion with ball in hand before delivering the ball. The resident should learn to roll the ball down the alley without throwing or lofting it, and make contact with pins without hitting gutters.
2. Physically handicapped residents should learn to push the ball off a specially designed ramp. Some can learn to take the ball from the ball return and place it on the ramp, as well as place the ramp for different shots. The blind residents should learn to use the guide rail.

The objectives of providing physical exercise and constructive use of leisure time are appropriate for all residents who participate.

ROLLER SKATING

Objectives. Roller skating is used to help develop the balance and motor coordination of the residents. Their sense of accomplishment is increased with mastery of skating skills, and they have a way to use their leisure time constructively. Residents need to learn the following skills:

1. Feeling comfortable with skates on.
2. Standing and moving about with a skate on one foot and the other foot on the floor.
3. Using side rails or rolling stand to initiate movement around the gym or day room.
4. Propelling themselves around the room.

---

[17] *Guidelines for Programing in Recreation and Physical Education for the Mentally Retarded.* Washington, D.C., American Association for Health, Physical Education and Recreation, 1968, p. 13.

[18] Plymouth State *Activity Therapy Manual. op. cit.,* pp. 7, 19, 21.

5. Balancing themselves well enough to walk or glide around the room on two skates.
6. Using alternate leg movements to move about on skates.
7. Attempting to skate to music.
8. Participating in a skating party with residents from other buildings.

Structure. Most ambulatory residents can learn and enjoy skating. From ten to 15 residents can be in a group for instruction. Fifty to 75 residents can participate in a skating party. Instruction is scheduled for twice a week for one hour at a time.

SWIMMING

Objectives. The swimming program for the physically handicapped (many retarded residents in institutions have physical handicaps as well as mental) is planned to meet the following objectives:
1. Build or maintain organic strength and vigor.
   a. Increase the range of movement within joints.
   b. Lengthen periods of sustained activity.
   c. Improve circulation.
   d. Promote deeper breathing.
   e. Improve control of body movements.
   f. Relax the body (sedative effect of immersion).
   g. Promote better elimination.
2. Improve the morale of the participants by:
   a. Socializing in fun activities with persons not physically handicapped.
   b. Developing a feeling of satisfaction in achievement.
   c. Satisfying their desire for physical activities (buoyancy effect of water enhances movement).
   d. Projecting thoughts beyond themselves to concentrate on the movement task.
   e. Reducing the appearance of the handicap.

Instruction in swimming is used to help all residents overcome their fear of water, and learn basic water safety skills, including:
1. Holding their breath for ten seconds.
2. Breathing rhythmically ten times.
3. Floating on their stomach.
4. Floating on their back.
5. Treading water.

All residents except the severely physical handicapped receive recreational benefits from swimming. The wide and varied range of swimming skills challenges even the more physically capable residents. Competitive swimming offers an opportunity for them to socialize and increase their ability to take the win or loss in a sportsmanly manner.

Structure. Therapeutic use of the pool is appropriate for any resident recommended by the doctor in charge. Swimming instructions are appropriate for all residents who are able to follow simple instructions and are somewhat mobile. Competitive swimming is appropriate for those residents with swimming skills on a competitive level and the desire to compete.

Each resident in the program should participate for one hour, including dressing time, and should be scheduled at least once a week. Therapeutic swimming can be provided for those residents who need one-to-one assistance in numbers no greater than 15 scheduled for the pool area at one time. Swimming instruction should be given to groups of ten or less per instructor. Competitive swimming should be in groups of six or less.

Creative Experiences: Arts and Crafts, Music, Dance and Drama

A second major aspect of recreation programming for the mentally retarded is in the area of cultural and creative activities. These can be adapted to meet the needs of residents at all levels of ability in institutional settings, or to provide engrossing and enjoyable hobbies for the mentally retarded in community life. In general, the same kinds of activities that normal children would engage in are provided for the retarded. However, as in the case of sports, it is necessary to teach them at a slower pace, to keep projects simpler and to provide a fuller level of supervision.

Arts and crafts may range from the use of crayon and paper in drawing, finger-painting, play with clay and similar unstructured kinds of activities, to more elaborate forms of painting or craft activities, such as block-printing, leatherwork, weaving and metalwork or ceramics.

Dance activities may range from simple singing games and rhythmic exploration, to more complicated folk and square dances, creative or modern dance—and, for older retardates, social dancing as a popular coeducational activity.

Dramatics may include puppetry, creative or informal dramatics or actually putting on plays. Since it may be difficult for many mentally retarded children and youth to memorize and deliver lines effectively, the emphasis may be on improvised dialogue in some dramatic ventures. However, it *is* possible to do much more elaborate dramatic productions with mentally retarded children. As an example, 65 children and young adults from Letchworth Village for the Mentally Retarded in Thiells, New York, a state institution, put on a full-scale performance of the musical "Oklahoma" before 3000 guests at the New York City Hilton Hotel. The individuals, with a chronological age of between eight and 35, and an I.Q. range between 30 and 79, prepared the show as a climax to a fund-raising campaign for the school. The residents rehearsed steadily for the performance for six months, and did an almost professional job of remembering their lines and cues.

Creative activities lend themselves to specific therapeutic uses. For example, simple musical activities may be used to promote reading readiness. In a year-long experimental program with 18 teenage boys with I.Q.s ranging from 17 to 56, at Northern State Hospital in Bellingham, Washington, such a process was carried out effectively.[19]

In a more general way, music may be used to provide a release for tension and emotional expression, to encourage and stimulate language and communication, to improve group interaction and enhance the self-image of residents. Additionally, it strives to improve the musical abilities of the residents, and to promote his sense of accomplishment and his ability to use his leisure constructively. At the Plymouth State School, it is presented in two forms: music therapy, and music education. Program content in each of these include the following:[20]

Listening Behavior

1. Sitting quietly and attentively listening to music played on a phonograph, tape recorder or instrument.
2. Improving the attention span until the resident can participate in a classroom setting for 30 to 45 minutes.
3. Discussing what has been heard.
4. Improving comprehension of instructions.
5. Giving creative interpretations of what has been heard.

Gross Motor Activities, Coordination and Rhythm

1. Developing basic movements of walking, marching, running, jumping, tiptoeing, hopping, galloping, skipping, and skating.
2. Clapping hands to strong rhythmic music.
3. Using rhythm instruments for marking simple and compound meters.
4. Participating in a rhythm band (playing when music begins, stopping when music stops, playing alternately and at different times).

Musical Games

1. Understanding the idea of the game by verbal or demonstrative instructions.
2. Taking turns.
3. Group participation.
4. Heading the group.

Singing

1. Humming.
2. Singing parts of songs.
3. Singing song in correct melody and rhythm.
4. Singing a song within the proper key.
5. Singing with the correct words.
6. Singing a complete song with a group.
7. Singing a complete song alone.
8. Leading others in song.

Ear Training

1. Recognizing various recorded sounds.
2. Differentiating stop and go.
3. Differentiating between high and low, fast and slow, loud and soft, musical and non-musical sounds.

[19] John De Blasio: "Teaching Pre-Academic Concepts with Music." *In* Larry L. Neal: *Recreation's Role in the Rehabilitation of the Mentally Retarded. op. cit.,* pp. 55–56.

[20] *Activity Therapies Manual,* Plymouth State School and Training School, Northville, Michigan, 1971, pp. 8–13, 19–20, 21–23.

4. Describing musical moods (happy, sad, funny, serious, etc.)

Instrumental Music

1. Playing simple musical instruments, (kazoos, hum-a-zoos, harmonicas, drums).
2. Learning the names of various instruments and recognizing them by sight.
3. Learning to play the more difficult instruments (tonettes, recorders, guitar, autoharp, piano).
4. Learning to play chords.
5. Playing by ear.
6. Reading music.

Use of Games

Games are extremely useful in recreational programs for retarded children, youth and adults. These may include quiet table games, more active equipment games, social games and mixers carried on in group situations and active outdoor or gymnasium games.

Games provide an important environment for the learning of social skills, as well as the opportunity to have fun in simple ways. Many retardates who have never really learned to play can have this experience for the first time in a game situation. Games provide the opportunity both to compete against others and to cooperate closely with others in a team effort. Specific games may require participants to learn and obey rules, to work with number concepts, to develop alertness, to practice memory or to dramatize roles.

Obviously, games that involve complex rules or highly developed skills are not appropriate for the mentally retarded. However, many basic games *can* be taught to educable or trainable retardates, with considerable success. It is important, in leading games, not to use those activities that depend on all participants functioning correctly. Thus, even if one or two players do not understand the point of a game, or are not able to carry it on successfully, it should be possible for the overall group to continue to play it with enjoyment.

Some institutions, such as the Rainier State School in Buckley, Washington, have published pamphlets in which they list the needed equipment, teaching procedures and time required to play specific games. Richard Endres, Patient Program Supervisor of the Brainerd State Hospital, Brainerd, Minnesota, has compiled a collection of basic games (relays, tag games, simple ball games, follow-the-leader and elimination games) which he has used successfully with the retarded.[21] Clearly, they represent one of the most useful and rewarding forms of program activities for this group—as well as a category which requires no special equipment or facility.

Social Activities

One of the most important elements of an overall program serving mentally retarded teen-agers and adults is the social program. Most retardates find it extremely difficult to mingle and be accepted by other people in their same age range who are not retarded. Often, their social skills and confidence are extremely limited because of this exclusion.

Therefore, it is essential to provide club activities, dances, parties, trip programs and similar activities to meet the important social needs of retarded youth and adults, and to prevent isolation and withdrawal. These may vary according to the setting. In an institutional program, such social activities should not only provide fun and social contact, but should contribute to the overall social development of participants.

At the Rainier School, for example, social recreation is used to develop social skills, and to learn to use leisure independently and creatively. Hough writes that "exchange dinners" between halls and units of the school are popular on a coeducational basis. Often these are followed by games, dancing and informal conversation. Proper table manners and social behavior are encouraged by the supervising staff. She continues:

A social atmosphere is also provided through parties and entertainment planned and carried out by staff and/or volunteer

[21] Richard Endres: *Modified Game Activities: Improvisation is the Key.* Brainerd, Minnesota, Brainerd State School, 1971.

groups. . . . The Residents' Canteen is another medium wherein skills learned . . . include: money handling, purchasing refreshments by name and cost, dancing, table games, social etiquette, group activity participation and interaction, and facility rules. Essentially, this is a place for the practice of skills. However, the recreation leader offers a reinforcing element by correcting inappropriate behavior, assisting each person who may have trouble with reading the name of an item he or she desires to purchase, and helping the person in recognizing the value of money. The program is primarily for use in one's leisure time and not structured as a class.[22]

Other social activities at the Rainier School are geared to the same objectives of achieving personal growth for teen-age retardates. For example, one program designed for the Placement Unit (youth and adults who might be discharged, but who lack the skills needed for community living) is the Holly and Cedar Leisure Time Activity Club. Hough describes this program as an extremely popular one, which deals not only with activity, but also with exploration and group discussion of the following areas:

Program content developed with the participants to include: grooming and care of clothing; personal hygiene; physical conditioning and posture; boy-girl relationships and dating procedures (with supervision); party and picnic planning; behavior problems discussions for correction and understanding of right and wrong; self-motivating hobbies; service projects; community based functions and other special items as brought up by the membership. . . . Special emphasis is made on the development of each individual's attitudes toward responsibility in work and play, as fellow men and women, and in general, life itself.[23]

Within this program, the development of potential leadership abilities receives special attention, and members of the club are encouraged to act as activity leaders and planners.

In the community, as indicated earlier,

many public recreation and park departments and voluntary agencies provide services for the retarded. As an example, the Nassau County, New York, Association for the Help of Retarded Children provides after-school and evening recreation for 200 retarded adolescents and adults in several locations around the county. Programs include eight bowling leagues which meet weekly in eight communities, and additional weeknight programs which include general recreation (ping-pong, social dancing, outdoor ball games when weather permits and dramatics). One group is organized as a club, electing its own officers and conducting its own agenda, and carrying out its own recreational events. In addition, social dances for adults, with music, refreshments, dancing and talent shows, are held each month for about 150 retarded adults.

Living Skills

Many recreation or activity therapy programs in state and private institutions include a strong component of special living skills. As indicated earlier, some of these—particularly those related to social behavior—are included in club and other social programs for teen-agers and adults. Not infrequently, special classes or workshops may be held in such activities as cooking, sewing or the repair of simple equipment.

As groups of retarded persons go out on trips, they learn to handle money and admission tickets, to find their way to needed facilities and to gain confidence in the community setting that will serve them in good stead at a later point. While these concepts and skills may be learned in a recreation activity, they are useful throughout the entire life of the participant. Having gained the ability to take a bus to a recreation event or sports program, the teen-age retardate has also gained the ability needed to take a bus every day to a job.

Camping Programs for Retarded

There is a rapidly growing interest in camping for the retarded. One of the

---

[22] Barbara A. Hough: "Activities for Youth." *In* Larry L. Neal: *Recreation's Role in the Rehabilitation of the Mentally Retarded,* p. 65.
[23] *Ibid.,* p. 66.

pioneer programs in this field has been Camp Confidence, the Northern Minnesota Therapeutic Camp—an independent organization intended primarily to provide year-round camping and outdoor recreation facilities for mentally retarded residents at Brainerd State Hospital, but which also serves groups sent by Daytime Activity Centers in the hospital's receiving area, and families of the retarded. Camp Confidence is unique, not only in its program but also in the way it has gained support and assistance from local businessmen, parents' groups and other auxiliary organizations, and even from a U.S. Army Reserve Engineer Battalion located in Brainerd.

Tent sites, picnic areas, cabins and a lodge have been constructed on a 140 acre wilderness site with over half a mile of lakeshore frontage. Program activities include winter sports (ice-fishing, snowmobiling and tobogganing, archery, swimming, boating, nature study and other activities suited to the natural setting. Richard Endres has outlined a number of categories to show how camps of this type may serve different classifications of mentally retarded persons, both institutionalized and living in the community. On a year-round basis, a number of the following programs might well be conducted simultaneously:

1. One-week programs for individuals considered capable of *independent or semi-independent community living*. Emphasis on outdoor education curriculum, with participants coming to camp approximately every six weeks.
2. Two- or three-day *vacation camping*. Primarily intended for hospital residents working in industrial program, who have little or no vacation opportunity. Less emphasis on outdoor education and more on recreational programs. Participation for such individuals suggested every three to four months.
3. *Day camping programs*. Primarily intended for children participating in child-development, special education classes at the parent facility (hospi-

tal). Instructors of child-development programs would serve as the major counselors for day camping experiences.
4. Two- or three-day *independent living skills camp*. Operated in separate units (away from the main camp complex), with six to eight individuals and one counselor living together with emphasis on home and camp living skills (cooking, clean-up, etc.).

In addition, as campers become proficient in various phases of the outdoor education curriculum, they might take part in two- or three-day *overnight tent camping* programs. Also, families of the retarded might enjoy meeting and camping together with similar families in a *family tent and trailer camping area*.[24]

For retarded children and youth living in the community, such special camping programs might serve as a preliminary experience which would then equip them to move into integrated camping programs with nondisabled peers. In writing about "habilitative camping," Marilyn Herb, Recreation Director of the Fairview Hospital and Training Center in Salem, Oregon, stresses the need to give campers real responsibilities in planning and carrying out program activities. Only if this is done, can camping produce the maximum results, in terms of positive social, emotional, physical and intellectual growth in retarded participants. The stress must be on the camper's abilities, not disabilities. She asks:

1. What responsibilities can be assumed by the camper?
2. How do these responsibilities affect the function of the camp?
3. Are duties and activities geared to camper abilities?
4. Who assigns these duties, you or campers?
5. Do your activities have carry-over values?
6. Are the activities new, or have campers been involved in like programs before?

---

[24] Richard Endres: "Northern Minnesota Therapeutic Camp." *Journal of Health, Physical Education and Recreation,* May, 1971, p. 75.

7. What is the potential for camper planning, executing, and evaluating programs?
8. Do activities stress anticipation, participation, and reflection?
9. How can activities be broken down to meet the needs of varied levels of participants?
10. Is the program the result of direct or indirect professional involvement?[25]

Scope of Therapeutic Recreation for the Retarded

This chapter has given examples of recreation programs and activities designed to meet the needs of the mentally retarded. How widespread *are* such programs? No fully comprehensive information has been gathered about all institutions and community programs. However, it is obvious that practices vary widely around the United States and in Canada today.

In many cases, inadequate staffing and funds have limited the total provision of care for severely and profoundly retarded patients in state hospitals. Often they are extremely overcrowded, and it is all that staff can do to keep up with their minimal physical needs. Aroused public opinion has, in some cases, resulted in improved funding and program development in such institutions.

As earlier figures made clear, the great bulk of mentally retarded individuals live in the community, and it is here that there is a marked need to improve the availability of recreation programs. Stracke, in a survey of 500 community recreation agencies in the United States, found that only 37 per cent of the 365 responding departments had assigned full- or part-time staff members to working with the disabled.[26] Mitchell and Hillman have commented:

> The overall picture of recreation services for the mentally retarded in municipal recreation agencies suggests that a wide gap

exists between the services provided and the services needed. Studies reveal that far too many recreation departments are not engaged in providing programs for which they should be basically responsible.[27]

Hillman stresses the need for improved coordination and intra-agency cooperation in the provision of services, as well as for improved research programs to determine needs and effective programs, better information services, training for staff, parent education and involvement and evaluation of participants. He writes:

> . . . the overall effort to provide information services related to recreation and mental retardation has been sporadic. The need to consolidate efforts and planning in this area is reflected along with other prevalent needs. . . . Vital to the delivery of any service is that of planning. The contributions to either comprehensive planning for mental retardation or planning for recreation services to the retarded have been scant. . . . The need to collect data on such topics as residential areas, transportation methods, buildings, commercial and public recreation areas, along with the demographic aspects of the population, is often completely overlooked.[28]

Berryman, Logan and Lander urge the need for research and demonstration programs in the following areas, if community and institutional recreation programs are to be improved throughout the United States:

1. Strategies for training and utilization of para-professional personnel to help reduce the current shortage of available trained manpower.
2. Methods of fostering inter-agency cooperation in the development of comprehensive recreation services to disabled children and youth.
3. Design and implementation of transportation services for disabled children and youth.
4. Community and parent-education pro-

[25] Marilyn Herb: "Habilitative Camping." *In* Larry L. Neal: *Recreation's Role in the Rehabilitation of the Mentally Retarded*, p. 53.

[26] Richard Stracke: "The Role of the Therapeutic Recreator in Relation to the Community Recreator." *Therapeutic Recreation Journal*, 1st Quarter, 1969, pp. 26–29.

[27] Helene Jo Mitchell and William A. Hillman, Jr.: "The Municipal Recreation Department and Recreation Services for the Mentally Retarded." *Therapeutic Recreation Journal*, 4th Quarter, 1969, p. 35.

[28] William A. Hillman, Jr.: "Federal Support of Recreation Services Related to Mental Retardation." *Therapeutic Recreation Journal*, 3rd Quarter, 1969, p. 10.

grams concerning the importance of early play experiences for disabled children.

5. Analysis of play and recreation activities in relation to sensory-motor, cognitive, and affective behaviors, and their development in the handicapped child.

6. Design and demonstration of methods for integrating disabled youngsters into recreation programs with normal peers.[29]

While this statement of research and demonstration applies to overall disabled population, it is especially meaningful for service to mentally retarded children, youth and adults. Within the community setting, a number of alternatives exist for serving the retarded. Programs may be sponsored by separate voluntary organizations or public recreation departments, or by joint efforts of both. When no program exists, and interested parents or community leaders seek to initiate one, a process of community education, identification of need, and organization, is required. Avedon and Arje have developed a handbook for sponsoring groups which presents useful guidelines for carrying on this process.

Guidelines for Developing Community-Based Programs[30]

1. *Assess retarded population and existing programs.* As a first step, it is necessary to determine the size and make-up of the retarded population, and the existing facilities and services within the area concerned. Usually such information can be gathered through the local chapter of the National Association for Retarded Children, public agencies such as the Board of Education or private agencies or welfare organizations serving the disabled.

2. *Assemble "framework" committee.* After determining the extent of need within a community, Avedon and Arje suggest that it is essential to develop a steering committee or "framework" of sponsors to plan and initiate action. This may include active parents of retarded children, representatives of community agencies, specialists in recreation and related rehabilitative services and similar individuals.

3. *Mobilize community interest and support.* To arouse community concern and promote involvement, it is desirable to have an initial, well-attended community meeting to discuss the need for, and ways of sponsoring an inter-agency program. Those to be invited might include representatives of the public school system, public recreation and park department, voluntary social and recreational agencies, civic clubs, government officials, churches and synagogues and the general public. If successful, this meeting should evoke concern, gain the support of community leaders and agencies in beginning a recreation program for the retarded and result in the formation of an advisory and programming committee to form the program and publicize and gather funds for it.

4. *Developing funding support.* Potential sources of financial support for such programs include: federal and state grants, Community Chest or other charitable funds, civic and service clubs, the municipal recreation and park department or the local chapter of the Association for Retarded Children. Not infrequently, money may be gathered from several sources (including fees from the families of retarded participants, if they can afford to pay them); at the same time, one agency may provide facilities free of charge, while another provides trained leadership, and another provides equipment or transportation. Special fund-raising efforts, such as rummage sales, car-

[29] Doris L. Berryman, Annette Logan, and Dorothy Lander: *Enhancement of Recreation Service to Disabled Children.* New York, New York University School of Education, Report of Children's Bureau Project, 1971, pp. 65–66.

[30] Elliott M. Avedon, and Frances B. Arje: *Socio-Recreative Programing for the Retarded, A Handbook for Sponsoring Groups.* New York, Teachers College, Columbia, Bureau of Publications, 1964.

nivals, theater parties or charity balls, may be used to raise initial funds, and thereafter repeated yearly.

An effective public relations program is necessary from the outset, both to support fund-raising efforts and to stimulate public awareness of the needs of the mentally retarded.

5. *Developing staff resources.* This is one of the most important considerations in getting a new program under way. Ideally, it is desirable to have the program directed by a recreation leader who has had direct experience with the mentally retarded and professional training in the field of therapeutic services. Since such persons are not always available, it is a reasonable solution to have the program directed by a qualified recreation leader, who is assisted by consultants or representatives of community organizations who are quite expert in the field of mental retardation—although not in recreation.

In addition, it is necessary to make considerable use of volunteers—since the ratio of staff to participants must necessarily be high, in working with the retarded. Young college students and even high school students often provide an excellent resource, since they are usually able to establish effective rapport with children. Other volunteers may be recruited from civic groups, women's auxiliaries, fraternal orders, religious groups or service clubs. A program of orientation, in-service training and on-the-job supervision should be established for all workers, professional and volunteer alike.

Programs should include not only a wide variety of activities, but also counseling and personal guidance for participants that will serve them in the various areas of development described earlier. Activities should include casual and unstructured participation, as well as some activities that require careful instruction and leadership. As much as possible, parents should be involved in planning the program and, to a degree, assisting in it, although one of the purposes of socio-recreative programming for the retarded is to free retarded children and youth from dependence on their families. When possible, program activities should be carried on in integrated settings with the non-disabled. This is most feasible when done with educable retardates, who are capable of functioning socially on a higher level.

This chapter has dealt with the nature of the mentally retarded, and presented a number of guidelines for developing recreation program services for this group, both in institutional and in community settings. It should be stressed that in many cases—particularly among the more severely retarded institutional residents—mental and social disability is complicated by other physical factors. A substantial percentage of such retarded persons have visual, auditory or other physical disabilities which hamper their overall development, and their participation in such programs.

The following chapter deals specifically with the nature of recreation service for various categories of physically disabled children, youth and adults. A number of its guidelines apply to the problem just cited—that of mentally retarded persons who also suffer from physical disability.

Suggested Topics for Class Discussion, Examinations or Student Papers

1. What are the unique characteristics of the mentally retarded that influence the planning of a recreation program for this special population?
2. Select a specific area of program activity, such as sports or camping, and show how it would be modified and planned, in order to meet the needs of the mentally retarded.
3. Develop a set of guidelines for the establishment of a community-based program of recreation service for the mentally retarded, including such elements as finance, public relations, leadership and scheduling.

Chapter 6

Recreation for the Physically Disabled

This chapter deals with major forms of physical disability as they affect both children and adults. Each type of disability is described, together with its effects on the individual afflicted, the consequent needs for recreation services and suggested program activities.

Physical Disability in American Society

As previous chapters have pointed out, it has been estimated that approximately one out of every seven persons in the United States today has some kind of serious physical disability. The range and extent of disability is great, varying from the severely disabled person who needs institutional care to the comparatively independent person who can hold a job and participate in the same activities as the normal person.

The specific types of disability are also extremely varied. Arthritis is a disease which afflicts more than 11 million people in the United States; for many it causes crippling or severe incapacitation. At least 10 million persons have some form of heart disease or blood vessel malfunction, the leading cause of death in the United States. It has been estimated that there are 250,000 persons in the United States confined to wheelchairs, 200,000 who

wear leg braces, and 140,000 with artificial limbs.[1]

In a sense, these statistics do not give the true picture of disability. The term brings to mind a cripple in a wheelchair or on crutches, or those who have lost one or more limbs, or who wear confining braces or prosthetic devices. Because of the lack of uniformity in defining the conditions of crippling and orthopedic handicaps, Fait points out that:

> . . . statistics of incidence are neither very meaningful nor very accurate. The number can be doubled or cut in half by the inclusion or exclusion of certain conditions.[2]

What this implies is that both the degree of physical disability and the *extent* to which it has proven to be a major limitation to the individual suffering from it vary very widely within *each* disability. The great majority of physically disabled persons live within the community, either with their families or independently. Many of them, even those with extremely

---

[1] *Outdoor Recreation Planning for the Handicapped.* Washington, D.C., Bureau of Outdoor Recreation, April 1967, pp. 2–3; and Kent Ruth: "Pleasure Travel is Becoming Easier for the Handicapped." *New York Times,* May 26, 1968, p. 2.

[2] Hollis F. Fait: *Special Physical Education.* Philadelphia: W. B. Saunders Co., 1972, p. 98.

serious physical limitations, are able to engage in a wide range of recreational and social interests. Unlike the mentally ill person who tends to be withdrawn and to avoid social contact or challenges that may be psychologically threatening, the physically disabled person is often eager to test himself among the nondisabled. And, unlike the mentally retarded individual, who has great difficulty in establishing a meaningful bond of friendship with his nondisabled peers, those with physical limitations are often well-integrated members of other social groups.

However, to provide adequate program service for the physically disabled, it *is* necessary to plan specifically for them, to provide programs geared to their needs and abilities, to modify activities and facilities and to provide sympathetic and capable leadership.

Goals of Recreation for the Physically Disabled

These goals are quite similar to those that have been described earlier for the mentally ill and mentally retarded. They include:

1. To provide rich and varied opportunities for the constructive use of leisure—both for those individuals who work, and those who do not, and thus have an excessive amount of free time.
2. To provide pleasure and creative satisfaction, and to serve as a form of personal enrichment and personality development.
3. To enhance the social independence of the individual and, where possible, give him satisfying group experiences in socially integrated settings.
4. To relieve the families of the disabled, both psychologically and in terms of time commitment, from the need for unremitting care for the physically disabled member of the family.
5. To help physically disabled persons compensate for their specific dis-

ability by mastering and finding personal achievement in other areas of activity, in which the disability is not an important factor.
6. To promote healthful physical involvement, and so to prevent further physical deterioration because of disuse.
7. To expand the disabled person's involvement in community life, and to complement other social, vocational, educational or civic involvements in a rounded schedule of activity.

As earlier chapters have pointed out, efforts to improve the lives of the physically disabled became widespread only in the 20th century, and after World Wars I and II, when public awareness of the needs of disabled war veterans led to a broad concern for the total rehabilitation of the physically disabled. Efforts were made to establish programs that would permit vocational and social reintegration into the mainstream of community life. In addition to programs established by the federal government, many municipal governments and voluntary organizations developed multiservice programs for the physically disabled. Among these programs have been a variety of recreation-oriented services.

A number of states have taken significant steps to provide needed recreation services for the disabled. In Massachusetts, for example, a state law was passed in 1958 to promote and foster recreation for the physically disabled and mentally retarded. While responsibility for this overall function was assigned to the Director of Special Education in the Massachusetts State Department of Education, it was specified that the responsibility for actually organizing programs would rest with recreation and park departments in municipalities throughout the state. The state reimburses local departments which provide day camping, swimming and various adapted indoor recreation activities for children and youth with a wide variety of disabilities.

In addition, there are a variety of voluntary organizations in American communities which have recognized the need of the physically disabled for recreation and are concerned with meeting their overall needs. As an example, the Easter Seal Society for Crippled Children and Adults is a national organization that operates through local chapters in cities throughout the nation. It provides special clubs and recreational programs in community centers, and also, in some cities, sponsors programs for the homebound physically disabled person.

In some cases, disabled adults themselves have organized to provide programs to meet their recreational and social needs. An excellent example is the Metropolitan Activities Club in Birmingham, Michigan. The members of this club range in age from 18 to 72, and all have serious physical disabilities; many are in wheelchairs or on crutches. Members of the Metropolitan Activities Club assume total responsibility for fund-raising and the organization of activities. These include bowling, basketball, swimming, square dancing, singing, arts and crafts and such special activities as parties and outings. Members also publicize their activities through a newsletter and yearbook, and through radio and television appearances.

On a national level, such organizations as the National Wheelchair Athletic Association promote specific forms of activity for the orthopedically disabled. Many other organizations designed primarily to serve the nondisabled, such as the Boy Scouts of America, also provide special programs for the physically disabled.

Although in many programs groups with various types of physical impairment are combined, it is helpful to be able to understand each major category of disability, in order to be able to plan to meet needs most effectively.

Recreation for Those with Orthopedic Disability

Orthopedic disabilities are those which prevent individuals from properly performing the motor and locomotor functions of their body and limbs. Such disabilities may be concerned with the functions of joints, tendons, bones, nerves or peripheral blood vessels, and may be caused by trauma, congenital conditions or infection.

Traumatic causes consist most frequently of amputation or peripheral nerve injury. Amputations may result from a number of reasons: accidents, illnesses such as diabetes, or surgery. Lack of development during the prenatal period, for a variety of causes, may result in a baby's being born without one or more limbs. Paralysis or motor loss in the muscles of the hips, lower trunk, legs, feet and arms may be caused by accidents effecting lesions in the nerves at the brain or attached to the spinal cord. If a person has lost the use of both legs, he is said to be *paraplegic;* if all four limbs, he is *quadriplegic.*

Congenital conditions causing physical disability include the following: *spina bifida,* a condition involving incomplete neurological development, which may cause loss of bowel and bladder control, or paraplegia; *congenital hip dislocation,* a malpositioning of the hip which weakens the leg and hip muscles, and which occurs more commonly among girls than boys; and *talipes,* a congenital condition commonly known as club foot. Other orthopedic conditions which tend to affect boys in the pre-adolescent or early adolescent periods are *coxa plana* and *Osgood-Schlatter* disease, both of which cause limping and pain in the legs or hips and may affect locomotion.

Infectious diseases which affect limb function include *poliomyelitis,* which may result in paralysis of one or more parts of the body; *osteomyelitis;* and *tuberculosis of the bone.* These diseases have been reduced considerably in incidence by vaccines and improved medical treatment, but they still affect many persons.

Despite greatly improved services for the physically disabled, severely orthopedic impairments have marked effects on the social, psychological and even economic lives of those with disability. Individuals who become handicapped by accident or illness must often find new ways of earning a livelihood, adjusting to the attitudes of family and friends and dis-

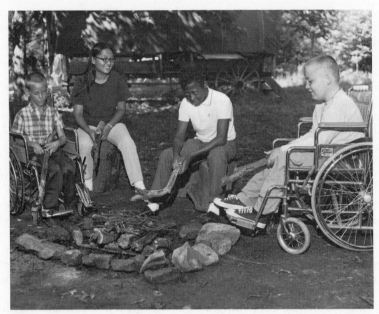

Disabled youngsters at Camp Kysoc, operated by the Kentucky Easter Seal Society at Carrollton, Kentucky, enjoy outdoor activities: building a campfire . . .

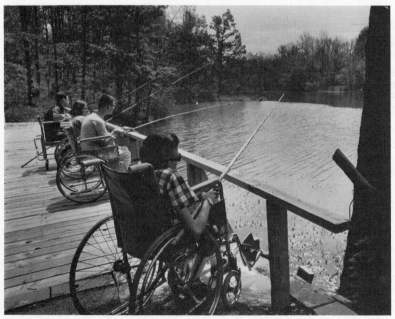

. . . fishing from a protected ramp . . .

covering new social and recreational activities to replace those which may no longer be possible.

Attitudes of rejection toward the orthopedically disabled still persist widely in society. The high value placed on physical appearance means that persons with crippling disease or missing limbs are often ostracized—either openly or in subtle ways. Particularly when the impairment

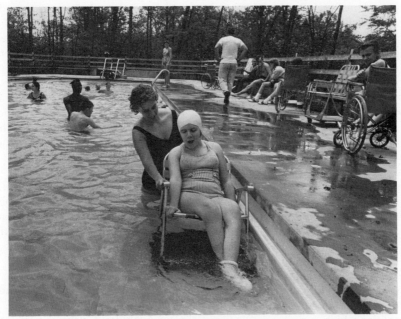

. . . and swimming in the camp's large, specially heated pool.

is sudden—as from an accident or severe illness—the problems of adjustment are extreme. Neser and Tillock write:

> A patient generally needs a period of time, which may range from nine to fifteen months, in order to translate his lack of physical improvement into the psychological acknowledgement that his disability is permanent. His attempt to integrate this knowledge often results in his entering a phase characterized by deep depression and mourning . . .[3]

Problems of the orthopedically handicapped are often accentuated by family attitudes. Financial difficulties resulting from the need for special care or equipment, as well as the need to devote considerable attention to the disabled child or youth, may cause family strain. Often parents or relatives of the disabled become overly cautious or overprotective, resulting in a state of dependence. It is essential that the orthopedically disabled person come to grips with his disability and be

encouraged to seek out activities in which he *can* perform successfully.

For patients in hospitals or rehabilitation centers who are recuperating from a serious accident or crippling illness, planned recreation programs may serve as a means of diverting attention from grief and providing constructive and rewarding ways of using time. It may lead to improvement in function and the development of *new* skills and interests which compensate for the disappearance of past abilities. Thus, it contributes to the physically disabled person's ability to accept his impairment, and to his growing independence and acceptance of his new status in life.

With intelligent modifications of activities and equipment, it is possible for the orthopedically handicapped to participate in a variety of sports, such as archery, bowling, table tennis, horseshoes, fishing or even such team games—dependent on the exact nature of disability—as soccer, baseball, softball, basketball or football. In a game such as soccer, in which the use of hands and arms is normally not permitted, except for the goaltender, a player who has normal use of his legs can function well. A one-armed player has

[3] William B. Neser, and Eugene Tillock: "Special Problems Encountered in the Rehabilitation of Quadriplegic Patients." *Social Casework*, March, 1962.

actually played major league professional baseball. Wheelchair basketball has become extremely popular, both in rehabilitation centers and community leagues, for players lacking the use of their limbs.

Other physical activities, such as fishing, hunting, swimming and dancing may readily be carried on by the orthopedically disabled. In the realm of social activity, the orthopedically disabled are able to enjoy group games, parties, carnivals and similar activities and events. With sufficient motivation, *every* form of creative activity, such as art, crafts, music, drama or creative writing, may readily be enjoyed by the orthopedically disabled. Even when an individual is so severely disabled that he cannot grip a paint brush with his hands, it may be strapped to his arm, or to a foot, or to his chin.

Specific descriptions of varied recreational activities which may be carried on by the orthopedically disabled are provided in the final section of this chapter.

Recreation for the Cerebral Palsied

Cerebral palsy is a condition affecting the motor control centers of the body, and is a result of lesions in various parts of the brain arising from injury, infection or faulty development. The condition is not regarded as an orthopedic disability, but is a neurological impairment.[4]

More than 600,000 children and adults are victims of this condition. It may occur before or at birth, or at any time later in life, although 90 per cent of all cases stem from natal or prenatal causes. These include maternal disease, severe maternal nutritional deficiencies, toxins, radiation therapy, incompatibility of Rh factors between parents or defective development of brain cells before birth and lack of oxygen to the developing brain (anoxia). Infectious diseases such as measles, mumps, whooping cough and encephalitis, or accidents involving a severe head injury, are responsible for the bulk of cerebral palsy cases that develop after birth.

The movement of the cerebral palsied

is impaired and awkward, and is often accompanied by postural malformations. Speech patterns are usually affected. The cerebral palsied may range from a complete inability to control muscular function, to a very slight lack of muscular coordination. Several types of functional dysfunction have been identified. These include: (a) *spastic,* characterized by jerky and uncertain movements and tightly contracting muscles; (b) *athetotic,* typically showing uncontrolled, sprawling muscular functioning; (c) *rigid,* with extremely tight muscles and limited, resistant movement; and (d) *tremor,* characterized by uncontrollably shaking limbs. Eighty-five per cent of all cases are either spastic or athetotic.

Cerebral palsy is classified as *mild, moderate* or *severe* in its impact. It may affect one or more parts of the body and often includes a degree of impairment in verbal ability, vision, hearing or intelligence, although the cerebral palsied person may be perfectly normal in these respects. Unless it is a mild case, the cerebral palsy sufferer has considerable difficulty in functioning socially and in being accepted by others. Drooling and jerky physical movements, constant facial grimacing and the overall physical appearance, as well as the hard-to-understand speech of many palsied individuals, tend to make normal social relationships extremely difficult. As a result, withdrawal and fear of social contact are common among many children, youth and adults with this impairment.

Although the condition cannot at present be cured, research has shown that intensive treatment, using a variety of modalities, can markedly improve the social, physical and intellectual capabilities of the cerebral palsied. The primary function of recreation services for the child with cerebral palsy is to promote normal growth and development by providing the kinds of experiences and activities that other children receive. However, because of the limitations of the palsied, it is essential to design activities carefully to meet his needs.

The first step is to become familiar with his total history, including the details of

---

[4] Hollis F. Fait: *op. cit.,* p. 84.

his home-life, the attitudes of his family toward his impairment, his medical history, his present physical limitations, his psychological make-up, his present social involvement and interests and other accompanying symptoms or conditions he may have.

In planning programs for the cerebral palsied, it is necessary to select activities which do not produce tension, and which do not require quick response or performance. While programs should not be overstrenuous, and frequent rest should be provided, it is important to provide physical activities to counteract the obesity and poorly developed motor skills characteristic of many cerebral palsied persons. Simple games, easy rhythmic activities and swimming are particularly desirable in working with this disability.

The United Cerebral Palsy Association of New York City is an example of a community-based voluntary agency which operates a day-care program for the cerebral palsied of all ages. Their recreation program, conducted under professional leadership, operates Monday through Friday in the evenings and during the day on Saturdays, serving teen-agers and adults.

Facilities operated by United Cerebral Palsy include two multipurpose rooms, arts and crafts shop, a music room, a library and apartments used for training the cerebral palsied in self-care and other life skills. Activities include arts and crafts, music, drama, table games, social events and trips, home-making projects, physical programs and discussion groups. They consist of approximately 40 per cent active programs and 60 per cent quiet, and are varied, according to age and the physical, mental and social levels of participants.

The heart of the adult recreation program consists of social clubs that meet weekly, each with between 20 and 25 members of both sexes. They meet in all five boroughs of New York City, and place emphasis on social events, bowling, creative writing and discussion groups and other common club activities. United Cerebral Palsy also operates a camping program to serve the cerebral palsied, and

conducts research, promotes legislation and disseminates publications in this field.

Recreation and Muscular Dystrophy

Muscular dystrophy is the name given to a group of chronic diseases whose main characteristic is the progressive degeneration of the voluntary muscular system of the body. It is a noncontagious illness which weakens the victim, who is eventually confined to a wheelchair and ultimately to bed. While its precise cause has not been determined, muscular dystrophy appears to result from an inborn metabolic defect—the lack of a specific enzyme essential for the conversion of food into tissues and energy.[5]

There are four main types of muscular dystrophy: (a) *Duchenne,* which begins as a rule between the ages of three and ten, affects more males than females, and is usually hereditary; (b) *juvenile,* which begins in adolescence and progresses slowly, sometimes reaching to middle age before it becomes severe; it is usually hereditary and affects both sexes equally; (c) *facioscapulohumeral,* which affects the facial muscles, shoulders and arms, and makes very slow progress, rarely shortening the life of the person afflicted, although it may cause considerable disability; and (d) *limb-girdle,* which occurs from the first to the third decade of life, and makes rapid progress, often causing death within from five to ten years.

The disease is not usually fatal in itself, although there are instances where it may cause heart failure. However, since muscular dystrophy patients cannot combat infections well, even the most trifling cold may result in suffocation and respiratory failure. It is estimated that there are over 200,000 persons affected by muscular dystrophy in the United States. Almost two-thirds of these are children, a high propor-

[5] Melville H. Manson: "Facts about Muscular Dystrophy." *Journal of Health, Physical Education and Recreation,* January, 1958, pp. 23–24; and C. Pearson: "Muscular Dystrophy—Review and Recent Observations." *American Journal of Medicine,* November, 1970, p. 634.

tion of whom die before reaching adulthood.

Recreation is extremely important for those afflicted with this disease. It helps to satisfy their basic human needs for recognition, creative expression, sense of accomplishment and group association. More specifically, it may be used to retard the progression of the illness, by strengthening those muscles which are still functioning well. Prolonged bed rest or confinement to a wheelchair can lead to limb atrophy and weaken patients unnecessarily.

Activities that are frequently used with those suffering from muscular dystrophy include arts and crafts, card playing, table games, informal music, modified sports and camping. Since the disease results in marked physical deterioration in its later stages, it is often necessary to modify activities and use ingenious devices to permit participation.

For example, a game like checkers may be played with the use of an instrument held in the mouth, to move the pieces across the board. Electric shufflers are used for card games, and racks have been constructed to hold the cards while they are played. Harmonica playing is often recommended because it is a good exercise for the lung muscles, and a device is available to hold the instrument in front of the player's mouth, so he need not use his hands. Arts and crafts may be simplified, and special devices used to hold tools or equipment. Sports activities are usually carried out with light, easily held equipment (whiffle bats and plastic balls), and with modified rules and court dimensions.

Recreation and Multiple Sclerosis

Multiple sclerosis is an organic disease which affects the nervous system in a variety of ways. Most commonly, it attacks the spinal cord, resulting in partial or complete paralysis of the legs and, at times, the trunk and arms. It is often mistaken for other illnesses, since its symptoms are varied and unpredictable; sometimes there are periods of remission, and even partial or complete recovery from the disease. Symptoms of multiple sclerosis include the

following: partial or complete paralysis of parts of the body; numbness; double or otherwise defective vision; noticeable dragging of the feet; loss of control of bowels and bladder; poor balance; speech difficulties; extreme weakness or fatigue; a pricking sensation in parts of the body; loss of coordination; or tremors of the hands.[6]

The disease is caused by a disintegration of the coating over the nerves, and the formation of scar tissue which causes interference with nerve impulses and subsequent malfunctioning. It usually occurs between the ages of 20 and 35, rarely appearing after 45, and is slightly more frequent in women than men. Multiple sclerosis differs markedly from patient to patient. Some individuals are able to maintain occupational and family responsibilities, and make an excellent adjustment to their illness. Others have severely crippling conditions followed by symptom-free periods. Still others are completely paralyzed and permanently incapacitated.

The National Multiple Sclerosis Society is an organization that serves persons afflicted with this illness in a variety of ways. It conducts research, provides medical and other referral services, and offers recreational and social programs through local chapters. Through clubs and organized social programs, it provides companionship (including home visiting for the severely afflicted), and organizes picnics, parties, theater programs and visits to sports and other entertainment events. There are comparatively few special recreation programs operated by voluntary or public recreation agencies for those with multiple sclerosis alone. Instead, they are normally served by programs geared to meet the needs of adults with a variety of physical disabilities.

Recreation and Cardiac Malfunction

Over 50 per cent of all deaths in the United States today are the result of heart

---

[6] *Multiple Sclerosis: The Crippler of Young Adults.* New York, National Multiple Sclerosis Society.

disease, a statistic which may be attributed both to the larger number of people who reach middle age today (owing to the elimination of other illnesses which attacked younger people in the past) and to changed styles of living. A second major factor is the high incidence of rheumatic fever among children, which causes cardiac damage in over two-thirds of those attacked.

Heart disease is generally classified under one of the following headings: (a) *rheumatic heart disease,* which usually occurs among children between the ages of six and 12, as a result of rheumatic fever which inflames and scars the heart valves; (b) *hypertensive heart disease,* which occurs as a result of high blood pressure or hypertension, or in association with arteriosclerosis (hardening of the arteries); and (c) *coronary heart disease,* which occurs most often among middle-aged and older persons who suffer from one or a series of heart attacks. Other causative factors include congenital heart disease resulting from birth defects, anemia which places a burden on the heart, and conditions brought on by such diseases or infections as diphtheria, myocarditis or endocarditis.

While the symptoms of heart disease are varied, their most significant impact on cardiac sufferers is that they impose an immense burden of fear. Heart disease carries the constant threat of death; while most individuals with cardiopathic conditions do not have the obvious impairments associated with other physical disabilities described in this chapter, they nonetheless are acutely aware of the danger of their condition. Thus, for both children or adults who are afflicted by heart disease, the normal urge to engage in physical recreation is frustrated.

Many children suffering from heart conditions are excessively restricted and become socially immature because they are shielded from any form of play and isolated from involvement with their peers. Fait writes:

Such children need to be counseled into a better course of adjustment, one which recognizes the restrictions essential but points

up the effective and enjoyable life which is possible within the limitations. . . .[7]

Similarly, it is important that adult heart sufferers be helped to take part in a regimen of safe but enjoyable recreational and social activities in order to prevent inactivity and social withdrawal. If they do not, they tend to become so obsessed with their illness that they are isolated and lack normal outlets for energy, as well as other forms of release, which may result in a high degree of emotional tension and actually promote heart disease. However, since heart patients require medical supervision and a specially planned program of activities, certain safeguards should be kept in mind:

1. Competition in recreational activity should be avoided or kept to a minimum, since it may cause a high level of emotional stress that is dangerous to the cardiac condition.
2. Children should not be permitted to overexert themselves in physical play, or in the duration of any sort of recreational activity, and should therefore be carefully supervised.
3. Individuals with heart conditions should be given frequent rest periods to prevent strain or exhaustion.
4. Environmental conditions, such as bad weather, heat or cold, may have an effect on cardiac patients; attention must be given to such factors, in planning recreation programs.

Associations serving heart disease sufferers have classified them in three categories, according to the degree of malfunction, and have used these classifications in recommending the amount and type of activity in which they may safely engage. Those in the *least serious* class are able to engage in active sports, such as swimming, softball, bowling, tetherball and similar pastimes, although care must be taken to avoid violent expenditures of energy or sustained periods of heavy activity. On the *middle levels of illness,* more moderate activity is required, and for the

[7] Hollis F. Fait: *op. cit.,* p. 119.

most seriously ill patient, only extremely quiet recreational activity, which can be carried on in bed or a sitting position, should be used. Since heart patients normally have full use of their vision, limbs and other body parts, they are readily capable of taking part in table games, cards, arts and crafts, music and similar sedentary activities.

Recreation for the Blind

An estimated 90 million Americans have some degree of ocular malfunction, with 3.5 million having a permanent non-correctable eye defect. Approximately one million persons lacking the ability to read ordinary-size newsprint are regarded as functionally blind. The legal definition of blindness uses the standard that an individual is blind if his vision is 20/200 or worse, meaning that, at 20 feet, he can see what a person with unimpaired vision can see at 200 feet. Based on this standard, there are an estimated 430,000 legally blind persons in the United States.[8]

Thus, although blindness is commonly thought of as the total lack of vision, in reality it may mean possessing varying levels of sight. Statistics on blindness are often inconclusive owing to varying legal and medical definitions of it. Nonetheless, it is obvious that it represents a major physical deficiency for persons of all ages in the United States. It is particularly important for those concerned with therapeutic recreation service because those affected by blindness do not usually suffer from other limiting physical impairments and tend to live a normal life span; however, the effect of blindness is to severely limit the individual's social integration and other life functions.

There are several causes of blindness: (a) *infectious diseases,* such as measles, scarlet fever, typhoid fever, etc.; (b) *accidents* causing injury to the eyes; (c) *functional disorders,* due to diabetes or

vascular disease; and a number of miscellaneous causes, including cataracts, genetic defects or poisoning.

As indicated, most persons who are considered legally blind have some degree of residual vision, and can distinguish light from darkness, see major forms or perceive movement. However, they are extremely limited in mobility and in many aspects of daily living, since so many routine activities are heavily dependent on visual perception. Sometimes they develop motor disabilities, poor posture and other physical impairments. The degree to which blindness affects the individual depends to some extent on when it developed. Some studies have shown that a person who becomes blind during the course of his lifetime tends to have more difficulty in adjusting than those who are born without vision. Another study has shown that individuals with no useful vision at all are better adjusted, particularly in group situations, than those with *some* vision.

As a result of blindness, many persons tend to become withdrawn, lacking in initiative and deficient in social relationships, particularly when they are overprotected, or when social opportunities are denied to them. Some blind persons develop anxiety and depression, while others become hostile; a variety of neurotic problems may develop as a consequence. That this is not the inevitable effect of blindness is demonstrated by the fact that many blind persons are able to lead full and happy lives, hold jobs, raise families and play meaningful roles in their communities.

Because services for the blind have frequently been inadequate, many blind persons are poorly developed physically. Often their locomotion, kinesthetic awareness and coordination are lacking. Approximately two-thirds of the visually impaired children in public schools are not given adequate physical education programs.[9] Often, without adequate physical

[8] *Facts About Blindness.* New York, American Foundation for the Blind, 1970; and Maxine Wood: *Blindness—Ability Not Disability:* Public Affairs Pamphlet No. 295-A, 1968, p. 3.

[9] Charles Buell: "Physical Education for Visually Handicapped Children." *Journal of Health, Physical Education and Recreation,* April, 1971, p. 63.

release, they develop a high level of tension. Many blind persons develop so-called blindisms, which are habits such as rocking, rubbing their eyes or waving their hands back and forth, which appear to stem from the repressed urge for physical movement.

All these factors reinforce the strong need of the blind for varied and interesting recreational outlets. Basically, such programs have three major purposes for the blind:

1. As an end in themselves—to satisfy the normal human needs and drives which the blind share with all persons.
2. As a diagnostic and evaluative tool—to determine the capabilities, weaknesses and needs of the blind individual.
3. As a specific tool in rehabilitation—which may be used to develop physical, social or intellectual growth, or to minimize overall disability.

Since many blind persons tend not to be employed, and, therefore, to possess great amounts of leisure, it is important that they be provided with the means of using this time productively and enjoyably. Thus, recreation can serve as a means of satisfying creative urges, releasing tensions, gaining self-esteem, promoting physical health and strengthening the socialization process. It is essential, in planning programs to meet the need of the blind, that this not be done *for* them, but *with* them. Ireland writes:

> A thorough understanding of the blind person is the only reliable basis upon which a recreation worker can set both a realistic and idealistic goal. What might be an ideal and yet realistic goal for one person might be wholly inadequate for the next person. The most important task of the recreation person is to assist the blind person to fulfill his desires and to be aware of his needs as fully as possible.[10]

---

[10] Ralph R. Ireland: "Recreation's Role in Rehabilitating Blind People." *Journal of Health, Physical Education and Recreation,* January, 1958, p. 44.

Blind persons today receive benefits in the form of education, rehabilitation services, Braille materials and income tax exemptions. Nearly all states have agencies which provide assistance with respect to homemaking, counseling for parents of blind children, vocational counseling, training and placement, and varied kinds of information services. With respect to recreation, most blind individuals are served through special organizations concerned with this category of disability rather than through public or voluntary agencies for the public at large.

Programs Serving the Blind

An example of a special school for the blind may be found in the Ontario, Canada, School for the Blind, a residential school which offers a three-phase curriculum: (a) academic; (b) social development; and (c) extracurricular. Out-of-school hours are supervised by residence counselors, who conduct Brownie, Guide, Cub and Scout groups. Such groups operate just as they would with sighted boys and girls, and in some cases share programs with similar groups in the community. The overall goals in the Ontario School for the Blind are:

1. To provide healthy, vigorous, outdoor living activities related to the Canadian cultural milieu.
2. To give the children practical skills necessary to cope with independent living outside of the school.
3. To develop the child's personality to the fullest.
4. To integrate the visually handicapped with seeing children as much as possible, and to guide them in handling themselves in such settings.

Trips and excursions are an important part of the program, and blind boys and girls in the school take part in track and field and wrestling meets, as well as in other clubs and associations in the community. Individuals are taught to travel, using the white cane for visibility, in order to facilitate independent mobility outside the school. Music in all forms, dramatics and other social and recreational activities are stressed for all residents.

A number of cities have special organizations that serve the blind. As an example, the New York Association for the Blind, also known as the Lighthouse, is a private, nonprofit, multiservice agency, serving approximately 3300 blind persons each year. It is funded through donations, grants, special funds and endowments, and offers the following social and recreational services: (a) a nursery-school-age play program, meeting twice a week; (b) a recreation program for rehabilitation clients, meeting four times a week; (c) a youth recreation program, meeting all day on Saturdays; (d) an adult education program in leisure activities, meeting two evenings a week; and (e) an older adult recreation program, meeting two evenings a week.

The facilities of the Lighthouse include bowling alleys, a swimming pool, social hall, kitchen and dining room, auditorium and stage, arts and crafts room, ceramics room, recreation hall and two residential camping areas. Since it is necessary to provide transportation for many of the participants in the program, it operates four station wagons and also uses private cars for this purpose. The Lighthouse also operates residential accommodations for both men and women in its training program, and has satellite programs elsewhere in the New York City area.

There are about 60 residential camps in the United States that are specifically designed to serve the visually impaired. One of these is Highbrook Lodge, a vacation camp for blind persons in northeastern Ohio, sponsored by the Cleveland Society for the Blind. It serves varied age groups, who attend four sessions of approximately one week each, and who pay fees based on their financial capability. Program activities include hiking, swimming, boating and fishing, bowling, horseback riding, baseball, wrestling and similar physical and social pursuits—many of which are planned by the campers themselves.

Recreation for the Deaf

The most commonly accepted definition of the deaf regards them as those whose sense of hearing is nonfunctional for the ordinary purposes of life. Complete loss of hearing is much less common than partial loss, in which sounds are garbled and unclear, or high or low sounds are lost. There are several ways of classifying deafness. It may be done according to the time the loss of function occurred: (a) *congenital deafness,* meaning that an individual was born deaf, as a result of prenatal or natal nerve destruction or injury, illness of the mother during pregnancy, incompatible Rh factors between parents or prolonged labor; or (b) *adventitious deafness,* referring to later loss of hearing caused by injury, infection or disease (measles, mumps, scarlet fever, diphtheria and meningitis are common causes), or psychogenic factors.

Deafness may also be classified as: (a) *nerve deafness,* usually congenital in origin, but sometimes resulting from accidents, illness or senility, and regarded as the more serious in its effects; and (b) *conduction deafness,* resulting from changes in the reception and conduction ear mechanisms. In many cases, both types of impairment may occur in the same individual. Finally, deafness may be seen more broadly as part of a concept of "auditory disorder," which is concerned with the total reception and interpretation of sound.

The effects of deafness are profound, since language and verbal communication are so important in all aspects of daily life. Since it is not a visible disability, people frequently show little understanding or sympathy toward the deaf, and tend to regard them with hostile attitudes, epitomized by the label "deaf and dumb," which is often attached to them. In fact, many deaf persons learn to speak quite effectively, and deafness does not imply any mental subnormality. In some cases, since spoken language is such an important factor in development, the deaf may be weak in the capacity for abstract thinking, and in some children who are born deaf, this may be a contributing factor leading to mental retardation.

Deaf persons generally have good motor skills, although poor balance and dizziness may exist when the impairment is related to semicircular canal injury or cerebral palsy. In some cases they may be slightly less skilled in touch perception; on the other hand, they frequently have faster reflexes than the person with normal hearing, probably because their level of tension is high, resulting from the understandable effort to compensate for the lack of hearing ability.

A primary objective of recreation and social programs for the deaf should be to integrate them with nondisabled peers. As in other areas of life, this poses a difficult problem because of the importance of verbal communication in most recreational activities.

Teaching the deaf or leading them in recreational programs requires careful attention to the means of communication. Involving them in games, dancing, or other group activities where directions must be heard, should be done carefully. In special situations where skilled leaders are working with the deaf exclusively, reliance may be placed on the manual method of spelling out words with "finger language." However, in mixed groups or with leaders not familiar with this method, lip reading is the more useful approach. Thus, the recreation leader should stand close to the persons he is working with, facing them directly, and should speak slowly and clearly, enunciating each word distinctly. He may also use hand gestures and other forms of direct demonstration, visual aids or diagrams, or may rely on persons with normal hearing in the group to assist deaf participants in learning activities.

Examples of Programs Serving the Deaf

Educational, vocational, social and recreational services for the deaf may be provided in a variety of settings, such as special schools or classes, voluntary organizations in the community or programs provided by public recreation departments. Special centers to serve deaf and blind children have been established in a number of cities with federal funding under Public Law 90-247. These assist local agencies with grants or contracts empowering them to provide diagnosis, evaluation, education, social services and consultants to parents and teachers.

An example of a special school for the deaf in New York City is the Lexington School for the Deaf, operated under the auspices of a board of trustees and the New York State Board of Education, with funding by the New York City Board of Education and private sources. This school serves some 400 students, almost half of whom are residents; all have auditory disability and some have multiple handicaps. Facilities operated by the Lexington School include a gymnasium, library, activity and game rooms, lounges, swimming pool, ballfields, playground, billiards room and arts and crafts shop.

The after-school recreation program includes a high proportion of physically active pursuits—all voluntarily participated in by students. It has been found that, once they have learned the basic rules, skills or strategy in a given activity, deaf children tend to participate extremely successfully in it. Particularly in sports or other activities where hearing is not an important factor, such as wrestling or competitive swimming, they are able to compete with others on an equal footing; occasionally, deaf competitors have won N.C.A.A. or A.A.U. wrestling championships. However, the school has experienced continuing difficulty in integrating its students in programs with nondisabled peers, a problem facing other community recreation agencies that seek to accomplish this goal.

Other Physically Disabling Conditions

In addition to the impairments described earlier, there are a number of other diseases or disabling conditions which may require specially designed therapeutic recreation service. These include, as examples, tuberculosis and diabetes.

TUBERCULOSIS. An infectious disease which affects the pulmonary system, tuberculosis may require long hospitalization in a sanitarium or rest home, together with sustained bed care and nutritious diet. Although it once was regarded as a major health problem, and often resulted in progressive disability and death, today it has declined markedly in incidence, particularly among children. However, it continues to appear on all age levels, and there is a substantial number of persons who have arrested cases. For such individuals, activity must be limited and precautions taken to prevent reinfection.

Recreation plays a vital role for those who are hospitalized in making the long period of hospitalization more bearable. It provides pleasure and interest, strengthens morale and helps the tubercular patient avoid depression and gain a sense of usefulness and involvement. It can also introduce new skills and interests to supplant those which must be given up by the patient. It may also contribute to the physical fitness level of the patient without unduly taxing his energies.

DIABETES MELLITUS. Diabetes mellitus is a disease in which the body is unable to properly ingest starches and sugars, owing to an inadequate supply of naturally produced insulin. The highest incidence of diabetes is among middle-aged persons, although approximately ten per cent of its cases occur among children. For the most part, diabetics can engage in a normal range of activities (some diabetics have actually been successful as professional athletes), and most can engage in the normal occupational, family and other community involvements of the nondisabled without danger. However, they tend to fatigue more easily than others, and care must be taken with respect to diet and regular medication. Therefore, camping or other residential programs serving the diabetic person must be specially designed to meet his health needs. When the condition is severe, it may require hospitalization and a sharply limited regimen of activity.

Modification of Activities for the Physically Disabled

The previous section has described the major areas of physical disability and the needs and types of programs provided for each. A number of categories of activity are now described, with specific illustrations of how each one is modified to meet the needs of physically disabled persons.

Physical Activities: Games and Sports

As indicated earlier, almost all the games and sports played by nondisabled persons can also be enjoyed by those with impairment. However, it is necessary in many cases to modify them with respect to playing conditions, rules and equipment, so that the disabled player can be successful rather than frustrated. Often, since such participants have had limited experience in physical activities, it is necessary to stress slow, careful, sequential teaching of basic skills.

SWIMMING. This is one of the most useful activities, because it can be adapted to the needs and capabilities of almost every type of disabled person. It is particularly suitable for those who have serious physical impairments. Grove writes:

Regardless of a person's mental or physical condition, buoyancy of the water allows him to move his most useless muscles. Water activities include movements, patterns and skills almost anyone can perform—if they are adapted to the individual.[11]

Swimming provides the disabled child, in particular, a kind of exercise and freedom of movement he cannot enjoy out of water. He is free of wheelchairs, special appliances or the support of his parents' arms, and is able to join his family or nondisabled friends in an enjoyable pastime which brings new confidence and pleasure. It offers the opportunity for the disabled to socialize with their peers in many programs.

11 Frances Grove: "Aquatic Therapy: A First Real Step to Rehabilitation." *Journal of Health, Physical Education and Recreation,* October, 1970, p. 65.

For most categories of disability, water should be heated to a warm temperature to avoid tension or chilling which may discourage the disabled child or youth from entering the water, or have an adverse effect on his impairment. There should be a fairly large area with shallow water to permit casual water play for children who have not yet gained confidence in the water. The pool should have a wide surrounding deck with a slip-proof surface. Steps with handrails leading into the water should be built with short risers and a wide step, to permit easy entrance or exit. In some cases, rails are fixed across the pool to permit participants to hold on and gain a feeling of security.

Daniels has suggested a number of guidelines for teaching swimming to the disabled:

1. The group method of instruction should be used whenever possible, supplemented by individual instruction when necessary.
2. All available teaching aids and equipment should be used to gain the participant's interest and encourage his attempting to learn to swim.
3. Instruction should be informal, with short teaching periods and frequent rest or opportunity for free play in the water.
4. Participants should be grouped according to their level of accomplishment or readiness for swimming, rather than by type of disability.
5. Each session should involve some progress or feeling of achievement, for all participants.[12]

Since fear of the water may be present in all nonswimmers, and especially so for the physically disabled, it is important for the swimming instructor to gain the trust of the participants and to help them relax in the water. Working in small groups, with aides personally helping those children who need special support, the first step is to accustom participants to being in the water, and help them lose their fear of it. The fun aspect of swimming

should be emphasized, and simple ball play, like water dodge ball, may be used to bring this about.

Artificial floats should be used for beginners; this is generally considered preferable to having them held by other persons. However, children using foam or inflated floats should be closely watched at all times, to prevent the accident that might occur if they slip from the supporting surface.

The selection of strokes depends on the specific disability of each participant. For persons with loss of arm function, an asymmetrical stroke, such as the side-stroke or trudgeon stroke, is often used. Learners who have had a loss of leg function, either full or partial, usually prefer symmetrical strokes, such as the elementary backstroke, breast stroke or dog paddle. For those individuals who cannot put their heads in the water, the body should be held at approximately a 70 degree angle, with the face lifted enough to be out of the water. If learners do not have use of their arms, a glide and flutter kick action may be used; swim fins help to give them added propulsion, and build up leg strength.

For more severely disabled persons, the emphasis at the outset may simply be on teaching breathing rhythms, and on beginning to learn to float. Even if they cannot learn to swim, just being in the water is likely to bring pleasure.

Swimming is particularly useful in working with blind children and adults, since it provides a degree of freedom that they do not normally experience on land. A slight elevation around the pool provides safety against blind persons accidentally falling in while walking around the deck. Swimming areas should be carefully roped off for those of different swimming ability, and ropes may be used to guard the blind participant from deep areas, or to help him find his way to the ladder. No particular stroke is to be preferred for the blind. However, since many of them fear to wet their eyes, they may prefer to learn a slow backstroke or breast stroke, with the head above the water. A safety precaution that is often helpful is the use of the buddy system. If diving

---

[12] Arthur S. Daniels: *Adapted Physical Education.* New York, Harper and Bros., 1954, pp. 227–229.

is permitted, the diving area should be carefully roped off from swimming areas in the pool, to prevent accidents.

ACTIVE GAMES AND SPORTS. Many different types of ball games may be used with the physically disabled. In order to permit such groups as the orthopedically disabled to take part in these activities, Pomeroy suggests a number of ways to simplify ball games:

1. Walking or wheeling may be substituted for skipping or running, when necessary.
2. A bounced throw or underhand toss may be used to replace a regular throw.
3. Positions such as sitting, kneeling or lying down may be substituted for standing positions.
4. The distances of bases or boundary lines, or of the dimensions of playing areas such as horseshoe courts, volleyball fields or baseball diamonds, may be reduced.
5. Lighter or more easily controlled equipment may be substituted for regular equipment.
6. Players may be restricted to a definite position or area on the playing field.
7. Players may be allowed to hit a ball any number of times, or to hold the ball longer in games like volleyball or basketball.
8. In games like baseball, if a child is unable to run, a runner may be used for him.[13]

Other devices may be used, such as increasing the number of players, permitting an extra number of strikes or modifying the rules. Those children who are not able to play, even under these circumstances, may act as umpires or referees, or scorekeepers.

Even with such modifications, it is usually desirable to build up the readiness of disabled children through low-organized games in which they learn the fundamentals of throwing or catching, kicking, running or dodging—before attempting to play more complex sports. All sports activities should be designed to emphasize the *abilities* rather than the *disabilities* of those taking part. They should stress maximum physical development, consonant with medical safeguards, and should emphasize the cooperative aspects of play. When competition is carried on, the pressure to win should be very low-keyed, and care should be taken to equalize teams according to ability.

For youth and adults with paraplegic conditions or amputations, but otherwise physically capable, one of the best organized sports programs is the wheelchair sports movement. A number of games and sports have been carried on by players in wheelchairs since World War II. In 1957, Benjamin H. Lipton, director of the Joseph Bulova School of Watchmaking, launched the first National Wheelchair Games in the United States A year later, the National Wheelchair Athletic Association was organized "for the prime function of establishing rules and regulations governing all wheelchair sports in the United States, except basketball, which had its own national association."[14]

Today, over 10,000 athletes engage in organized wheelchair sports competition throughout the United States. In addition, 56 other nations sponsor similar programs. There is a "Paralympics" which takes place around the time of the regular Olympics, at which teams and disabled individuals from various nations compete in wheelchair sports. Some of the specific events include archery, bowling, track and field (including javelin, shotput and racing, swimming, weight-lifting and basketball. Participants are placed in one of five classes according to their degree of disability, and competition in each of the sports is classed according to different levels of ability. In each event, modifications or devices may be used to adapt the rules to the needs of wheelchair competitors. Thus, in throwing events such as the shotput, an official shotput circle is used, but a stop-board or attendant may be used to hold back the contestant's chair from going outside the circle.

Wheelchair basketball is extremely popular; in some cases, teams of physically

---

[13] Janet Pomeroy: *Recreation for the Physically Handicapped.* New York, The Macmillan Co., 1964, pp. 306–307.

[14] Benjamin H. Lipton: "Wheelchair Sports: Its Role in the Rehabilitation of the Physically Disabled." *Therapeutic Recreation Journal,* 4th Quarter, 1970, p. 9.

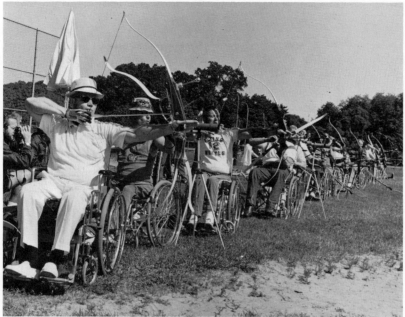

Being in a wheelchair need not be a handicap! Participants release their arrows at an archery contest organized by the National Wheelchair Athletic Association . . .

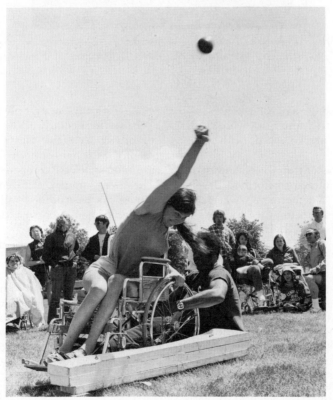

. . . while another young lady competes in the shot-put, with a special guard to control the movement of her chair.

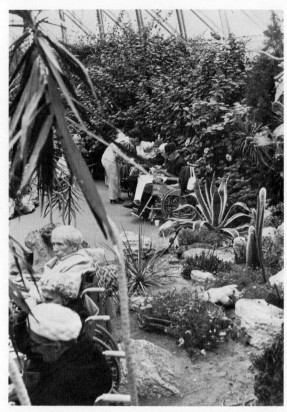

In Vancouver, British Columbia, Canada, aged patients from a nursing home are treated to an outing in a lovely conservatory operated by the city's Department of Parks and Public Recreation.

disabled compete against nondisabled players who are also in wheelchairs. N.C.A.A. rules are followed, with minor exceptions.

An obvious benefit of wheelchair sports is that participants are helped to develop self-confidence. Furthermore, wheelchair sports events tend to improve society's attitude toward the physically disabled. Stein writes:

> Their accomplishments and feats through sports and athletics can do much to inform the public, to educate it, and to attack those rigid attitudinal barriers which promote the continuation of hardened categories. The ideology of sports rests in what one does, and upon ability, not disability.[15]

[15] Julian W. Stein: "Why Sports?" *Performance*, Washington, D.C., President's Committee on Employment of the Handicapped, October-November, 1971, p. 5.

Realistically, many physically disabled persons, particularly those with such conditions as cerebral palsy, muscular dystrophy or severe orthopedic impairments, are *not* able to compete on this level. However, many different sports and games can be modified still further to permit enjoyment for even the most limited players.

For example, *archery* may be carried on with lighter bows and at shorter distances. When shooting, a person on crutches should lean forward on one crutch, while a person in a wheelchair should turn his wheelchair sideways and shoot from that angle. Even a person with only one hand or arm may take part in archery by having the bow fixed to a post anchored in the ground.

Bowling. Bowling is enjoyed by many disabled persons. Again, lighter balls and pins may be used, and shortened alleys.

Individuals in wheelchairs may be permitted to swing the ball back and forth more than once, to give it extra momentum, or they may use a specially constructed metal rack to release the ball. Players on crutches may stand at the foul line. Bowling is also carried on with blind players, who use a guide rail in approaching the foul line. A sighted person assists by telling the blind player what pins he must shoot for, and by keeping score. A Blind Bowlers' Association was formed in 1951. It assists in the formation of leagues, and conducts tournaments through the mail.

Dual Games. These games, which are usually carried on between two players, such as badminton, billiards, table tennis, tennis or shuffleboard, may all be carried on successfully with the disabled. In tennis, for example, the court may be smaller and several players may be put on the court at a time, to make up for their limited mobility. When advisable, players may use shortened rackets or hold the racket further up the handle; players with one arm begin the serve with the ball on the racket. In this or other racket games, like badminton, even double arm amputees may take part by having the racket strapped to their arm stump.

Table tennis has been adapted in several ways for the physically disabled. Special paddles have been made which permit poorly coordinated players, such as those with cerebral palsy, to play the game. Patients with scoliosis and in a body cast, or children with Legg-Perthes disease, or with dislocated hips, can all take part in table tennis using high stretchers that support them. Those in wheelchairs can play, provided that there is enough room around the table for them to maneuver. Similar adaptations are made for other dual games.

Golf. This sport has also been used successfully with physically disabled players. A small and less demanding course can be developed, with players using an electric golf cart to get around. In some cases, miniature or "putt-putt" courses are used for the disabled. Depending on the disability, players may use lighter or shorter clubs, and may vary the

stance or grip in order to be able to stroke successfully.

In addition to such sports, many other forms of physical activity are useful with the disabled, including dancing, rollerskating, fishing, quiet games and camping and nature activities.

Dancing. Dance is a major form of activity which is used in many hospitals for the mentally ill, but which may also be adapted to the needs of the physically disabled. Essentially, three forms may be presented: (a) *creative dance* in any of its forms, such as modern dance, ballet or children's rhythmics; (b) *social dancing,* also known as ballroom dancing; and (c) *folk* or *square dancing,* which is usually conducted as a group activity. It is an extremely useful form of activity because it combines physical exercise with an emotionally or artistically expressive quality.

Creative dance may readily be adapted for the physically disabled, depending on the nature of the impairment. Deaf men and women students at Gallaudet College in Washington, D.C., have formed an outstanding modern dance club which gives many performances throughout the year; despite their not being able to hear music, deaf people are able to "feel" the rhythm through floor vibrations, and to use visual cues to coordinate their movement. Dance is uniquely important for the deaf because, as Peter Wisher, professor of physical education at Gallaudet College, points out:

> Because of the reduced influence of sound in the lives of the deaf, perception of visual images increases in importance in all phases of education and daily living. This dependence on the visual serves to emphasize the importance of movement, which is an important aspect of communication. . . . Consequently, the area of the dance may have relatively more importance in the lives of the deaf than of the hearing.[16]

Children with varied disabilities also enjoy creative dance, particularly when

[16] Peter R. Wisher: "Dance and the Deaf." *Journal of Health, Physical Education and Recreation,* March, 1969, p. 81.

it is presented in an unstructured way, with free and spontaneous movement of the body to music or other rhythmic accompaniment. Blind children, in particular, profit from this form of activity, since it encourages them to learn space relationships and to move about freely and expressively—as opposed to their usual cautious and restrained movement.

Simple folk and square dances, in lines, circles or squares, can also be mastered by the physically disabled. Obviously, dances at a high tempo or with complicated foot movements should be avoided. However, the blind, the deaf and other disabled individuals can do a wide range of such traditional dances and find pleasure in their lively rhythm and social involvement. When a group with mixed disabilities is taking part in folk and square dancing, it is helpful to pair them off so their abilities complement each other. In other words, if a deaf teen-ager is partnered with a blind teen-ager, as a *couple* they have both *vision* and *hearing,* and can help each other master the dance.

Wheelchair square dancing has become a popular activity for many orthopedically disabled persons. They are able to do many of the same dances that are done by the nondisabled, but certain modifications need to be made. Since a wheelchair is considerably wider than a person and cannot revolve or turn in as narrow a course, it is necessary to enlarge the dance area and to slow down, or allow longer musical sections, in order to perform each part of the dance. Since wheelchairs cannot move sideways, forward-and-back movements should be substituted where appropriate. Other actions, such as the swing, do-si-do or promenade, can all be done in modified form by wheelchair square dancers.

Fishing. Fishing is an extremely popular recreational activity for all age levels in the general population and may be used successfully with disabled groups. It depends on the availability of fishing waters, although it is always possible to provide transportation to nearby lakes or fishing piers at the seashore. The activity may be more or less vigorous, depending on the capability of the participants, rang-ing from sitting by a stream or pier holding a handline, to actual bait-casting, surf-casting or more difficult forms of fishing.

QUIET GAMES. Quiet games and hobby activities are extremely useful with the physically disabled, partly because they may be carried on with extremely limited skills, and partly because they lend themselves either to individual or small group participation.

Table games, including cards, chess and checkers, dominoes, Parcheesi or equipment games like Nok Hockey or Skittles, are extremely useful. Special equipment may be designed for those with manual limitations, particularly with cerebral palsy and similar conditions. This may include holding racks for cards, electric shufflers or devices with which to move chessmen or checkers; as crude an instrument as a stick held in the mouth may be used to move pieces. Braille playing cards have been designed for the blind, and board games with raised squares that can be felt are also helpful. Other quiet games include social games and mixers, usually played while sitting in a circle.

Hobby activities may be carried out in a variety of settings, such as social clubs, hospital wards in rehabilitation centers, or even as individual activities for those confined to their homes. These usually involve special interests like collecting (stamps, coins, records, dolls, postcards, etc.), or the development of a particular skill or craft. Hobbies may be pursued as group projects, and often lend themselves to hobby shows or demonstrations, at which the disabled can show what they have accomplished.

ARTS AND CRAFTS. Probably more than any other major category of recreation, arts and crafts lend themselves to adaptation for individuals at all levels of ability. Like hobbies, they may be carried on individually or in group settings, and may range from the most simple projects to extremely advanced activities. They offer an excellent outlet for creative expression and the constructive use of energy. In addition, since the work produced may be used to decorate a home or hospital ward, as gifts to friends or family or may be exhibited in shows, they help to bring about a strong sense of personal accomplishment.

One major area of activity is the graphic arts: sketching, water-color and oil painting or print-making. For those with adequate vision and manipulative skills, these may be approached just as with nondisabled persons. For those with more limited dexterity, it may be necessary to devise special holders for crayons, charcoal or brushes.

Clay modeling, soap carving and papier-maché work are also useful for the physically disabled. These may be approached on an extremely rudimentary level or may involve advanced projects. They may include carving or modeling animals, dolls, puppets and similar projects. Ceramics represents a more advanced medium, which may be carried on using the mold process or, with those capable of using hands effectively, with the potter's wheel or by building slabs or pinch-pots. There are many other craft activities that can be suited to the physically disabled, many of which improve manual dexterity and coordination.

The emphasis in using arts and crafts should be on creative expression rather than on developing useful or impressive products. Participants should be allowed considerable choice in selecting their products, and should be able to move at their own rate. Although it may be convenient for the leader to use prestructured craft materials, such as "paint-by-the-numbers" kits, these reduce the value of the activity for participants. As much as possible, they should be creating their *own* works.

Musical Activities

Music is one of the most varied and useful activities in meeting the needs of every type of disability. It can be conducted on every level from the simplest to the most complex, and has value both as a "listening" and as a "doing" activity. It may involve single individuals or large groups in choral or instrumental programs. It engenders a feeling of compan-

ionship and group solidarity, and at the same time is an expressive art that brings emotional pleasure and release. In one state hospital manual, the following description of the values of music is provided:

In general, music can elevate the depressed patient, calm the hyperactive one, create a desired mood, dispel unpleasant sensations, unite a disparate body of people. By appealing to the senses, the mind is released from inhibitions and out of the environment both physical and mental, into a more appealing world. . . . The interrelationship of the members of the group to each other and to the therapist develops a special aura of its own quite different from other more structured therapies in atmosphere and affect.[17]

Essentially, there are three phases to the program of music as it may be provided for the physically disabled: (a) listening; (b) singing; and (c) instrumental music.

1. *Music listening.* This can range from listening to recorded or taped popular or classical music, to having visiting performers entertain in large hospital situations. Sometimes listening may involve music appreciation sessions, with discussion of the background of the music—whether it be classical, jazz or folk.
2. *Singing.* This may involve informal folk singing, or community songfests, as well as choruses, madrigal groups or other forms of performing units. Young children are likely to enjoy action songs, while older persons will prefer songs that were popular years ago. Singing for disabled persons may simply be a casual recreational activity—preferably with an accompanist at a piano or accordion—or it may become an important area of personal growth and emotional release. In general, all those with physical disability, except the deaf,

[17] *Program Media.* Manual of Rehabilitation Therapies Department, Spring Grove State Hospital, Catonsville, Maryland, September, 1970, p. 6.

may take part, although some individuals with major speech defects (such as the severely cerebral palsied) may have some difficulty in singing. It may actually be used to *improve* voice production.

3. *Instrumental music.* Obviously, this requires skilled leadership. Often, if the recreation leader is not able to direct instrumental music programs, and there is no skilled music therapist available, it is possible to get volunteers from the community who have a high degree of skill in instrumental music. This may range from rhythmic sessions with children or beginners, using simple percussion or other rhythm instruments, to instruction on beginning, intermediate or advanced levels for players of all ages. Since the key factor in playing music is the use of hands and arms, and particularly finger dexterity, individuals with other types of disability are usually able to play wind, string or percussion instruments.

Dramatics

This represents another extremely useful and enjoyable kind of recreational experience in which the physically disabled may take part. It is easily adapted so that people with different levels of ability and almost every type of impairment may take part, with great satisfaction. In part, this is because it can take so many different forms, and be approached on so many different levels. It provides, more than any other medium, the opportunity to play roles, express emotions, ventilate fears and hostilities and find release from tensions. Individuals who normally stammer severely are often able to speak with fluency and ease when playing a dramatic role.

The rehabilitation therapies manual of a large state mental hospital comments on the role of drama in working with psychiatric patients:

It is a method of diagnosis as well as a method of treatment. One of its character-

istic features is that role-acting is organically included in the treatment process. It can be adapted to every type of problem, personal or group, of children or adults. . . . The psychodrama is human society in miniature, the simplest possible set-up for a methodical study of its psychological structure. Through techniques such as the auxiliary ego, spontaneous improvisation, self-presentation, soliloquy, the interpolation of resistance, new dimensions of the mind are opened up, and what is most important, they can be explored under experimental conditions.[18]

While emotional catharsis is not as significant a part of the need of physically disabled persons, it is obvious that many of them have psychological problems stemming from their disability. The blind, deaf, paraplegic or otherwise severely impaired person frequently is withdrawn, isolated, unsure of his own role in society, lacking in confidence and unable to relate easily to others. Dramatics—because it is *make-believe*—provides a vehicle through which he can *safely* express himself, making his feelings and needs known to others, and through which he can temporarily leave his *own* identity to play other roles.

Special Events

These represent an important aspect of recreation programs for the physically disabled in all kinds of settings. They provide an opportunity for working together with others to plan events, or simply to enjoy the entertainment offered. Special events may be informal last-minute activities, or elaborately planned parties, carnivals, concerts, shows, dances, sports programs, celebrations or trips.

In addition to providing recreation for physically disabled persons in a rehabilitation center or community-sponsored program, special events may be used to educate the public about programs serving disabled people. By holding an open house, or inviting outsiders to come to a party, carnival or other event, it is possi-

---

[18] *Ibid.*

ble to show them what disabled persons are like and dispel their misconceptions, and to build more positive links with community groups.

Hooper, Mullen and Kennedy suggest varied special events which may be offered in nursing homes:

> A monthly birthday party, celebrating for each birthday in that month; holiday parties such as Hallowe'en or St. Valentine's Day. . . . Talent and fashion shows, teas, bazaars, open houses, hobby shows and entertainment programs can be scheduled throughout the year. Trips and outings can be arranged in many instances, in small groups by car or by bus when proper permission is granted.[19]

While these suggestions apply specially to the elderly, they also are useful for other types of residential situations.

In Veterans Administration hospitals, special programs frequently include visits by performing groups from the community, who will put on musical, dramatic or dance programs or provide other special entertainment for large numbers of patients. In hospitals in large cities, professional performing companies will often appear on their nights off, and professional athletes may also give talks, demonstrations or clinics. When physically disabled persons plan their own programs, such as carnivals, festivals, large-scale picnics or barbecues or talent shows, these events should be carefully organized. As much as possible, the disabled persons themselves should form committees (such as program, publicity, finance, clean-up or special arrangements committees) and do the actual work of running the event.

When trips and special outings are planned for the disabled, careful arrangements need to be made with respect to: (a) arranging transportation; (b) getting permission for those who will be traveling (either from parents, or, when necessary, medical approval) ; (c) screening all par-

ticipants to determine whether the trip will be appropriate for them; and (d) making arrangements at the place that will be visited, to ensure that they are prepared to accept and have suitable accommodations for a group of physically disabled persons.

The value of such programs is that they provide novelty and special interest to the lives of the physical disabled, and help to keep their morale high. They tend to maintain constructive ties with the community, and promote socialization and group involvement. For patients in a rehabilitation center, trips and outings have the very special value of helping them learn to get around in the outside world and to develop the kinds of practical skills they will need when they are discharged.

Camping and Nature Activities

Day camping, resident camping and nature activities in general are among the most successful and valuable programs provided for the disabled.

Usually, such activities provide an opportunity to live, play and work with others in an environment that promotes good fellowship and understanding of the outdoors. Group interaction is a strong benefit of camping programs, and participants are enabled to learn new skills and recreational interests which may serve them in good stead.

There are special camps in the United States today which serve epileptics, diabetics, cardiac patients, the blind, deaf, mentally retarded, convalescent patients and other categories of physical disability. Such programs usually require a high staff-to-patient ratio, and often make considerable use of volunteers. Day camping programs are usually easier to operate, because of the extensive care that many disabled persons require, which makes overnight or residential camping much more demanding. Frequently in such settings, campers who are given responsibilities for self-care or for helping to do chores for their bunks or in the dining

---

[19] Langdon Hooper, Dorothy Mullen, and Irene J. Kennedy: *Recreation Service in Connecticut Nursing Homes for the Aged.* Hartford, Connecticut, Connecticut State Department of Health, 1968, p. 17.

area, gain a new degree of independence and social functioning, and make dramatic gains in personal adjustment.

Camping programs may be scheduled in a variety of ways:

1. Day camping, in which a group of physically disabled children or youth attend a program near their home regularly. To be considered a "day camp" program, as opposed to an ordinary vacation playground program, it should be a full-day activity, including lunch, should have some involvement with nature and the outdoors, and should be organized in groups. As opposed to an ordinary summer playground program, day camping involves formal registration and regular attendance, and usually has a carefully organized program with trips and outings to places of special interest.

2. Resident camping for the physically disabled is usually sponsored by organizations concerned with a specific disability, such as cerebral palsy, blindness or orthopedic impairment. Frequently such camps have one- or two-week sessions; in some instances they are sponsored by public recreation departments, in which case they usually serve children or youth with different types of disabilities.

3. Nature activities, either in a camping program or as part of any recreation program, might include any of the following: hiking and exploring natural settings; camping and campcraft, such as putting up tents, sleeping in the outdoors, knot-tying or camp cookery; campfires and related activities; nature-related crafts, such as shell and rock painting, building bird feeders or flower and leaf pressing; or the study of nature: vegetation and wildlife, effects of erosion, conservation projects and gardening activities.

In addition, water activities, such as boating, fishing, swimming or water games, are usually extremely popular. If a lake or beach area is being used, extreme caution must be taken with the physically disabled, since such areas are not as easily supervised as a swimming pool (because of the rapidly changing depth of the water or surf, or the difficulty in seeing beneath the surface). Safe swimming areas should be clearly marked off with ropes and closely watched, with a high ratio of staff to participants.

The ideal camp situation is one in which the physically disabled are integrated with the nondisabled. However, for many, their limitations are such that they cannot keep up with the full range of activities enjoyed by the nondisabled, and are not yet ready for the degree of independent self-care required in such a setting. For them, a segregated camp setting is preferable, in order to build the necessary skills and help them gain confidence. For some physically disabled children, there may be a progression through the following stages: (a) day camp, in which they begin to gain skills and confidence; (b) resident or overnight camp, for the disabled alone; and (c) resident or overnight camp, for both disabled and nondisabled children.

A number of examples of special camps for disabled children and youth are described elsewhere.[20] Usually, information about them can be gained from major organizations serving the disabled, which have chapters in metropolitan areas.

Modification of Facilities for the Physically Disabled

A final important area of concern in providing recreational opportunities for the physically disabled is the elimination of architectural barriers that prevent those with impairment from using parks, playgrounds, community centers or a variety of other special recreation facilities. This problem, which does not affect the mentally ill or retarded, *does* affect hundreds of thousands of individuals, young and

---

[20] See pp. 104, 111, etc.

old, who are in wheelchairs or on crutches, or who have limited powers of locomotion. A 1967 report by the Bureau of Outdoor Recreation made this need clear:

> It is clearly evident . . . that great numbers of disabled persons are not receiving the benefits of our nation's recreation resources. The severity of their disabilities, architectural barriers, non-acceptance by society, and slowness of the recreation profession to adjust its programs and facilities to their needs all have contributed to a serious lack of opportunity.[21]

A number of national and statewide organizations concerned both with architectural design and engineering requirements, and with recreation and parks, has taken strong action in this field. Today, the Bureau of Outdoor Recreation requires that all comprehensive state outdoor recreation plans, prepared as a prerequisite to participating in the Land and Water Conservation Fund program (federal subsidy for open space and recreation facility development), consider the needs of the disabled. In recent years, increasing numbers of federal or state agencies have developed guidelines, or laws have been passed, to ensure that public facilities be designed and built along lines that will permit access and use by the disabled. The United States of America Standards Institute has published a pamphlet suggesting ways to adapt facilities so that they can readily be used by the physically disabled. This includes such passages as:

> Steps are augmented by paths and ramps for wheelchairs; doorways are made wider and easier to open; grab-bars are placed in restrooms, drinking fountains are lowered; stepdown curbs are modified; and so forth.[22]

---

[21] *Outdoor Recreation Planning for the Handicapped. op. cit.,* p. 1.

[22] "U.S.A. Standard Specifications for Making Buildings and Facilities Accessible to and Usable by, the Physically Handicapped." In *Outdoor Recreation Planning for the Handicapped, op. cit.,* p. 6.

Specific design details are now established in a number of states for park and recreation facilities. For example, the New York State Council of Parks and Outdoor Recreation published a handbook of design standards for various types of facilities, in order to make them accessible to the physically disabled. These standards must be followed by all municipalities that wish to qualify for state or federal assistance. Examples of such standards follow:

1. Parking facilities should have special parking stalls designed for wheelchair users. The parking area should be close to the recreation site and paved with a nonslip surface. An opening of 30 inches should be maintained between guardrails to permit a wheelchair to pass.
2. Walking trails should have a minimum width of 48 inches, in order to be accessible to disabled persons. They should be smoothly graded without steep inclines, and with sufficient area to turn around at various places on the way. Ramps should be used where necessary. Doors of buildings should have a minimum clear opening of 32 inches, with the threshold close to the floor.
3. Food service areas should have special service areas in at least one concession where wheelchair users may be served and seated. Public telephones mounted on poles at appropriate heights make it possible for wheelchair users to make calls unaided.
4. For toilets to be made accessible, ramps with sufficient width should be installed to reach stations that are above-grade. Urinals should be floor-mounted, no higher than 19 inches above the floor, and equipped with horizontal handrails. Handdriers, soap dispensers and mirrors should be at levels accessible to wheelchair users.

Many other detailed guidelines indicate the ways in which recreation and park agencies should plan specifically to provide access for the disabled. Swimming facilities can be made more useful by providing a paved walk leading to the swimming area. Sloping handrails or ropes mounted on posts make it easier to get into the swimming facility. Bathhouses should have enlarged dressing room facilities with a bench, guardrails and outward swinging doors for wheelchair users.

Spectator areas, picnicking and camping sites and boating sites should have similar modifications or design features. Fishing areas should have a paved surface at the water's edge, with a protective handrail to make the sport safe for the physically disabled. Auditoriums should have seats missing in some rows, with a level surface, so wheelchair users may sit there rather than in crowded aisles or at the back of the hall.[23]

A number of playgrounds, parks and other facilities have been designed for special use by the physically disabled. For example, a unique playground was developed for disabled preschool children at the New York University Medical Center's Institute of Rehabilitation Medicine. Planned by the well-known architect, Richard Dattner, it includes a ladder leading to a tree house (which may also be reached by ramps), a waterfall, table-top sandboxes and similar features which contribute to children's varied play opportunities and overall development. A special playground with large animal forms and modified equipment has been developed by the Child Study Center in Fort Worth, Texas.

A number of states have experimented in this field. Georgia, for example, has created a state park designed specifically for use by the disabled and their families. Located within the larger Fort Yargo State Park, this facility includes the following features:

> . . . the park adjoins a lake whose sloping beach makes possible the construction of walks and ramps of moderate incline. Boat

docks . . . serve small, flat-bottomed fishing boats that can be boarded safely, and pontoon boats . . . available for persons in wheelchairs. Planned recreation activities include organized resident camping, nature walks, swimming, picnicking, fishing and bicycling.[24]

Travel has always imposed special problems for the physically disabled. Such states as Oregon, New Jersey and Michigan have constructed new rest areas along the highways with special aids for disabled persons, or have stipulated that restaurant chains or lodging chains with concessions along major thruways must provide facilities to meet the needs of disabled persons. The construction of all major state buildings—including university dormitory, classroom and student service units—is increasingly being geared to serve disabled persons, a need that was almost completely ignored in the past.

Finally, other facilities or types of equipment are being used to ensure that the physically disabled are more fully involved in recreation programs of all sorts. More and more agencies are using special buses, equipped with hydraulic lifts, to transport children and adults in wheelchairs. Elevators are being designed with slow closing speeds, and with controls and alarm boxes set at appropriate heights on their walls. Nature trails are being developed in a number of national parks to serve the blind, with special guide ropes and Braille signs pointing out natural features. Audible balls with clicking devices inside them have been developed to permit the blind to play popular ball games.

In many other ways, attention is being given to meet the needs of the physically handicapped for varied recreational opportunities. However, much progress needs to be made, particularly in terms of improving public attitudes toward accepting the physically disabled in recreation and park settings, and having a larger number of recreation and park administrators accept this as a high-priority program concern.

[23] *Outdoor Recreation for the Physically Handicapped.* Vollmer-Ostrower Associates and New York State Council of Parks and Recreation, August, 1967.

[24] Kent Ruth: "Pleasure Travel is Becoming Easier for the Handicapped." *New York Times,* May 26, 1968, p. 3.

Suggested Topics for Class Discussion, Examinations or Student Papers

1. How does the problem of providing recreation for the physically disabled child or adult differ sharply from that of planning for the mentally ill or retarded individual?
2. Select a specific area of physical disability, such as the blind or orthopedically impaired. Based on the special needs of this population, outline a set of goals and then a model program of recreational activities, including administrative guidelines for service.
3. Discuss the need of specially designed or modified facilities to serve the disabled, and give examples of how present facilities frequently limit their participation.

Chapter 7

Recreation and the Aging

This chapter deals with the aging population in American society today. It discusses statistics of aging and retirement, the nature of the aging process and the special problems that face older persons in modern culture. It examines the role of government on various levels, and analyzes various types of settings where recreation and related social services are provided for older persons.

The Aging in American Society

Who are the aging in our society? There are approximately 20 million Americans today who are 65 or older. This number is nearly twice that of 20 years ago, and constitutes about ten per cent of the entire population. It has been estimated that the number of Americans over 65 will be 32 million by the year 2000. *Time Magazine* states:

> Even today the population over 75 in the United States is increasing at two and a half times the rate of the general population. If the average life-span is significantly further increased, the population would indeed become aged, a trend which should be accelerated by a drop in the birth rate.[1]

Within the population over 65, the ratio of women to men is about four to three. This disparity increases with age.

About 70 per cent of older Americans live in their homes or with relatives, while about 25 per cent live alone or with a nonrelative, and about five per cent live in institutions.[2]

Why is the aging population a matter of special concern for those involved with health and welfare services in the United States and Canada? This population's role in society has been rapidly shifting as a result of increased life span, changes in the nature of family structure and social attitudes, population shifts in our cities and other economic and psychological factors. Great numbers of older people today lead isolated, unhappy lives. They are often relegated to a position of inferiority within a youth-oriented culture. They are stereotyped and misunderstood, and often shunted aside following retirement from business or family responsibility; they reach the point where their lives become empty and meaningless and they deteriorate both physically and psychologically.

This is not an inevitable part of aging. It happens only because society permits it to happen. In order to understand it, it is necessary to examine the following: (a) the process of human aging; (b) the social and psychological implications of aging; (c) the economics of retirement and aging; (d) needs and problems of

---

[1] "The Prospects for Living Even Longer." *Time,* August 3, 1970, p. 52.

[2] "European Countries Meeting Problems of the Elderly with Burgeoning Programs." *New York Times,* January 27, 1971, p. 43.

older persons; and (e) the role of recreation and related services in programs for the aging.

The Process of Human Aging

First, it must be understood that aging is a universal process, although it varies greatly from person to person. It is generally regarded primarily as a physiological development, although it obviously has social and psychological components as well. *Gerontology* (study of the aging process and of aged persons in society) and *geriatrics* (the branch of medicine dealing with medical problems of the aged) have both contributed greatly to our understanding of this developmental stage of life.

Although the age 65 is considered to be the beginning of old age, the process is not strictly age-correlated and can vary tremendously among individuals, with some persons beginning to show signs of aging in the 40s or 50s, and others remaining extremely vital and alert well into the 80s. In general, the process of aging includes the following physiological changes:

1. Slowing of biological functions.
2. Breakdown in functioning of body systems.
3. Reduction in physiological reserve.
4. Altered structure of cells, tissues and organs.

These changes produce decreased efficiency in the functioning of the body systems and begin to bring about progressive disabilities related to the heart and nervous system, the five senses (especially vision and hearing) and the motor abilities of older persons. Aging persons increasingly have health problems; it has been estimated that, of the approximately 19 million older persons who live in community settings, only 20 per cent are free from illness.

The exact nature of the aging process is still not fully understood; one medical researcher writes:

The biology of aging is no better understood today than was the circulation of the blood before William Harvey.[3]

However, within this limited understanding, geriatrists have concluded that physiological changes occur because of both internal and environmental causes. One of the obvious factors that are important in influencing the process of aging is the availability of competent medical care. Yet, a recent National Health Survey found that one in four persons aged 65 and over had not been to see a physician for two years or more—a reflection of the inadequacy of our social concern and practical provision of services for the aging in society.

It is necessary to recognize that many persons have false stereotypes about the older people in American society which are usually detrimental to this segment of our population. In an effort to correct these stereotypes, the National Council on Aging has formulated ten basic concepts of aging. These are:

1. Aging is universal.
2. Aging is normal.
3. Aging is variable. The way in which each person ages is unique. The process is influenced by the individual's life pattern of work or activity, rest, human associations, diet, exercise and mental attitude.
4. Dying is inevitable, something which is hard to accept for most people.
5. Aging and illness are not necessarily coincidental. It is possible to enhance one's chances for a healthy old age through improved living habits.
6. Older people represent three generations; it is necessary to identify the variable characteristics among these generations.
7. Older people can and do learn. Learning patterns may change, the speed of learning may diminish, but the basic capacity still exists.
8. Older people can and do change. The radical changes in their pattern of life make readjustment essential. The com-

---

[3] Alexander Comfort: *In* "The Old in the Country of the Young." *Time,* August 3, 1970, p. 52.

mon idea of inflexible old age is in most cases inaccurate.

9. Older people want to remain self-directing. The idea that they need to be told what to do is highly inaccurate.
10. Old people are vital human beings. They have certain incapacities, but they can develop existing capacities to lead a productive, rewarding life.[4]

Problems Facing Older Persons

The aging process has been seriously affected by recent social changes in the lives of older persons. These relate chiefly to the problem of enforced retirement and exclusion from meaningful roles in community life, and shifting patterns of family structure.

COMPULSORY RETIREMENT. Early retirement, which has become widespread in American life as a result of pension and Social Security plans, and Civil Service or personnel regulations in most businesses, has enormous implications for older persons. For many, retirement from work brings a loss of prestige and status. In a society which places great emphasis on work and productivity, being cut off from a job commitment means a drastic change in life style. Coupled with the general tendency in our society to value youth and denigrate age, it means that older persons who no longer play a meaningful role in society tend to have a feeling of uselessness and to lack a sense of self-worth and dignity.

Linked with this is the problem of economic insecurity. The major sources of income for the elderly retired person are Social Security, employment pensions, welfare programs, savings and assistance by members of their family. However, retirement almost always decreases income, and Social Security or pension benefits have no cost-of-living clauses to compensate for the inflationary trend in the economy.

Certain expenses, such as medical costs, tend to increase sharply for older persons and, as a consequence, many older persons face an economic nightmare today, with their meagre incomes barely stretching to meet basic needs of existence. It has been estimated that one out of four older persons in the United States is living at a poverty level.[5] A United States Senate Panel on Aging concluded in the late 1960s that the retirement income problem had reached a crisis stage, with 200,000 Americans over 65 entering the poverty class, while all others in the population were improving in economic status.[6]

SHIFTING FAMILY ROLES. Traditionally in American society, several generations lived together, and older persons continued not only to receive the affection and support of their children or grandchildren, but also to play meaningful roles in family life. However, with the shift toward urban and suburban living in apartments or one-family development houses, increasing numbers of older persons are living alone in small apartments or single-room units. This is particularly crucial for women who have lost their husbands; the life expectancy of women at birth is 74, thirteen years greater than that of men.

Thus, many aging persons are faced with the problem of living alone, without family and with few friends, and are often unable to take care of themselves properly. Particularly in run-down areas of larger cities, where they are often victims of thieves or muggers, old people tend to be afraid to leave their homes, and thus they are deprived of the opportunity for social involvement. The need for companionship does not diminish for older persons, and with the breaking of other ties and the increased amount of leisure time at their disposal, their loneliness becomes all the more difficult to bear.

STEREOTYPES OF AGING. Frequently, older people behave in ways which younger people find childish, or senile.

For example, many older people seem to live in the past and refuse to change, or even to be concerned with what is happening in the present. While this is some-

[4] Report of National Council on Aging. Reprinted in *Recreation,* February, 1963, p. 67.

[5] "The Old in the Country of the Young." *op. cit.,* p. 49.
[6] Robert Lindsey: "Many Aging Face an Economic Nightmare." *New York Times,* January 30, 1971, p. 28.

times considered an evidence of senility, it is quite understandable. For many aging persons, the present is bleak and unpleasant, and they would *rather* live in the past. Childish behavior is also frequently considered to be a symptom of aging. However, this may be regarded in many cases as the result of a self-fulfilling prophecy; when older people are expected to be childish, and when they are treated in this way, they naturally behave helplessly or petulantly.

Similarly, the tendency toward complaints about being ill, that often verge toward hypochondria, may readily be understood. Dr. Ewald Busse, director of the Duke Study Center, comments that, when someone keeps criticizing the older person unjustly, and:

> . . . makes him feel unwanted, uncomfortable, he may retreat into an imaginary illness as a way of saying, "Don't make things harder for me. I'm sick and you should respect and take care of me." It is clear from our studies that if the older hypochrondriac's environment changes for the better, he will too. He will again become a reasonable, normal person.[7]

Increasing numbers of older persons *are* finding difficulty in adjusting to their status in life. In response to psychological, economic and social stress, many problems crop up. One of these is alcoholism. Although this is not commonly thought of as an older person's disease, the fact is that since 1958, the death rate due to alcoholic disorders has risen over 52 per cent for white males between the ages of 60 and 69, and 114 per cent for white females in the same age bracket.[8]

Similarly, suicide appears to be a special problem of aging persons. Statistics indicate that the suicide rate in most countries increases with age. The rate of self-inflicted death among white American males over 65 is three times that at the ages of 20 to 24; among white females, the ratio is two to one. In addition, research suggests that many deaths among aging persons are incorrectly attributed to accidental causes because the nature of suicide among them is not clearly understood.

Researchers have concluded that many older persons, rather than directly injuring themselves, place themselves in vulnerable or life-threatening situations, which tend to increase the possibility of their demise. It suggests that a significant segment of the older population no longer *wishes* to live, and in effect, withdraws from previous active roles played in life.

This point of view has been expressed in a theory of adjustment in aging that was formulated in the early 1960s, known as "disengagement" theory.

Disengagement Theory

Cumming and Henry, who developed this theory, perceived aging as an inevitable mutual withdrawal or disengagement by older persons from others in the society. Withdrawal may be initiated on either side, and the aging person may withdraw dramatically from some groups of people, while remaining relatively close to others. It:

> . . . may be accompanied from the outset by an increased preoccupation with himself; certain institutions in society may make this withdrawal easy for him. When the aging process is complete, the equilibrium which existed in middle life between the individual and his society has given way to a new equilibrium characterized by a greater distance and an altered type of relationship.[9]

In essence, the theory suggests that society should accept the needs of older persons for a "dramatically reduced social life-space," and permit them, in effect, to disengage themselves from meaningful life relationships and move into roles of greater isolation. Disengagement theory

[7] Ewald Busse: *In* "The Old in the Country of the Young." *op. cit.,* p. 51.

[8] "Alcoholism Leading Cause for Jailing Older Persons." *Geriatric Focus,* Knoll Pharmaceutical Company, January, 1969, p. 1; and "Characteristics of Aged Alcoholics Studied." *Geriatric Focus,* April, 1968, pp. 1, 3.

[9] Elaine Cumming and William E. Henry: *Growing Old: The Process of Disengagement.* New York, Basic Books, 1961.

would not encourage attempting to keep older persons alert and active by providing them with programs of recreational, social and service activities. However, a number of leading sociologists and gerontologists have not been willing to accept this point of view. A Harvard sociologist, Chad Gordon, writes:

> Disengagement theory is a rationalization for the fact that old people haven't a damn thing to do, and nothing to do it with.[10]

The Activity Approach

In contrast, many authorities on aging favor an activity approach, which sees successful adjustment as dependent on the ability to find substitutes for the life activities carried on in previous years, or to maintain such activities for as long as possible.

Both the "disengagement" and the "activity" approaches to adjustment have been criticized because they fail to take into account the wide individual differences in mode of adjustment, and deal with only one aspect of this process. Reichard has carried out research on the aging process, in which she identified at least five different kinds of adjustment to aging.[11]

As one example of the falsity of certain stereotypes regarding the aging, one might point to the widely held belief that older persons normally no longer engage in sexual intercourse—and the dependent view that any older person who does is therefore "different." Recent research carried out at the Center for the Study of Aging and Human Development at Duke University indicated that between 40 and 60 per cent of different groups of subjects aged between 60 and 71 years reported that they still engaged in sexual intercourse with some frequency. Additional research has revealed that considerably older persons continue to have sexual rela-

tions successfully; such behavior seems to involve a continuation and modification of earlier life patterns.

The basic point is that life does not *stop* when one reaches 65 or 75 years of age. The same needs and interests tend to continue; many of the weaknesses or problems demonstrated by older persons stem from their difficulty in adjusting to social, psychological, economic or physiological change. In order to help the elderly to make such adjustments successfully, it is obviously necessary to develop programs and assistance within the following areas:

1. Provision of economic security, an element essential to all other aspects of aging.
2. Health assistance, including both community-based and hospital medical care—readily available and nondemeaning.
3. Practical assistance with housing and maintenance problems—living units for aging persons are today being included in larger, low- or middle-income housing projects, along with plans for assisting older persons who live by themselves in such developments.
4. A sense of importance and contribution to society, to supplant the loss of past work.
5. The opportunity for meaningful social relationships with others.
6. Interesting and challenging physical and mental activities, appropriate for their age level.
7. A position of respect and dignity in society.
8. Direct help to those who are able to maintain their living independence in the community, and carefully planned programs of maintenance and treatment for those who cannot.

Recreation's Role With Aging Persons

Within this total context, it is obviously important for older people to have a range of interesting and appropriate rec-

---

[10] Chad Gordon. *In* "The Old in the Country of the Young." *op. cit.,* p. 54.

[11] See *Retirement Roles and Activities.* Washington, D.C., Report of White House Conference on Aging, 1971, p. 20.

reational opportunities available to them, both to fill their long leisure hours and to meet, in a positive way, some of their important personal needs. What exactly are these needs, and what contribution does recreation make to them? They fall into the following six areas:

IMPROVES PHYSICAL HEALTH. A number of studies have established that recreation of a physical nature makes a significant contribution to the physical condition of the aging, particularly in terms of cardiac function.[12] Moderate and enjoyable exercise frequently means that individuals need not take certain drugs for release of tension, and it helps to prevent unnecessary deterioration of the body and progressive breakdown of the body systems. There is evidence that the satisfaction derived from accomplishment and continued physical activity is linked to human longevity.[13]

IMPROVES EMOTIONAL WELL-BEING. Meaningful involvement in social, physical and creative recreational activities tends to improve the state of mind of most aging participants. It takes their mind off the preoccupation with themselves, their illnesses and their problems, and provides a sense of accomplishment in performance. Generally, it contributes to a positive outlook toward life.

RE-AWAKENS CREATIVE IMPULSES. For many older persons, the recreation programs found in a home for the aging, or community-based senior center, offer opportunities in the arts, music, theatre or literature that awaken or revive creative impulses not felt for many years. Again, these stimulate intellectual functioning and emotional well-being and encourage a sense of vitality and energy.

ENCOURAGES SOCIAL INVOLVEMENT. Obviously, recreation can provide an atmosphere which is conducive to developing friendships and to overcoming

isolation and resulting loneliness. For many older persons who have been widowed or divorced, such programs may even result in friendships between the sexes which develop into marriage. There is a surprisingly large number of such marriages among elderly persons who meet in recreational settings, although match-making is not, of course, their primary purpose.

PROVIDES MEANINGFUL ROLES. As described earlier, an important need of many older persons is for significant roles in society, to supplant job or family responsibilities which have disappeared. For many aging persons, projects undertaken in recreation programs include giving assistance to the homebound or hospitalized, to children needing adult guidance, or similar ventures. Sometimes projects involve political campaigning, work in ecology or providing advice to minority group members who are beginning a business and need help from experienced, retired businessmen. The opportunity to contribute to society and to feel of real value to other human beings is of great importance to aging persons.

OFFERS THRESHOLD TO OTHER SERVICES. While recreation offers an important area of experience in itself for older persons, it is also valuable in that it often paves the way for their making use of other vital social services. Frequently, aging persons come initially to a center because of its recreational and social programs. As they become aware of other services, such as health care, legal aid, budget planning or other advisory assistance, they tend to make use of them.

Recognizing all these benefits, the purpose of this text is to focus most heavily on the values to be derived directly from participation in recreational activities, as a vital part of living for older persons. Their importance should not be underestimated, according to the United States Public Health Service:

. . . an activities program is the environment of challenge, of achievement, and hope. An activities program can help a person along on the road to recovery [the reference is to nursing homes]. It brings with

---

[12] See, for example, James S. Skinner: "Exercise, Aging, and Longevity." In *Proceedings of 8th Annual Meeting, International Congress of Gerontology,* 1969, p. 47.

[13] "Physical, Mental, Social Predictors of Longevity." Report to International Congress of Gerontology, cited in *Geriatric Focus,* October, 1969, p. 1.

it a dignity of life. It creates a purpose for living—to go on, to do more, to achieve more.[14]

Many studies and reports affirm the ultimate value of recreational participation for aging persons. Havighurst, a leading researcher in the field of social adjustment, has observed that "there is a high degree of relationship of leisure values with personal adjustment."[15] Ford concluded that: ". . . older people who are no longer working have high morale and personal satisfaction when they voluntarily participate in activities which afford them status, recognition, and achievement."[16]

A concrete evidence of the increasing importance that is being given to recreation for the elderly is found in a summation of the application of federal funds under the Administration on Aging grants program for states and municipalities. Out of millions of dollars spent in 1968, 34 per cent was used to support recreation and leisure time activities, including 250 senior center programs—a higher percentage than that granted to any other form of service for older people living in communities.

Programs Provided for Aging Persons

Recreation services are provided for aging persons in a variety of institutional or community settings, including the following:

1. Senior Citizen's clubs or centers.
2. Golden Age clubs.
3. Special residential centers, such as leisure villages or housing projects.

4. Hospitals or nursing homes.
5. Programs for the homebound.

The following section includes a description of programs offered in each of these types of settings. Since only five per cent of aging persons in the United States live in institutions or nursing homes, the greatest number of those who are to be served are in community settings. Typically, such persons must seek out Senior Citizen's clubs, Golden Age clubs or other community center programs designed for older persons.

Senior Centers

These are described by Anderson, who carried out the first nationwide study of such programs, as:

> . . . places where older persons come together for a variety of activities and programs, ranging from sitting and talking or playing cards to professionally directed hobby and group activities. Some centers also provide counseling services to help the individual make better use of personal and community resources; some assume responsibility for encouraging community agencies to provide more help to senior citizens.[17]

Senior centers are considered to be agencies which meet for substantial periods of time several days a week, and which have professional staff direction and offer more than one form of service. Usually, they operate in their own facilities and may be sponsored by a variety of types of agencies, such as municipal recreation and park departments, housing or welfare agencies or religious federations. In contrast, *Golden Age clubs* are usually thought of as social or recreational clubs for older persons, operating under volunteer or nonprofessional leadership, and meeting once or twice a week, or even less frequently.

[14] *Activity Supervisor's Guide, A Handbook for Activity Supervisors in Long Term Care Facilities.* Washington, D.C., U.S. Department of Health, Education and Welfare, Public Health Service, 1969, p. 5.
[15] Robert J. Havighurst: "The Leisure Activities of the Middle-Aged." *American Journal of Sociology,* LXIII, 1957, pp. 152–162.
[16] Caroline S. Ford: "Working with Older People: A Guide to Practice." St. Louis, Missouri Gerontological Society, Vol. IV, 1967, p. 323.

[17] Nancy N. Anderson: *Senior Centers: Information from a National Survey.* Minneapolis, Minnesota, Institute for Interdisciplinary Studies, American Rehabilitation Foundation, 1969, p. 1.

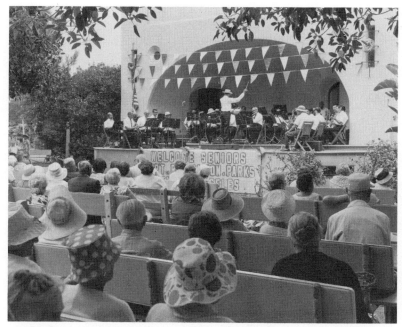

Many communities offer varied programs for senior citizens. Here, retired persons enjoy a band concert at a Senior Citizens' Outing sponsored by the Los Angeles Department of Recreation and Parks.

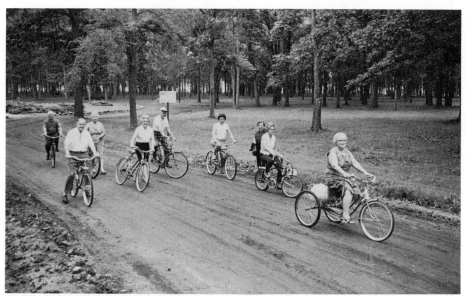

In Flint, Michigan, hundreds of Golden Agers belong to a city-sponsored bicycling club . . .

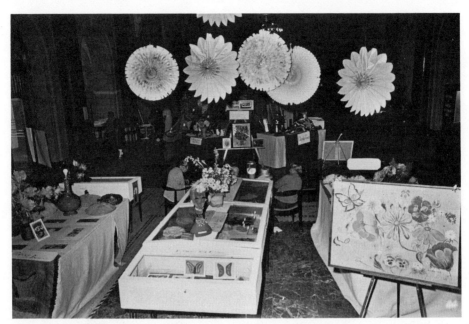

. . . and, in Washington, D.C., Senior Clubs cooperate in sponsoring an annual hobby show where members may show and sell their handicrafts.

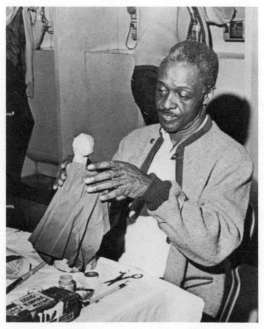

Some city recreation departments, like the Chicago Park District, sponsor special projects which serve the homebound with crafts and other individual activities.

In her study of 1002 senior centers, Anderson found that the average responding agency was reaching one-third of the estimated target population in its community. All agencies provided *recreational programs;* 73 per cent offered other *community services,* and 60 per cent offered *counseling services* as well. Slightly over one-third of all responding senior centers offered all three types of services.

FRANKLIN H. PIERCE CENTER. One example of a senior center may be found in Flint, Michigan, where the Franklin H. Pierce Center provides several hundred older persons with a wide variety of social activities, games, classes, musical activities, physical conditioning and weight-watching programs and special trips and outings. This center was built with funds from the city of Flint, and is assisted by the city in its operation. It offers scheduled programs five days a week, and also has special activities on weekends. The Flint municipal recreation department operates a Senior Citizens Services Division, which uses the Pierce Center as a headquarters, and operates other programs throughout the city, including the publication of a special newspaper for senior citizens.

Among the program activities offered in the Pierce Center for Senior Citizens are the following: card games and instruction, craft classes, men's and women's choruses, dancing, golf, shuffleboard, lectures, library services, supper club, bingo, a "Married 50 Years and Over" Club, and a special program of recreation for stroke-afflicted persons, which seeks to rehabilitate these individuals physically and socially. On a city-wide basis, the Flint Recreation and Park Board provides the following services to aging persons:

1. Publication of the *Senior Citizens News.*
2. Sponsorship of the Genesee County Senior Citizen Orchestra.
3. Publication of news releases for all news media regarding aging and senior citizens' programs.
4. Development of a discount card program, giving reduced rates and prices to older persons.

5. Sponsorship of a bicycle club, ecology club and over 80 club.
6. Planning of one-day bus trips and more extended vacation trips for older persons.
7. Sponsorship of other special events, including citywide dances, parties, luncheons, tournaments and similar programs for senior citizens.

This center is fairly typical of programs operated by both public and voluntary agencies in communities around the United States.

ATWATER SENIOR CENTER. A second example, the Atwater Senior Center, operated by the New Haven, Connecticut, Department of Parks and Recreation, breaks its programs down into several different categories. These include the following.

I. Organized Group Programs
  A. Groups with Definite Enrollments
    1. Interest groups, such as Christmas decorations, oil painting class, sewing, arts and crafts, singing, reading and discussion groups, knitting and cards.
    2. Committee meetings, including those responsible for birthday parties and socials, programs, membership, nominations, public relations, refreshments, telephone services, trip planning and similar functions.
  B. Organized Group Activities without Definite Enrollment
    1. Regularly Scheduled Activities
      a. Events at the Center, such as bingo parties, card parties, community singing, coffee hours, concerts, dancing, films and travelogues, lectures, luncheons, meetings and evening entertainments.
      b. Events away from the Center, such as annual Mass for deceased members of the club, entertainment by members at hospitals and homes in the vicinity, or trips to resorts, New York City, Cape Cod, Senior Citizen's conventions,

a glaucoma center, boat trips, country fairs, foliage festivals and similar outings.
C. Special Events
  1. Fund raising, including raffles, rummage sales, food and cake sales, and a Christmas bazaar.
  2. Fairs, special performances and holiday parties.

In addition to these services, the Atwater Center provides a substantial number of special services to individuals. These include consultation and referral services with senior citizens, which may include informational meetings, or direct consultation, examination or assistance related to such concerns as: health (glaucoma and diabetes checkups), visiting nurse services, Social Security advice, Housing Authority assistance, and counseling on tax exemptions, food stamps and similar matters.

SEMINARS AND SERVICES. Senior centers *must* offer considerably more than bingo, cards or social dancing if they are to meet the realistic life needs of older persons. Such programs should help to support and improve the lives of older persons, particularly those in large cities who are isolated or dependent. For example, the Los Angeles Parks and Recreation Department sponsors a series of seminars directly related to the needs of older persons, on such topics as "consumer protection," "dental care," "fraud schemes" or "housing." These are scheduled at ten centers specifically designed to meet the needs of older residents, and at over 75 other facilities where programs for senior citizens are part of the overall departmental programs. In addition, Los Angeles sponsors a Senior Citizens' Federation, which unites all older people in the metropolitan area in joint efforts to meet their needs in such areas as recreation, health and housing services, legal aid, Social Security, legislation and similar concerns. It sponsors major citywide events for older persons, many of which attract thousands of aging participants.

Operating in cooperation with the Mayor's Departmental Council on Aging, the Detroit, Michigan, Department of

Parks and Recreation provides an extensive program of services for senior citizens. In addition to its own centers, it sponsors several in cooperation with the United Auto Workers, a labor union which has traditionally taken a strong interest both in recreation and in the needs of its retired members. The Detroit Senior Citizens program places strong emphasis on developing leadership among older persons, having them serve as volunteers or paid leaders in programs and encouraging their involvement in public service.

Like Los Angeles, Detroit provides many informational and similar services to older persons; these are related to reduced rates for transportation, food, housing, library service, special resident camping for senior citizens, golf, fishing and other special programs available at limited cost.

In numerous other cities throughout the country, recreation and park departments are providing services for elderly and retired persons, operating chiefly through senior centers and Golden Age clubs. In many cases, as in New Haven, Cleveland and Milwaukee, the club members themselves assume a great deal of responsibility for planning and carrying on programs, and for providing volunteer leadership to help homebound elderly persons.

How effective are such programs in meeting the needs of retired people in the community at large? It seems clear that they are providing a valuable service, but that far too few older persons are being served by them. For example, in 1970, the Federal Administration on Aging assembled a directory of 1200 senior centers throughout the entire nation. If one were to estimate the average regular attendance of such centers, it would probably not be more than 100 or 150 members, although larger numbers of retired persons are registered and may attend special events. Thus, it seems probable that not more than 180,000 older persons (less than one per cent of all persons over 65 in the United States) are regularly served by senior centers.

The United States Commissioner on Aging, John B. Martin, commented in 1970:

In time, the senior center may come to hold a place in the older person's life equivalent to the central role now played by the school in the lives of children.[18]

In view of the extremely limited budgets of most senior centers, and the fact that only about one-third of them have full-time directors, it seems clear that vigorous steps need to be taken to strengthen the Senior Center and Golden Age club movement.

Other Programs for Retired Persons

In addition to those who live independently in the community, large numbers of retired persons now reside in special-care facilities. These serve the full gamut of the aging population, with fairly well-to-do and physically capable people often living in retirement villages, retirement

hotels or high-rise apartment complexes, and persons who are ill, infirm or socially dependent living in hospitals or long-term care units—usually referred to as nursing homes.

With the increased number of older persons requiring such care, and with funding available from the government to support the indigent, hospitals and nursing homes for the aged and chronically infirm have become a major form of service. In many cases, state departments of health have recognized the need to police these carefully, because of unscrupulous operators, with limited professional background or competence, who have entered this field primarily to reap profits from it. In a number of states, regulations have been established which *require* nursing homes to provide activity programs for residents. One of the more diligent states is Connecticut, where the State Department of Health has established the following code for approval of nursing homes:

---

[18] John B. Martin: In *Retirement Roles and Activities. op. cit.,* p. 25.

Standards for Certification
of
Therapeutic Recreation Program
by
Connecticut State Department of Health

I. PHYSICAL REQUIREMENTS
   A. There shall be adequate space to accommodate recreation program in the form of recreation rooms and/or day spaces.
   B. There shall be separate facilities for administration of program, and for storage of supplies and equipment.
II. ADMINISTRATION
   A. There shall be a professional recreation director or a person having equivalent experience and training, who shall direct and supervise the recreation program in the institution. This program director shall be approved by the State Department of Health. Upon approval, two weeks' in-service training is required, and will be arranged by the State Department of Health.
   B. The program director will be other than a regular employee of the institutional staff, and will wear street dress.
   C. The program director will be required to work the number of hours per week as determined by the licensed capacity of the institution as follows:

5– 14 beds	10 hours per week (at least 3 days)
15– 29 beds	20 hours per week (5 days)
30– 59 beds	30 hours per week (5 days)
60–120 beds	40 hours per week (5 days)

   For *each* additional 60 beds or fraction thereof, 40 hours per week is required.
   D. The program director shall generally work Monday through Friday, except for special program events on holidays and weekends or evenings. Work schedule shall be filed with the State Department of Health.
   E. The State Department of Health shall be notified immediately when any change in program director occurs.

III. RECORDS
  A. Monthly reports shall be submitted *by the 10th of each month* to the State Department of Health and shall include:
    1. Advanced Monthly Program Calendar
    2. Current month's Patient Participation Record
    3. Budget breakdown on program costs.
  B. Four additional records shall be kept on file at the facility:
    1. Patient Interest and Progress Record
    2. Volunteer Interview Record
    3. Volunteer Sign In Record
    4. Clergy Sign In Record
IV. PROGRAM REQUIREMENT
  A. The program shall be planned from *individual patient/resident needs and interests.*
  B. Activities shall be regularly scheduled and planned monthly in advance.
  C. There shall be diversified group and individual activities to include *per week:*
    1. *Art or Craft Program*
      a. Individual art or crafts for patient/resident at bedside where indicated.
    2. *Games* such as bingo, horse racing, bowling, and shuffleboard.
      a. Participation should be encouraged in special interest or small group games such as cards, checkers, chess and dominoes.
    3. *Cultural Activity*—music, literature, drama, adult education.
      a. Individual interest to be pursued and encouraged.
    4. *Religious Assembly*—conducted by clergy and/or volunteers.
      a. Individual pastoral and lay visits should be encouraged.
    5. *Personal Services*—to include letter writing, reading to, library service and patient/resident visitation.
  D. At least two of the following activities shall be scheduled per month:
    1. Film
    2. Birthday Party
    3. Entertainment program
    4. Special event such as holiday party, picnic, bus trip, or carnival.
  E. Special Interest or small hobby group activities shall be provided.
  F. The program shall be evaluated and revitalized periodically with new ideas and/or adaptation of standard activities.
  G. Work activity, community service, out trips, group discussions, current events, story telling, puppets, marionettes, skits, variety shows, and fashions, as well as hobbies should be incorporated in general programming when interest and capabilities so indicate.
  H. Effort should be focused to secure volunteer assistance for all programs and especially for personal patient/resident contact as friend to friend.
    1. Interviewing, screening and orientation of volunteers is necessary.
    2. Supervision, evaluation, and coordination of volunteer efforts is required, with staff as well as with general program.
    3. Recognition of volunteer assistance should be encouraged by administrator and staff of facility.
V. GENERAL INFORMATION
  A. Renewal of certification will occur yearly from date of initial accreditation.
  B. Approval may be withdrawn by the State Department of Health at any time should the institution fail to meet the requirements outlined in the above specifications.
  C. Approval will be automatically revoked within 30 days after the resignation of a program director. Re-certification must be made in the name of program director replacement.
  D. Special seminars for program directors will be offered periodically by the State Department of Health, which program directors shall attend.
  E. Program Directors should avail themselves of continuing training and educational opportunities through professional organizations and educational institutions.

Programs in Nursing Homes

It should be made clear that such programs are comparatively new, and even in states where regulations have been set in motion, enforcement is often lax. In many cases, aides, nurses, attendants or volunteers conduct recreation programs, under the direction of a professionally qualified part-time consultant.

As an example of the limited extent to which many extended-care facilities provide recreation, a study of nursing homes in the state of Kentucky was reported in 1970.[19] One hundred and nine institutions licensed by the State Department of Health were surveyed. Of these, 47 replied, and only 24 indicated that they had an organized recreation program for residents. In *no* case was a qualified recreation director or therapist responsible for programs, and in only four settings did respondents feel that the recreation activities provided for residents were adequate to meet their needs.

What *are* the elements of effective recreation programming in nursing homes?

SUITABLE ACTIVITIES. Since many residents are bedridden, confined to wheelchairs or otherwise limited physically, it is necessary to avoid physical activity of a strenuous nature. However, it certainly is possible to provide games that require a moderate amount of activity for those residents who are able to take part. Similarly, although many older persons in extended-care facilities may have limited mental capabilities, others are perfectly capable of enjoying activities that require verbal or intellectual participation.

In general, activities fall into the following classifications:

1. *Arts and crafts*—particularly activities such as knitting, needle-point, crocheting or similar crafts which do not require elaborate shops or complicated equipment.
2. *Music*—both as a participating activity (group singing, rhythm instruments or small ensembles) and as a form of entertainment.
3. *Dramatics*—in the form of skits, recitations, pantomimes or creative dramatic programs.
4. *Dance*—with social, folk and square dancing involving those residents who are physically able to take part, and with simple rhythmic movement involving even patients in beds or wheelchairs.
5. *Religious services*—including Bible readings, hymn singing, meditation

or rosary programs, or more formal worship services. Volunteer groups frequently come from the community to assist in such activities, and then extend their involvement to include personal visiting and other recreational activities.

6. *Films*—may include travelogues or popular movies shown to all residents, or home movies or slides of residents' families, which may be viewed individually in their bedrooms or dayrooms.
7. *Other activities*—include special interest groups such as *hobbies* (gardening, cooking, scrap book collections or photography), *social programs* (such as parties, bingo, birthday events or discussion groups), *games* (adapted bowling, golf, shuffleboard, horse racing and toss games are examples) and *trips and outings*.

Programs should be geared to serve the needs of patients who are bedridden or limited in mobility as well as those who can get around easily. Services such as beauty parlor or other self-care or personal activities must be brought to those residents who are confined to their rooms. Even if a resident can benefit from no other activity than friendly visiting and conversation, it is important that this be provided. Often, patients who have few interests and who resist involvement at the outset, gradually begin to participate more fully.

Recreation in a nursing home implies far more than just spending leisure time enjoyably; instead, it is part of a total concept of patient care. Miller has written:

Social rehabilitation of patients in a nursing home setting is effected through a treatment program that includes medicine, nursing, physical therapy, religion, occupational therapy, social work services and recreation. With optimal patient function the goal of the long-term care facility, recreation plays a particularly important part in the totality of professional disciplines. Consequently, the administration of a progressive nursing home is committed to the

[19] Martha Peters and Peter J. Verhoven: "A Study of Therapeutic Recreation Services in Kentucky Nursing Homes." *Therapeutic Recreation Journal*, 4th Quarter, 1970, pp. 19–22.

encouragement and development of the imaginative recreation service.[20]

Within such a setting, the recreation director must work closely with those in the other rehabilitative disciplines, as well as the director of volunteers. This policy is in keeping with the position of the American Hospital Association, which "encourages the active . . . use of volunteers in all long-term care facilities, provided that in proprietary institutions the volunteer's services are those that clearly benefit patients and do not serve to add to the institution's profits."[21]

Miller points out that therapeutic and diversional programs must be planned in terms of various levels of patient capability. Such activities as music, reading, gardening, crafts or games may be used individually or on a group basis, in order to help integrate individual patients into the overall community of patients. In addition, programs for the entire patient population, such as religious services or celebrations, music or dance performances, or other entertainment events, may provide colorful highlights for all residents.

Patients with organic brain damage may enjoy simple, rhythmical musical activities, simple crafts or repetitive exercises, parties or similar events. On the other hand, those patients who may have suffered physical impairment but whose brain function is sound, will enjoy more sophisticated programming, including discussion groups, art and music appreciation, more complicated games and entertainment on a higher level.

Recreation personnel in nursing homes frequently complain that the service they provide is not understood, or supported, by other members of the staff. Therefore, Miller suggests that the administrator should assist the recreation personnel in maintaining satisfactory intra-staff relationships:

> . . . by interpreting the recreation program to other departments, seeking cooper-

ation of the nursing and housekeeping departments as to scheduling to provide ample time for activity programs and by lending the weight of her position to experimental projects. The administrator also assists the staff in organization of written material of an administrative nature, e.g., development of manual and resources file.[22]

Activities must be scheduled at hours of greatest leisure, and must avoid conflict with nursing care or medical treatment. It is usually possible to provide some individualized programs in the morning, but afternoons usually offer the largest segment of completely free time; therefore, most group activities are scheduled after lunch. In some homes, with supper over early, individual activities or special events may also be planned for the early evening hours. As much as possible, patients should be involved in planning, both in terms of choosing desirable activities for the program, and in actually carrying out parties and other special events.

Programs in "Retirement Villages"

In general, residents in homes or hospitals for the aging are people who have suffered fairly serious physical or mental impairment, and who are not able to live independently in the community. Many retired persons, who have *not* suffered impairment and who are financially capable of independent living, have chosen in recent years to live in retirement villages or communities which have been established specifically to attract older persons.

This concept, which began on the West Coast, has since gained popularity throughout the United States. Generally, it consists of homes or garden apartment developments which have been specially designed for maximum convenience and safety. Only persons beyond a certain age are normally eligible to enter such communities. They may do so by purchase of property, on a rental basis, through a condominium or cooperative arrangement or a variety of other financial procedures. Since they may be extremely expensive,

---

[20] Dulcy B. Miller: "Nursing Home Setting." *Parks and Recreation,* January, 1967, p. 38.
[21] *Ibid.,* p. 39.

[22] *Ibid.,* p. 54.

they tend to appeal chiefly to elderly couples who are financially independent.

Although they vary considerably, in many leisure villages medical and other services are made readily available as part of group plans. In some, meals are served in dining buildings as part of the overall plan; properties are maintained by central services, and housekeeping services may also be provided. Because of the convenience they offer, as well as the safety (most villages have elaborate security, and some are actually walled villages), retirement communities have become extremely attractive to many retired persons. Davies writes:

> By the tens of thousands they are flocking to new retirement homes, often leaving behind the clamor of cities, frequently moving to warmer climates for community living in villages and high-rise facilities tailored to their particular tastes. They are looking for people of similar ages and interests, for convenience, for peace and security and sometimes for a less expensive existence.[23]

Often the primary motivation is the need to be with other older persons. As American society has become more stratified on the basis of age, many retired persons find comfort and reassurance in such a setting. One psychologist comments, "The older you get, the more you want to live with people like yourselves. You want, to put it bluntly, to die with your own."[24]

Typically, such retirement communities have extremely active recreation programs. These may include use of golf courses, swimming pools and other major recreation facilities, as well as a wide variety of clubs, classes, hobby groups and events throughout the year. Increasingly, they are employing social or recreational directors to conduct these programs, and usually a members' council serves in making policy and helping to carry out programs.

Programs for the Aged with Serious Disability

Frequently, aging is accompanied by serious disabilities, such as blindness, deafness or confinement to a wheelchair. In many cases, these conditions require institutionalization, but frequently, disabled elderly persons are able to live in the community. However, it is necessary for them to receive help. Often, groups of members of Senior Citizens' clubs, as described earlier, provide "meals on wheels" programs, friendly visiting services or a "daily hello" program, in which a safeguard checkup is carried out each day by volunteers who telephone incapacitated club members who are living alone.

In larger cities, special programs may be operated for aging persons with special disability. For example, in New York City, the New York Association for the Blind sponsors summer camps which have special weeks set aside for the elderly blind. Since more than 50 per cent of all blindness occurs in the 65-and-over age bracket, it seems probable that an increased number of community programs will be developed in this area.

Overall, it is apparent that the role of government on all levels must be expanded if the needs of aging persons in American society are to be met more adequately. What *are* the major functions of government with respect to aging persons, at present?

Role of the Federal Government in Aging

The federal government has provided varied forms of help for older persons in the United States for several decades. Since 1935, when Social Security was established, it has provided retirement income for a large number of elderly persons. The Medicare program, enacted in 1965, greatly relieves the burden of medical costs for the aged, by helping to pay hospital bills, bills for stays in extended-care facilities and medical bills for those who live at home. In addition, it has set standards for the care received in various

---

[23] Lawrence E. Davies: "The Retirement Village—A New Life Style." *New York Times,* January 18, 1970, p. 1.

[24] *Ibid.,* p. 48.

types of facilities licensed to serve the aged.

In general, Medicare has had its heaviest impact on the improvement of health services for lower socioeconomic groups in the United States. A second major contribution has been the passage of the Older Americans Act of 1965:

> The act is designed to develop needed services, opportunities and facilities for older persons by: 1) establishing an Administration on Aging in the Department of Health, Education and Welfare, to serve as the Federal focal point and clearing house of information on all matters of concern to older Americans; 2) providing grants to the States to develop services for older persons; and 3) providing grants to public and private agencies for demonstration, research, and training. Titles III, IV and V provide grants for planning, service and training programs. The Title III grants are made directly to State agencies on aging which, in turn, provide funds to public and private non-profit organizations to operate approved programs.[25]

As indicated earlier, many of the programs initiated by this program have had recreational elements. In some cases, they have given support to community services for aging persons, particularly senior centers and multiservice programs. In others, such as the Foster Grandparents Program, initiated by the Administration on Aging and supported at the outset by the Office of Economic Opportunity, older persons have been paid to work full or part time with disadvantaged children. In other programs, such as employment projects, funded by the United States Department of Labor, older persons have been placed in jobs as community aides—many with recreation responsibilities.

Under Title IV of the Older Americans Act, many research programs and demonstration projects have been funded. These have tended to focus heavily on the process of successful aging, and the kinds of community services required to promote healthy adjustment in later life. The goals of such projects have been described by the Social Rehabilitative Service of the

Administration on Aging in the following terms:

> Each project focuses on the older American and a specific factor which contributes to his living a wholesome, meaningful and satisfying life—as free as possible from fear, loneliness, and undue disappointment. The need for differentiating the problems of various sub-groups of older persons and of tailoring solutions to the needs and resources of the community and of the particular persons to be served are also recognized in the projects funded under Title IV.[26]

State Programs for the Elderly

An important section of the Older Americans Act was Title III, which authorized allotments to states for the purpose of supporting programs to serve the elderly. In order to receive grants, it was required that states organize statewide agencies and develop plans for serving the aged, which would be approved by the Secretary of Health, Education and Welfare. By January of 1969, 49 states had developed full-time leadership and program staffing intended to promote statewide services for aging persons. An analysis of state reports from 1969 showed that more than four million elderly persons resided in communities where Title III federal funds had been provided, on a matching basis.

Within these communities, the following statistics were reported in 1969:

1. Nearly 300,000 elderly persons participated in recreation and leisure activities.
2. Nearly 83,000 elderly isolated persons received telephone and visiting services.
3. About 52,500 older persons participated in "life adjustment" education activities, including consumer education, health education, and retirement preparation.
4. Thousands of others were trained to work in behalf of others, and were placed in full or part-time jobs.[27]

While this overall program has thus met the needs of only a small fraction

---

[25] *The Older Americans Act in New York State: A Progress Report*. Albany, New York, New York State Office for the Aging, 1967.

[26] *Aging*. Washington, D.C., Social Rehabilitation Service of Administration on Aging, U.S. Department of Health, Education and Welfare, January, 1969, p. 6.

[27] "Three Years of Progress Under the Older Americans Act." In *Aging. op. cit.*, pp. 5, 6.

of aging persons, it has obviously been a move in the right direction. With its assistance, a number of states have moved ahead aggressively to provide recreation programs and services for aging persons. Among these have been Michigan and Connecticut.

MICHIGAN. The state government of Michigan has organized a special Commission on Aging which coordinates the issuance of funds from Title III. This Commission has sponsored a Michigan White House Conference on Aging, which has sought new solutions to the problems of the state's 762,000 elderly citizens, and which has also formulated recommendations for federal aid to the elderly. The state's attitude is reflected in the statement of Governor William Milliken, made to the 1971 Conference on Aging:

> In this youth-oriented culture of ours, we have sent too many of our older citizens to a kind of early death—a quiet limbo where they will live out their remaining years without becoming a burden to our pocketbooks or our consciences.[28]

Michigan provides aid to communities in establishing low-cost housing and developing community centers for the aging. Such centers customarily provide a wide range of services, including free community education at local schools (several Michigan school districts are leaders in the field of school-sponsored adult education and recreation); telephone calls, visitations and similar services for elderly shut-ins; counseling; trips and other varied social activities. The state provides funding to the Institute of Gerontology at the University of Michigan and to Wayne State University, to conduct research or hold workshops on problems of the aging.

Large numbers of senior citizens in Michigan have become actively organized in promoting services to meet their own needs. The level of participation in center-sponsored social and recreation programs, some of which are assisted by the Michigan Recreation and Parks Association, is high. A newspaper for the aging published in Flint, Michigan, boasts:

Not many communities in the United States can say they have senior citizens who are bowling, swimming, iceskating, hiking, golfing, and riding bicycles after they have reached their 75th birthdays. Flint can.[29]

CONNECTICUT. For a number of years, this state has been a leader in recognizing the importance of recreation in programs for the aging. In 1960, with the support of funds from the Public Health Service of the United States, the Connecticut State Department of Health employed a recreational consultant to supervise the organization of recreation programs in institutions, hospitals and nursing homes. This consultant, Dorothy Mullen, has accomplished a number of major objectives, among them having the State Department of Health establish standards of physical, program and staffing requirements for institutions serving the chronically ill and aging.

Under Mullen's leadership, the state has also provided a variety of consultative services to improve patients' activities programs. Each year, several meetings of the Program Directors' Association are held, and training centers have been established where recreation workers receive two weeks of intensive training in this field. Connecticut has also placed emphasis on the use of skilled volunteers, and has established a yearly conference which serves both to recognize the important contribution made by volunteers, and to provide them with needed skills training.

Such efforts on the part of the states are generally reflected in programs in major cities within them. For example, the New Haven Department of Parks and Recreation has assumed a major responsibility for providing programs for the elderly. Its programs include a number of senior centers and a "Mobile Workers Outreach Program" (which assists elderly persons in a number of low-income housing units), a "Meals on Wheels" program, a "friendly visiting" program, an Annual Senior Clubs Council Hobby Show and Fairs and many similar activities.

New Haven is the center of many state-

[28] "Report of 1971 Michigan Conference on Aging."

[29] Gertrude Cross: *Senior Citizens News.* Flint, Michigan, Department of Recreation and Parks, 1971.

wide meetings on the aging, and of special conferences of the Connecticut Council of Senior Citizens. Overall, it has tackled many aspects of the aging problem, and has used a number of approaches, ranging from direct service to legislation and research in retirement preparation, to improve programs for the aged.

Within its centers, New Haven offers religious services, crafts, health counseling and community services, lectures, trips and various other recreational activities to meet leisure needs. It publishes a periodical, *Senior Citizens News,* and has promoted the need for courses in gerontology, seminars, workshops and in-service training programs at nearby community colleges. Overall, its program represents one of the most comprehensive municipal efforts to serve the aging in the country.

In many other states and cities, innovative programming for the aging is being carried on. However, two elements thus far have not been sufficiently developed to ensure fully adequate services. These are: (a) a full understanding of the dynamics of aging, and the kinds of services and pre-retirement preparation needed to ensure the most healthy and happy kinds of adjustment to old age; and (b) strong public concern that will support programs designed to meet the needs of aging persons and make it possible for them to find new roles in retirement.

Research on Aging

A considerable portion of the research that has been carried on with respect to aging has dealt with the problems of geriatic patients in institutional settings—in part because hospitals and extended-care facilities provide subjects and controlled environments for scientific investigation, and in part because funding has been made available for research on this level.

The trend of such research has been to show that much of the deterioration of older persons is not organic in nature, but results from the circumstances under which they live.

Woodrow Morris, Director of the Institute of Gerontology and Dean of the College of Medicine at the University of Iowa, has concluded on the basis of a number of studies that senility is not inevitable, but represents for many a "cultural artifact." Morris emphasizes the importance of economic, social and intrapersonal stresses that lead to insecurity, confusion and strong feelings of rejection and isolation. These, and not organic brain damage, are the real causes of the radical deterioration of many aged persons, in his view.[30]

It has been found, in a number of experimental projects, that "feasible, confused, deteriorated and withdrawn" geriatric patients have made dramatic improvements as a result of recreation programs geared to promoting social interaction. As simple a remedy as "beer and tender loving care," applied in a conscious program of recreation and social activity, has made remarkable changes in the life situation of badly deteriorated patients. Their self-awareness, general ability to function and cooperation with hospital staff have all been markedly improved in such programs. In many cases, the development of such programs has made it no longer necessary to prescribe drugs to geriatric patients.[31]

Obviously, such research findings have important implications for the administrators of extended care facilities. Lissitz writes:

> The senile comprise about 60 percent of all residents and patients in nursing homes, homes for the aged, and geriatric hospitals. Requiring special supervision, care, stimulation and motivation, they represent a serious challenge to the capacity of extended care facilities.[32]

If, as these investigations suggest, social activities and carefully planned remotivation programs are able to improve the status and functioning of senile patients, they are worthy of much fuller use, as part of the practical treatment of institutional geriatric mental patients.

[30] Woodrow Morris: *In* "Senile Psychoses Termed 'Cultural Artifact.' " *Geriatric Focus,* May, 1967, pp. 1, 3, 5.

[31] "Beer More Effective than Drugs as Psychologic Prop to Elderly." *Geriatric Focus,* September, 1970, p. 5.

[32] Samuel Lissitz: In *Geriatric Focus,* February, 1967, pp. 1, 5.

However, the broader question of what *causes* deterioration among older persons within the community itself is obviously the more important one. If it is possible to scientifically determine the basis for successful aging, and to create the circumstances in community life that will help middle-aged persons make the transition to old age—recognizing its inevitable social, physical and economic stresses—then it will be necessary for a far smaller number of individuals to be consigned to the "senile ghettos" which serve so many of them today.

Preparation for Retirement

Some researchers have pointed out that the very fact of free time poses a major challenge of adjustment to retired older persons. Pfeiffer and Davis, of Duke University, have concluded that, because of the strong work orientation in American society, a great number of older persons find extreme difficulty in accustoming themselves to the constructive, creative and guiltless use of the leisure that usually accompanies aging. They conclude:

> In order to avoid serious dissatisfaction, our society must provide either more training for leisure in middle age, or more opportunity for continued employment in old age.[33]

Increasingly, universities and major industries are devoting themselves to the problem of preparing older persons for retirement and for constructive adjustment to aging. For example, Fordham University has a training program for pre-retirement leaders, supported by a grant under Title V of the Older Americans Act. This curriculum deals with:

1. Topics relating to retirement, including health care, financial planning, where to live, legal affairs and taxes, and how to spend leisure time.
2. Basic conference and discussion skills, problem-solving techniques.

3. Practical training in leading pre-retirement education sessions, and opportunity to evaluate ongoing programs.

Major business concerns, including utility companies, banks and oil companies, as well as industrial unions and government agencies, have taken part in this training program. A number of other universities have developed similar programs. Their concern is not only the study of the aging process as it presently exists, but to explore the possibility of extending the life span markedly—based on new forms of medical care. If and when this occurs, scientists agree, it will be necessary for us to develop entirely new approaches in our social structure and economy, and in personal and family attitudes toward the elderly.

Current gerontological research speculates that the average life span may be extended to the age of 96 in the United States and other nations, at some time in the decades ahead. If this occurs, or even if a more modest gain in the life span occurs, the problem of the aging in society will become even more acute. Morris writes:

> The most significant problem for the future will be the evolution of new roles for the older adults—roles that have a reasonable connection with the mainstream of American society. . . . We must decide whether the elderly are to be encouraged to form a major subgroup with its own values and organizations, or to remain part of our society.[34]

He suggests the following as an essential set of components in a program for the elderly: (a) a mixture of work and nonwork activities; (b) improved pre-retirement preparation; (c) extension of the opportunities for community service; and (d) new opportunities for retirement income. In addition to these elements, Walter McKain, Chairman of the Committee on Retirement Roles and Activities of the 1971 White House Conference on

---

[33] Eric Pfeiffer and Glenn C. Davis: "Free Time Poses Problems to Elderly in our Society." *Geriatric Focus,* February, 1971, p. 1.

[34] Robert Morris: "Future of the Aged in a Changing Society—Testimony before U.S. Senate Sub-Committee on Aging." *Geriatric Focus,* March, 1968, pp. 1, 6.

Aging, has stressed the need for more research in aging, more legislation to improve old age benefits, improvement in long-term care facilities, expansion of senior centers, improved health care and preparation of more specialized personnel to serve the aged.

Aging persons themselves are beginning to mobilize to fight for improved benefits for the retired. Some six million elderly have joined politically oriented groups, such as the National Council of Senior Citizens and the American Association of Retired Persons, to lobby for improved legislation and better social services. As an estimated 17 per cent of all registered voters, the elderly have the strong potential for exerting considerable influence on government.

However, even if better programs to serve the aging are put in motion by government, this will only serve part of the problem. *Time Magazine* comments:

> The ranker injustices of age-ism can be alleviated by governmental actions and familial concern, but the basic problem can be solved only by a fundamental and unlikely reordering of the values of society. Social obsolescence will probably be the chronic condition of the aged, like the other deficits and disabilities they learn to live with. But even in a society that has no role for them, aging individuals can try to carve out their own various niches. The noblest role of course, is an affirmative one—quite simply to demonstrate how to live and how to die.[35]

[35] "The Old in the Country of the Young." *op. cit.,* p. 54.

It seems clear that, within an increasingly mechanized society and with more and more stringent union and Civil Service regulations, the amount of available work is not going to expand, and the work life of a great number of people will not be lengthened. Therefore, the fact of retirement is a reality that must be faced. Clearly, the task of providing a meaningful set of involvements in life which will hold the interest and provide the potential for creative and rewarding involvement for older persons, is going to be the responsibility of those providing senior center, institutional and other programs of special care. Recreation will continue to be a major element in such programs. Broadly conceived, it will not be "thumbtwiddling" or bingo alone, but a full range of cultural, social, creative and similar activities—including structured opportunities for older persons to provide meaningful volunteer services to society.

The real challenge will be for recreation professionals to establish their expertise in this area, and to do so by *action* rather than words. The trend toward providing professional education for administrators of multiservice programs for aging persons in college and university recreation departments is a healthy one. However, the recreation and park profession itself must develop a fuller sense of responsibility in this field, and must expand its programs markedly in the years ahead. Many millions of older persons are still unserved and provide a clear challenge in terms of the need for leisure programs and allied social service.

Suggested Topics for Class Discussion, Examinations or Student Papers

1. What are the unique problems of the aging in modern society that differ sharply from those of the past? How can recreation and related services play a significant role in meeting the needs of older persons?
2. To what extent *are* the needs of aging persons being met today, with respect to leisure? What social and governmental policies would help to improve this situation?
3. Outline a model program of recreation and related services for a specific type of institution, such as a nursing home or senior center.

Chapter 8

Programs for Socially Deviant or Dependent Youth

This chapter is concerned with the role of recreation in institutional programs designed to serve socially deviant children and youth. It deals with such settings as homes and special schools for children who have come from broken homes, or have a degree of personal disturbance that makes it difficult for them to function adequately in the community or in regular schools. It also includes correctional institutions for those who have been in difficulty with legal authorities, and special programs designed for the growing number of drug-addicted youth in our society.

The concept of social deviance includes such special problems as juvenile delinquency, drug addiction, alcoholism, aggressive and hostile behavior, truancy, sexual promiscuity and similar problems. While deviation may take a variety of such forms, this chapter deals primarily with those groups in society that are regarded as requiring special care or rehabilitation, because they are socially maladjusted, and unable or unwilling to conform to the demands of society.

Delinquency is the most common cause of such commitment. This has been defined in many ways. One state police manual describes the juvenile delinquent as ". . . a child of more than seven and less than sixteen years of age, who does any act which would be a crime if done by an adult, is deemed guilty of juvenile de-

linquency."[1] Other codes list a variety of minor offenses as the basis for a charge of delinquency. Commonly, children below the age of 16 or 18 who are "incorrigible, ungovernable, or habitually disobedient and beyond the lawful control of parents or other authorities,"[2] are subject to juvenile court action and may be committed to institutions for care of deviant youth.

The problem of juvenile delinquency was described by the President's Commission on Law Enforcement and Administration of Justice in 1967 as the "single most pressing and threatening aspect of the crime problem in the United States." It found that one out of every nine children is referred to juvenile courts for an act of delinquency before his 18th birthday. To illustrate the seriousness of this problem, 52 per cent of those charged with burglary, 45 per cent of those charged with larceny, and 61 per cent of those charged with auto theft are juveniles.

The Causes of Social Deviance

The causes of delinquency are the subject of debate. There are basically two schools of thought—one which sees it as

---
[1] *New York State Police Manual,* 1971, p. 109.
[2] *Ibid.*

a psychological or psychogenic problem, and another which sees it primarily from a sociological or cultural viewpoint.

The psychological view regards habitual antisocial or criminal activity as an outcome of defective personality structure, stemming from feelings of inferiority, poorly developed control mechanisms or inadequate or disturbed family relationships. The typical delinquent has a relatively weak ego, is highly insecure and has a strong tendency toward aggressive and hostile behavior.

The sociological view of delinquency sees it primarily as the result of cultural and environmental factors. This view is supported by evidence that there is a much higher percentage of delinquent behavior in low-income areas—marked by slum housing, poor schools, broken or unstable families and the lack of desirable adult models—than in middle- or upper-class neighborhoods. It rejects the notion that juvenile delinquency indicates a disturbed or disorganized personality, and suggests instead that the youthful lawbreaker may be a member of a cultural group that deliberately rejects "establishment" values and regulations, and determines its own code of peer behavior.

Talcott Parsons suggests that the problem is chiefly one of masculine identification. In this view, delinquents are protesting against female domination and affirming their own masculine self-image through antisocial behavior.[3] Block and Neiderhoffer regard delinquency as the result of inadequate societal processes for helping adolescents become adults; in their view, gangs engage in criminal activity as a way of stating their independence and adult identity.[4]

Merton explains socially deviant behavior as a form of protest by disadvantaged and racial minority youth. He writes:

When a system of cultural values extols . . . certain *common* success goals *for the population at large,* while the social structure rigorously restricts or closes access to . . . these goals for a *considerable part of the population* . . . deviant behavior then results on a large scale.[5]

The theory that the baffled aspirations of lower-class youth are responsible for delinquent gang behavior was most fully developed by Cloward and Ohlin. They established a set of categories of urban youth gangs, including *fighting* gangs who derived their status chiefly from making war on the community and on other gangs, *criminal* gangs concerned mainly with financial gain through theft, racketeering and similar activities, and *retreatist* gangs, who are involved chiefly with drugs, sex and alcohol as forms of escape.[6]

Recently, writers on juvenile delinquency have tended to minimize the role of play and recreation in the prevention of antisocial behavior. However, there has been considerable evidence that there is a meaningful relationship between the leisure and recreational patterns of many youth gang members and their criminal activities. This relationship takes two forms.

1. Play itself frequently is used in antisocial ways; leisure becomes the time in which early delinquent patterns are established. Tannenbaum writes:

In the beginning, the definition of the situation by the delinquent may be in the form of play, adventure, excitement, interest, mischief, fun. Breaking windows, annoying people . . . playing truant—all are forms of play. . . . To the community, however, these activities may and often do take on the form of nuisance, evil, delinquency, with the demand for control . . . punishment, police court.[7]

It seems probable that the relationship between the play impulse and delinquent

[3] Talcott Parsons: *Essays in Sociological Theory.* Glencoe, Illinois, Free Press, 1954 pp. 304–306.

[4] Herbert Bloch and Arthur Neiderhoffer: *The Gang: A Study in Adolescent Behavior.* New York, Philosophical Library, 1958, p. 17.

[5] Robert K. Merton: *Social Theory and Social Structure.* Glencoe, Illinois, Free Press, 1957, p. 105.

[6] Richard A. Cloward and Lloyd E. Ohlin: *Delinquency and Opportunity: A Theory of Delinquent Gangs.* New York, Free Press, 1960, pp. 20–30, 161–186.

[7] Frank Tannenbaum: *Crime and the Community.* New York, Columbia University Press, 1938, pp. 17–20.

activity is particularly high among middle-class and wealthy youth:

> In the case of the low-income teen-age thief, often the drive represents a craving for possessions that the parents can't afford or simply won't consider buying. . . . But for the youth from a better and even high-income background, the stimulus is curiosity, a desire for "kicks," and escape from boredom . . . they want a thrill.[8]

Often, what begins as random or occasional behavior related to minor theft, gang fighting, drug experimentation or sexual exploitation, gradually becomes more consistent and serious. When a child is arrested and brought before a juvenile court, and particularly when he is sent to a youth house, the pattern of behavior becomes fixed. The behavior traits of the young offender become more firmly established. Ultimately, what began as casual, impulsive play, becomes serious criminal behavior.

2. A second important element of the relationship between recreation and juvenile delinquency lies in the fact that youthful offenders typically have not learned to use their leisure in constructive and creative ways. It has been found that their family life usually lacks shared recreational pastimes, and that they usually avoid taking part in organized community recreation programs.

As a consequence, many socially deviant youth have extremely narrow recreational interests. A former reformatory warden has written:

> Among the inmates of correctional institutions there are many who have no knowledge or skills which will enable them to make acceptable use of their leisure. Most of them lack the avocational interests of the well adjusted. They cannot play, they do not read, they have no hobbies. In many instances, improper use of leisure is a factor in their criminality. Others lack the ability to engage in any cooperative activity with their fellows; teamwork is something foreign to their experience. Still others lack self-control or a sense of fair play; they cannot engage in competitive activity without losing their heads. If these men are to leave the institutions as stable, well-adjusted individuals, these needs must be filled; the missing interests, knowledge, and skills must be provided.[9]

Types of Institutions

There are many different types of institutions which serve socially deviant children and youth. These include both public and private residential treatment centers. While a certain number may chiefly serve children who come from broken homes or otherwise unacceptable environments, the majority are for children and youth who have already displayed antisocial tendencies and have been in trouble with the authorities. In the past, such institutions were usually known as reform schools. More recently, they have come to be called training schools or residential treatment centers. Several different types are:

1. State youth camps, frequently set in rural surroundings, with an emphasis on conservation work and outdoor living.
2. Cottage schools or homes operated by public, religious or voluntary agencies.
3. Institutions serving emotionally disturbed youth, who have also frequently been involved in delinquent behavior.
4. Youth houses or "remand" centers which serve to hold young people until their cases are ruled on by the courts.
5. Other penal institutions, ranging from minimum to maximum-security prisons, for older inmates.
6. Narcotics treatment centers.

As a rule, those who are sent to such institutions do not come to the attention of the authorities until their behavior has become seriously antisocial. Society's solution to the problem has been to place such offenders in treatment centers—ostensibly for rehabilitation rather than for punish-

---

[8] *New York Times,* December 1, 1968, p. F-1.

[9] Garrett Heyns: "Penal Institutions." In *Annals of the American Academy of Political Science.* September, 1951, pp. 71–75.

ment. The Children's Bureau has described, in cooperation with the National Association of Training Schools and Juvenile Agencies, their goals in the following terms:

> The word "treatment", as used in training schools today, means help given to the child—the total effort made by the school to rehabilitate the child and the after-care services in his home community. It denotes helping a child by providing a new and more satisfying experience in community living, together with any special services that he may need. It includes a proper diagnosis of the child's problems and a plan of care based on that diagnosis. It implies providing an environment in which all activities are directed to getting the child ready for a successful return to community living.[10]

Many special homes are operated by voluntary and religious organizations, which serve children assigned to them through specified commitment procedures. When they accept children sent by the courts, they may charge the state as much as $10,000 to $12,000 a year for each child—a sum three or four times as much as the cost of a college education. In one such institution, the annual cost per child is as high as $18,000.

In general, institutions serving juvenile delinquents have high recidivism rates. Almost 75 per cent of those discharged from youth training schools or other correctional institutions are rearrested within five years.

What this suggests is that, in many cases, treatment centers for the socially deviant are defeating their own purpose. Many young people who enter such institutions leave after a year or two far more hardened to society and knowledgeable in crime techniques than when they entered. Amos writes:

> The ineffectiveness of our institutional programs is partly to blame . . . because many of the youngsters who return to their neighborhoods carry with them the added

sophistication of a one-year course in delinquency, manipulation, conning, utilization of the sub-cultural codes, and assume roles of leadership and influence among other youngsters in their areas.[11]

Young people who enter such institutions often have immature expectations regarding authority figures, stemming from earlier parent-child conflicts. They have confused self-images regarding their own worth, vocational goals, personal skills and sexual identification. Usually, they are listless and tend toward the passive use of free time; yet they have a great deal of pent-up energy and hostility. They tend to have a low level of tolerance for failure or frustration, and desperately need to acquire skills, training and a sense of accomplishment. Although they come to the institution to be rehabilitated, the bulk of their time is often spent in learning about better ways to commit crimes, and establishing relationships with their peers on the basis of their own toughness and resistance to societal values. Barker and Adams write:

> They often react against the dominant value structure and develop the feeling that anything that is valuable and acceptable for the dominant culture is wrong for them and vice-versa.[12]

This sense of alienation and resistance is understandable. The mere fact of the institutional setting is one that militates against the resident's responding to even the most intelligent and constructive treatment. MacIver writes:

> Technically, the institution is a place where the youth is sent for friendly guidance and training, but for the youth himself, it is a prison, a punishment. He is cut off from all familiar associations. He is under restraints that he bitterly resents.[13]

---

[10] See Ruth Cavan: *Juvenile Delinquency*, Philadelphia, J. B. Lippincott Co., 1969, p. 26.

[11] William E. Amos: "The Future of Juvenile Institutions." In Ruth Cavan, (ed.): *Readings in Juvenile Delinquency*. Philadelphia, J. B. Lippincott Co., 1969, p. 26.
[12] Gordon Barker and W. Thomas Adams: In Ruth Cavan, (ed.): *Readings in Juvenile Delinquency. op. cit.,* p. 435.
[13] Robert M. MacIver: *The Prevention and Control of Delinquency,* New York, Atherton Press, 1966, p. 163.

Within this context, then, it is essential that the program be one that provides a variety of needed kinds of experiences and human relationships. These should include counseling services, group discussions and therapy, academic education, vocational classes, work experience and recreation.

Goals of Recreation in Treatment Centers for the Socially Deviant

In many ways, the goals of recreation in youth camps and other correctional or treatment facilities are much like those found in hospitals, nursing homes or similar institutions. However, they include certain unique elements:

1. Recognizing that institutional life represents an unnatural and limiting kind of living arrangement, a primary purpose of recreation is to improve morale, to help make the setting more bearable and enjoyable. The lack of freedom, and a high level of anxiety, tension and boredom, can all be alleviated by a well-organized program of enjoyable activities.
2. A second purpose of recreation in the institutional setting is to help individuals learn new recreational skills, discover talents and interests, and generally learn to use their leisure in socially acceptable and constructive ways.
3. Recreation provides a means of improving the social adjustment of participants; through it, they are helped to develop constructive social relationships with adults or with their peers, to learn to become cooperative group members and to accept social rules and values of sportsmanship and responsibility.
4. Generally, recreation may help the individual participant gain a more favorable self-concept and a sense of accomplishment and personal worth, as well as the knowledge that he is using his free time in a productive and acceptable way.
5. By providing a release for energies

and drives that are pent up in the prison situation, recreation may help to reduce the danger of friction and hostility; sports and creative and social activities are particularly useful in this respect.

While recreation—like other rehabilitative services—is an important part of the institutional program, it is clear that it can accomplish little by itself. Decker writes:

Recreation is not a cure-all. It does not prevent, control or cure unacceptable behavior. But it does have an important role in the total rehabilitation process. . . . If a program is well-planned and adapted to the participants, they can be guided and assisted in learning self-control and self-discipline, engaging in cooperative enterprises, building more constructive social relationships, and acquiring interests that replace undesirable past interests.[14]

Recreation in Correctional Institutions

Despite the growing awareness of these purposes for recreation in correctional institutions, in many youth camps, training schools or prisons, the provision of recreation services is extremely limited. In part, this stems from a concept of such institutions as places meant for the *punishment* rather than the *rehabilitation* of inmates. While this viewpoint is gradually being replaced by more constructive views, the fact is that a brutal and harsh attitude toward offenders has characterized American penal institutions until comparatively recently.

Among the more brutal measures employed in the recent past were the following:

In North Carolina, a decade or so ago, men were thrown naked into solitary confinement cells, where guards used high-pressure water hoses from time to time to "knock them up against the wall."

In Maryland, inmates were disciplined until recently by receiving a meal only once every 72 hours.

[14] Larry E. Decker: "Recreation in Correctional Institutions." *Parks and Recreation,* April, 1969, p. 32.

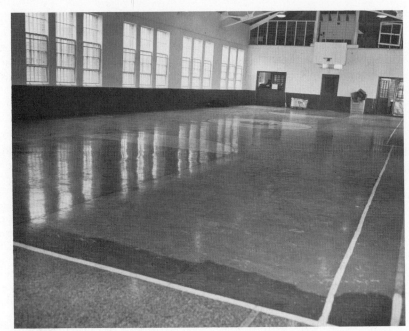

Increasing numbers of penal institutions are providing sports facilities and programs. The Chillicothe, Ohio Correctional Institute has gymnasium facilities . . .

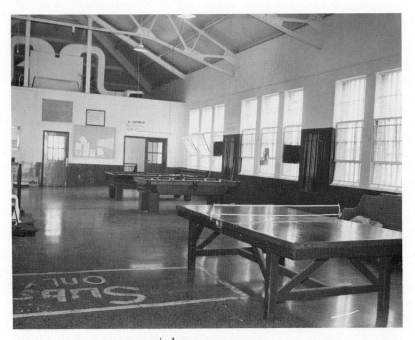

. . . indoor games rooms . . .

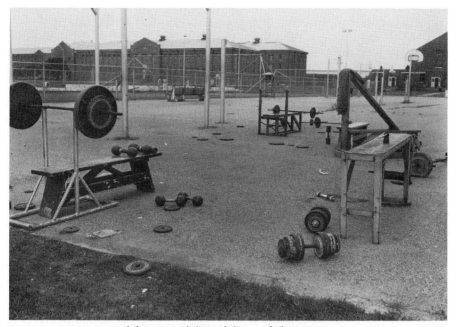

. . . an elaborate weight-training and fitness program . . .

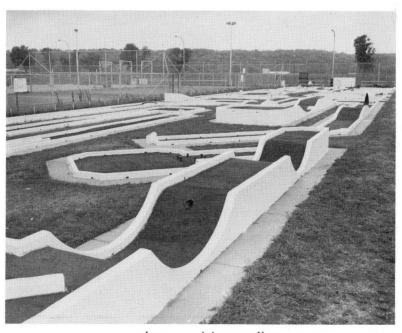

. . . and even a miniature golf course.

In Pennsylvania, until the mid-1950s, recalcitrant prisoners were placed for long periods in dark, damp underground holes.

In Arkansas, until the late 1960s, men were whipped on the bare buttocks with rawhide straps (flogging was practiced in 26 prisons as recently as 1963), and some were tortured by having needles pushed under their fingernails.[15]

Given this record of extreme harshness, it is understandable that meaningful educational, vocational, counseling and recreational services have been slow to enter many youth correctional institutions or adult prisons. However, even where there is a desire to provide such services, staff limitations and overcrowded facilities have made it difficult to do so. The former Attorney General of the United States, Ramsey Clark, has pointed out that 95 cents out of every dollar spent in prisons is for custodial care, and only 5 cents is spent for rehabilitation services.

Many youth houses and prisons throughout the United States are extremely overcrowded and lack badly needed programs to carry out rehabilitation goals. Several examples may be drawn from institutions in New York City—probably no better and no worse than those in other large cities.

A report based on a nine-month study of correctional facilities and prisons concluded that:

> Intense overcrowding, inadequate personnel and poorly designed facilities have resulted in turning detention facilities into settings less humane than our public zoos.[16]

The city's commissioner of correction commented of youth houses and "remand" centers that extreme overcrowding had an overwhelmingly negative effect, and made it almost impossible to provide needed programs:

> Pressure-cooker living has very abrasive effects. Programs relieve tensions. You keep people busy and you've got a safety valve. With idleness, things are pent up and you

insure hostility. We're supposed to be rehabilitating people, but we're so thinned out that rehabilitation has to take a back seat.[17]

Typically, a world of "fear, violence, filth and degradation" was described by prisoners who answered an uncensored questionnaire about conditions in the Tombs, a municipal house of detention for men. The use of force by guards, the lack of adequate medical care, schooling or other services, plus extreme overcrowding, made this facility a "dungeon of fear," in the words of one prisoner. In other centers, the shortage of caseworkers, teachers and recreation personnel limits programs markedly. Rikers Island, a reformatory jammed with almost twice the number of inmates originally planned for it, is marked by beatings, sexual abuse and suicides; observers have described it as an "island of idleness." There, writes one reporter:

> . . . teenagers can associate with accused felons and spend the day talking about the best kind of drugs to take, the most lucrative crimes, their real or imagined sexual experiences and the people they've beaten up. There is time, lots of time, for them to plan great crimes because their days are not disrupted by such unpleasantries as education, work, or sports. They get three meals a day and a place to sleep.[18]

Correctional institutions often are so understaffed and overcrowded, with minimal facilities and equipment, that it is almost impossible to provide truly meaningful recreation activities. In youth shelters, problems of racial antagonism, impulsive acts of violence, forced homosexuality and the knowledge that they are in a "temporary" state until court action is taken on their cases, all make it extremely difficult to operate effective recreation programs. The turnover of staff members is high, and the salary range—considerably less than that for teachers or other

[15] "Prisons Curb Brutal Discipline; Find Relaxed Controls Effective." *New York Times,* May 15, 1971, p. 14.

[16] Peter Kihss: "Albany Report Calls Jails Crime Breeding Grounds." *New York Times,* November 10, 1969, p. 30.

[17] Michael T. Kaufman: "Detention Centers 60% Over Capacity." *New York Times,* January 22, 1970, p. 39.

[18] Joseph Feurey: "Idle Rikers Teens Get Crime 'Tutoring.'" *New York Post,* February 20, 1970, p. 22.

professionals—makes it difficult to acquire capable recreation leaders and youth counselors.

It is obvious that sufficient support has not been given to this area of rehabilitation service in most institutions. Decker comments that, within the corrections field, there has been comparatively limited acceptance of the need for professionally staffed recreation personnel. He summarizes the findings of a recently completed Recreation Planning Study for the Oregon State Division of Corrections, which indicate some of the reasons why recreation programs in correctional institutions are inadequate:

1. The role and values of recreation are not emphasized.
2. There is no professional staff member trained in recreation.
3. The emphasis is on custodial care and security.
4. Professional guidance and assistance in recreational services are not readily available to the staff.
5. Where recreation programs do exist, they often are instituted with little planning and few long-range objectives in mind.
6. The administrative climate is not conducive to evaluation and change.
7. The professional recreator's efforts have not been directed toward explaining and increasing the role of recreation in the institutional setting.[19]

Despite this generally negative picture, there are a number of excellent programs of recreation in youth institutions throughout the United States. Among the leading states to have moved vigorously into the improvement and reform of their correctional institutions are Ohio, Illinois, Georgia and California.

Effective State Programs

Probably the leading example of a state which has taken action to reform and vitalize its correctional program is Illinois. There, in 1968, Governor Richard Ogilvie moved to merge separate state departments or boards dealing with youth

offenders, adult correction facilities and penal institutions into a single state department with cabinet-level representation.

> This reorganization was designed to spearhead a shift from a limited, punitive corrections program to one dedicated to rehabilitation and based on community involvement in the rehabilitation process . . . effective vocational training and counseling, improved youth activities, decent capital facilities—in short . . . a real rehabilitation effort.[20]

As part of this effort, Illinois took the following actions in the years immediately following 1968: (a) it raised its correctional budget sharply; (b) it established a strong central administrative staff to provide research, long-range planning, program analysis, policy evaluation, public information and medical and professional services; (c) it established a larger, full-time Parole and Pardon Board; (d) it developed a variety of new community-based programs, including four halfway house community centers for parolees, six new work-release centers, ten group homes for youth parolees, a special services unit in Chicago to provide counseling and job placement for youth parolees and a new pre-release program to aid adults about to be discharged; (e) it developed several new minimum security facilities with emphasis on vocational and educational treatment programs; and (f) it expanded professional counseling, and vocational and educational services in all facilities.

Within two years, the recidivism rate dropped sharply for youth and adults who had access to the new programs and procedures. Among juveniles, the rate dropped from 51.4 per cent in 1969 to 35.3 per cent in 1970—a decline of almost one-third.

Illinois State Training School for Boys, St. Charles

This medium security facility, serving an average daily resident population of

---

[19] Larry E. Decker: *op. cit.,* p. 31.

[20] Richard B. Ogilvie: *First Annual Report, State of Illinois Department of Corrections.* 1970, p. 3.

approximately 500 to 600 boys, provides extensive academic and prevocational programs, as well as medical, dental, religious, recreational, psychiatric, psychological and social services. It is the largest facility for delinquent youth in the state. In an effort to overcome this disadvantage, it has been divided into smaller operational units with separate staffs and program identities, housed in clusters cottages. Each such unit develops its own statement of rehabilitation goals and methods of achieving them. Intensive use is made of group living experiences, student council programs, planning and advisory roles in policy-making, along with more traditional forms of individual and group therapy.

Overall, the school's physical education and recreation program is operated under the direction of the Recreation Division, staffed by a director of recreation, an assistant director, an occupational therapist and a staff of physical education instructors. Facilities include a gymnasium and indoor swimming pool, 12 combination basketball, badminton and volleyball all-weather courts located near the cottages, 13 softball diamonds with backstops, a football field, a running track, a baseball field and four tennis courts that double as ice skating rinks during the winter months.

In addition to formal physical education, health and first aid instruction, the Illinois State Training School at St. Charles sponsors the following recreational activities:

1. Varsity sports competition with other schools or boys' clubs, for highly skilled participants.
2. Intramural competition, including leagues and tournaments in all seasonal sports, carried on among the cottages.
3. Weekly swimming participation and instruction in small groups for nonswimmers.
4. Weekly movies of 35 mm first-run features, and talent shows by service organizations, colleges or other entertainment groups.
5. Ice skating during the winter and roller skating during the summer, using outdoor facilities.
6. Monthly birthday parties, special holiday parties (including trips to neighboring communities or special activities) and special events for Halloween, Labor Day, Thanksgiving and other holidays.
7. A hobby shop program, including lanyard, leather, clay, raffia and other craft activities.
8. Individual units may also sponsor special interest clubs; among the activities provided have been swimming, chess, Spanish, guitar lessons, physical fitness, tailoring and horseback riding.
9. Drum and Bugle Corps, and other musical activities.

Although each of the units provides somewhat different approaches to treatment, the following statement is typical of the overall institution's philosophy, and the framework in which recreational activities are carried on:

The Rehabilitative Environment. It is the intended purpose of this Unit to create an accepting, warm, non-threatening, humane, and enriched environment in which the delinquent youth can learn that the world is not overwhelmingly hostile and alien. However, unlike the therapeutic setting in which the neurotic child or adult would likely be placed, this environment is not to be permissive. It is to be highly structured. A sense of authority is to be consistently maintained. The consequences of the delinquent youth's behavior, whether positive or negative, are to be clearly defined. An integral part of this environment is the creation of learning situations in which the delinquent youth can:

1. Ventilate his anger constructively.
2. Modify undesirable behavior and learn age-appropriate means to satisfy his desires and wants.
3. Learn the rewards of socially desirable behavior and deferred gratification of needs.
4. Experience the rewards of close, nondelinquent interpersonal relationships.
5. Correct distorted perceptions so that he

can deal more effectively with the demands and stresses of life.[21]

At other institutions operated by the Illinois Department of Corrections, there are similar approaches and programs. In one center, the Reception and Diagnostic Center for Girls, and in the Illinois State Training School for Girls, at Geneva, Illinois, cottages engage in similar activities—with the difference that a variety of coeducational activities are provided. One of the most common problems facing the staff in training schools or treatment centers for adolescents is that of homosexuality, which—apart from its moral connotations—may lead to friction and a variety of problems of a disciplinary or control nature. Obviously, one of the best ways to minimize this is to provide outlets for coed recreation—either sports and games, trips and outings or similar events. At the Geneva school, at least four such social events co-sponsored with other all-male juvenile facilities are held each month, two on the Geneva campus, and two away. In addition, varied cultural programs, such as a campus choir, drama club, gardening program and similar activities, have been introduced—some carried on with the assistance of community groups.

Ohio Department of Mental Hygiene and Correction

Another state which has taken vigorous action to improve its correctional institutions is Ohio. Here, until 1954, there were three separate departments with related responsibilities: the Division of Mental Hygiene, responsible for all mental institutions; the Division of Correction, responsible for all penal institutions; and the Division of Juvenile Research, Classification and Training, responsible for juvenile institutions. At present, these functions are combined within a single Department of Mental Hygiene and Correction.

This administrative structure has facilitated the development of programs concerned with psychiatric criminology. A special division operating under this title is responsible for providing care for the criminally insane, sociopaths and sex offenders.

Both in experimental new facilities operating under this division, and in institutions run by the Division of Correction, recreation is offered along with academic and vocational programs, and religious, psychological and other social services. As an example, in 1970, a new treatment center for psychosocially handicapped young offenders was opened at Junction City, Ohio. This psychiatrically-oriented 135-bed center operates a large multipurpose gym-auditorium, classrooms, vocational shops, appliance repair shops and hobby rooms, along with a library and conference room. The center is divided into four living units, consisting of either individual rooms or six-man dormitories. Each unit has a day-room for recreation, group therapy and other activities.

The Junction City Treatment Center has the advantage of small size, a treatment-oriented staff (with a high patient-staff ratio of approximately one-to-one), and a relaxed, flexible atmosphere. An individualized treatment program is tailored to each man's needs; it normally includes academic and vocational training, recreation, work assignment, development of an avocation or hobby, group therapy and similar forms of rehabilitation. Recreation is provided by activity therapists who offer a variety of sports, hobbies, social activities, music, art and similar programs. The institution's size and approach allow the inmate-patients and staff to get to know each other on a very personalized basis. In fact, staff and inmate-patients eat their meals together and mingle freely and informally throughout the institution.[22]

Probably more typical of the Ohio correctional system is the Chillicothe Correctional Institute, a medium security facility serving an inmate population of approxi-

[21] *Statement of Rehabilitative Objectives and Approaches,* Unit III. Departmental Manual, Illinois State Training School For Boys, St. Charles, Illinois, 1971, p. 2.

[22] *Eight Years of Progress in Psychiatric Criminology.* Ohio State Department of Mental Hygiene and Correction, 1970, p. 11.

mately 1100 men. The associate superintendent of this facility describes its recreation program in the following terms:

> The Institute has a rather large number of men who are advanced in age or who are physically handicapped and for this reason we must structure many of our recreational programs toward sedentary spectator activities. However, we do provide facilities for participant sports such as varsity and intramural softball and basketball, tennis, miniature golf, weight-lifting, horseshoes, shuffleboard, badminton, volleyball, billiards, table tennis and checkers.[23]

A strong effort is made to involve the community in the Chillicothe Correctional Institute's recreation program, both to strengthen the program and to inform community residents about prison life. During the past year, for example:

> . . . four hundred and twenty-five teams were admitted from the outside community to participate in games in our gymnasium and on our ball-fields and tennis courts. These teams participated both against each other and against our own varsity teams made up of our inmate population . . . an estimated 4,000 persons from outside areas gained access to our Institute last year for the purpose of providing recreational activities for the men.[24]

In addition to this heavy emphasis on sports—which comprises the bulk of the recreational programming for many penal institutions—weekly and holiday motion pictures are provided for the inmates, and live entertainment, such as musical or dramatic performances, is provided by outside groups in the prison auditorium about once a month.

In general, recreation programs in most penal or correctional institutions around the country are extremely limited. In one survey of women's penal institutions in the United States, Canada and Puerto Rico, it was found, for example, that a number of prisons or reformatories had no organized programs at all. Of 17 responding institutions, only six had formal educa-

tional requirements for the director of recreation; in others, degrees were not required, and staffing responsibilities were heavily assumed by male guards or female supervisors. In this survey, the most frequently found activities tended to be *active games,* such as softball, volleyball, badminton, croquet, basketball, tennis, horseshoes and tumbling, and *quiet activities,* such as cards, bingo and shuffleboard. It was concluded that the women's penal institutions with the most clearly defined purposes, and with leadership assigned to specific recreation directors, tended to have the most extensive and well-organized programs.[25]

Recreation in California Youth Authority Institutions

Traditionally, the California Youth Authority has used recreation in varying degrees as a rehabilitative tool, with primary responsibility for planning and organizing physical education and recreation programs assigned to instructors in recreation and physical education. Additional recreation programs within living units in state youth institutions have been provided by group supervisors or youth counselors assigned to living units. Programs have varied considerably in different institutions, depending on group workers' interest and talent in the recreation field; the absence of any stipulation requiring group workers to have formal training in recreation has led to inadequate and unimaginative programs in many Youth Authority centers.

In 1964, the Youth Authority requested the State Department of Education and the State Department of Parks and Recreation to conduct a survey of its institutions in order to determine the adequacy of existing recreation and physical education programs. The survey team recommended that the roles and duties of the staff members responsible for recreation in institu-

[23] Letter from M. D. Marsino, Associate Superintendent, Chillicothe, Ohio, Correctional Institute, January 5, 1972.
[24] *Ibid.*

[25] Diane Peoples and Russ Walkup: *Survey of Women's Penal Facilities.* Unpublished report, Ohio Reformatory for Women, Maryville, Ohio, 1970.

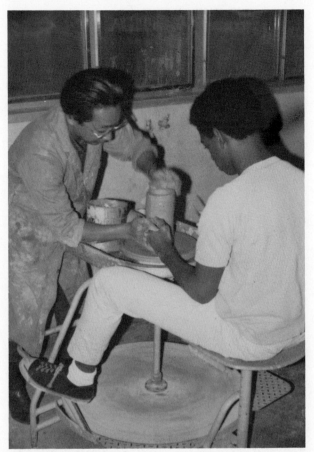

Youth at the O.H. Close School for Boys, operated by the California Youth Authority, take part in crafts programs, including ceramics . . .

tions be defined and developed through the medium of a demonstration project.

In 1966, the Youth Authority initiated a new treatment team approach which has since been adopted as a standard program method in all of its institutions. It was decided to carry out an in-depth recreation demonstration project at two recently opened schools in Stockton—the O. H. Close and Karl Holton Schools for Boys. With funding by the van Loben Sels Foundation, an 18-month project was conducted at these two schools, from January, 1968, to June, 1969.

Under the direction of the Institute for the Study of Crime and Delinquency in Sacramento, California, the overall objective of this project was:

To demonstrate whether a dynamic total recreation program, implemented by pro-

fessionally trained recreation consultants, would have a significant impact as a rehabilitative technique for institutionalized delinquent youth. These related questions were also explored: How much recreation is desirable in a juvenile institution? How much time can an institution afford to spend on recreation in view of all of the other elements of treatment?[26]

It had the following specific aims:

1. To organize and implement an in-service training program in recreation leadership for Youth Counselors.
2. To experiment in the use of Youth Authority wards as "Recreation Staff Aides."

[26] Robert E. Myers, Jr., and Cleveland Williams: *Operation Recreation: A Demonstration Project at Two California Youth Authority Institutions.* Sacramento, California, California Youth Authority, 1970, p. 2.

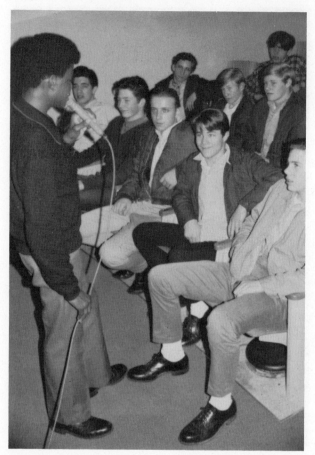

. . . informal dramatics and discussion groups . . .

3. To develop a community "Recreation Volunteer" program.
4. To evaluate the desirability of employing a professionally trained recreation specialist in all Youth Authority institutions.
5. To develop a recreation intern program by providing recreation field work placements in Youth Authority institutions for undergraduate majors.
6. To test and evaluate various recreation equipment and supplies.
7. To produce a recreation handbook for use primarily by the institution line worker, and to develop a standardized recreation budget.[27]

The demonstration project that was put into effect had a number of major components. Initially, it placed two trained rec-

reation specialists in the Close and Holton Schools as consultants. They devoted six months to preparing for the program, and the training and orientation of staff members, including inmate Ward Aides. Ward recreation committees were set up, which involved the boys in the planning of their own recreation programs.

Volunteer programs were coordinated by the recreation consultant, with a considerable number of volunteers being recruited from nearby high schools, a college, churches, civic clubs, labor unions and similar organizations. A recreation internship program was established, with student interns from San Jose State College assuming responsibility for volunteers and other special phases of the program. In addition, recreation activity specialists were employed to conduct activities requiring specialized skills.

---

[27] *Ibid.*

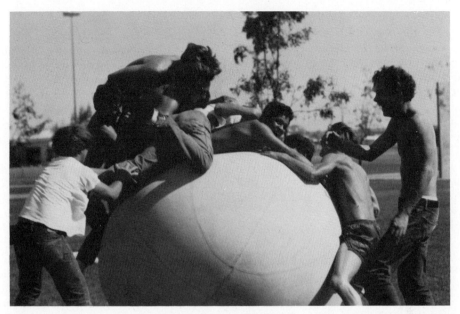

. . . and outdoor games and sports, including, as shown here, rough-and-tumble team stunts.

NEW APPROACHES TO RECREATION PRO-GRAMMING. In the past, programs had been nondirective in nature, and often dependent on spontaneous participation:

A typical occurrence would find youth counselors, upon seeing a group of boys milling about, attempting to direct them into activities such as table tennis or shooting baskets. This approach used recreation as a management rather than a rehabilitation tool. There was little recreation planning of a systematic nature. . . .[28]

In developing a more carefully planned program, a survey was carried out to determine how many leisure hours were available to the boys in the two schools. The survey indicated that wards had about 30 hours per week, the bulk of this coming on Saturdays and Sundays. It was therefore decided to concentrate school-wide recreation activities on these days. Recreation consultants conducted training sessions for staff, wards and volunteers. Hall recreation committees were formed, which developed monthly recreation program calendars. Typically, they developed such projects as:

COEDUCATIONAL EVENTS. Coed swim parties, including a swim, a barbecue and a dance, were held, inviting girls who were on parole in the Sacramento area. Coed sports nights were held, including activities such as table tennis, checkers, cards, volleyball, billiards and dancing; girls from nearby schools in Stockton were invited to these events.

OTHER PARTIES. These included carnivals, shows, holiday events, play-days and picnics and barbecues, spaced throughout the demonstration project.

Schoolwide activities included the establishment of music and dance, arts and crafts and talent shows. Social dancing classes were held; the school's glee clubs and "rock" bands, and outside groups, put on performances.

Extensive intramural sports leagues in basketball, tackle football, flag football, and other instructional or competitive events in boxing, golf, gymnastics, handball, soccer, kickball, wrestling and volleyball attracted large numbers of participants. Other developmental activities, such as physical fitness and weightlifting, were introduced successfully. In addition, hobby activities, such as a camera club and a slot-car program, were carried on.

[28] *Ibid.,* p. 9.

The demonstration project in recreation service in the two Youth Authority schools was subjected to a careful evaluation in three major areas: (a) the degree of staff and ward participation in recreational activities both in the institution and the community; (b) the effect of recreation on relationships among the boys and between the boys and staff members; and (c) staff and ward attitude toward the value of recreation. Evaluative questionnaires were filled out by wards and staff members on all levels, and careful records kept on the various elements in the project.

Findings of the Project

1. The project had a significant impact on the attitudes of the wards in residence at both the O. H. Close and Karl Holton Schools. Analysis of questionnaire responses showed that most of the wards' commitment offenses had occurred during their "free time." Many boys indicated that active recreation programs in the community would have provided positive outlets for their leisure needs, and that the project had helped them become more aware of organized recreation and its advantages.
2. It was found that the shifting of program emphasis to weekends, which had formerly been unscheduled, meant that many hours of "dead time" were now being filled with meaningful activity. A realignment of staff schedules was recommended by the project staff, in order to provide additional coverage in the living units during weekends and holidays.
3. The report concluded that trained leadership was essential to the planning of successful recreation activities, and that staff members primarily concerned with security or casework responsibilities had neither the time nor the ability to consistently plan and carry out dynamic and imaginative programs.
4. It concluded that recreation programs are most successful when community resources and volunteers are used. The contributions of skilled and interested volunteers from the community provided an element of vitality, and assured the wards that others cared about them—an important therapeutic message.
5. The interest of wards in institutional recreation programs was stimulated when they had a chance to plan them and select equipment and supplies; this supplanted an attitude of apathy or even defiance when programs were imposed by authority.
6. Facilities were shown to be markedly inadequate for a well-rounded recreation program, and were primarily geared to housing and security needs; thus, much improvisation had to be done to ensure the use of facilities.

In general, it was concluded that the best programs were those which were carefully planned, structured and carried out. The project showed that Ward Aides and college recreation internes could be extremely valuable in carrying out a total recreation program. Although a handbook for recreation service was prepared at each of the schools, it was found that these were of limited value, in terms of their applicability to other correctional situations. A final interesting finding was that white youth felt that recreation would be more useful to them when they were discharged than black or Mexican-American youth. It was concluded that this was because minority group youth felt that their home communities offered extremely limited recreation facilities or programs, and thus, what they had learned in the program could not readily be carried over into community life.

Examples of Other Programs

A number of other examples might be cited of superior programs in correctional or youth-care institutions. In many cases, these are found in youth homes operated by voluntary or denominational agencies.

One such illustration is provided here: the Dobbs Ferry Children's Village, in Dobbs Ferry, New York. This institution cares for neglected, emotionally disturbed or socially maladjusted boys whose families are unable to provide adequate care for them.

It has an extensive program of sports, musical and dramatic activities, hobbies, trips and special events. In addition to these regularly-provided activities, it has experimented with a number of unique programs which have been extremely successful in involving children with limited recreational backgrounds and interests.

One of these programs has involved nature activities. Children's Village operates an extensive nature study and hobby program, including 32 different organized activities, such as the study and observation of mammals, reptiles and amphibians, plants, birds, insects and other arthropods. While studying mammals, for example, the children collected nearly 30 assorted skulls and portions of skeletons, usually of skunks, raccoons, opossums and birds, found in the woods adjacent to the Village. They restored and mounted these artifacts, became involved in field trips and in a variety of other experiences related to natural science and animal life.

The institution also maintains an extensive winterized zoo, with a variety of birds, and domestic and small wild animals. Many of the children are involved in the care of these animals; this experience has been found to be of great value in working with emotionally disturbed children, who often have difficulty in relating to their peers, and in accepting other types of responsibility.[29]

A second major project of the Children's Village has been the development of unique outdoor recreation areas. Working under the direction of professional staff members, children have built an elaborate Indian village, with tepees, totem poles, archery ranges and similar facilities. Materials were bought from government surplus stocks or donated. The Indian village has become the site of many interesting activities related to Indian lore, including arts and crafts, tests of courage, music, dance and other programs based on Indian rituals. In addition to this project, children have also built a space center, an Army camp center, a pioneer fort and a Western town. Each of these facilities is used for varied forms of outdoor recreation activity, including camping out, pageants and similar program features.

Need for Improvement of Correctional Programs

Despite these examples, it should be stressed that the majority of correctional institutions do *not* provide adequate recreational programs, or for that matter, adequate rehabilitation services overall. This is particularly true of prisons for adult offenders. One authority, the Police Commissioner of the City of New York, has characterized the nation's prison systems as a "total failure." He describes the criminal justice program as a "perpetual-motion machine," in which police arrest felons and send them into the courts, which send them into prisons, which in turn send them out into the streets to be re-arrested:

> We do no more for the criminal in jail than we do for animals in the zoo. We cage them and feed them. The average citizen has seen prison purely and simply as retribution. The uglier and grimier and older the prison, the more it has seemed to the average citizen to be a fine and splendid prison.[30]

What is needed is a widespread revolution in public attitudes, and the infusion of large sums of money to replace vengeance with rehabilitation in the correctional system. If this does not happen, jails will continue to be nothing more than "warehouses for contaminated goods," and prison riots, crime and the rate of recidivism will continue unabated.

---

[29] Howard Romack: "Children's Village Experiments." *Parks and Recreation,* April, 1969, p. 39.

[30] "Murphy Attacks Nation's Prisons as 'Total Failure.'" *New York Times,* January 29, 1972, p. 33.

This point of view is strongly supported by Ramsey Clark, who points out that the present sum of less than two billion dollars a year spent in all correctional programs (federal, state and local) should be doubled. However, he stresses that the mere increase of expenditures in this field will not solve this problem; it is necessary to develop entirely different approaches to law enforcement and corrections. He urges the following priorities:

1. A philosophy of avoiding detention wherever possible through prevention efforts, community treatment, and probation supervision.
2. Recognition that the needs of each individual are different. Corrections programs should be carefully tailored to individual needs.
3. The creation of new substantive rights of persons convicted of crime that would require government to fulfill basic human needs in the following areas: a) health and social services; b) safety from assault, forced homosexuality, corporal punishment of solitary confinement; c) communications, including the free access to family, friends, advisors and attorneys, and the right to write and read freely; d) improved educational and vocational training programs; and e) job placement services.
4. The creation of new procedural rights for prisoners.
5. An intensive effort to move offenders to the community where they will live, making use of the following: a) improved probation and parole programs; and b) a network of work-release, prerelease guidance, and halfway houses, with small, unmarked community facilities that will assist discharged or paroled prisoners in making the transition to responsible and law-abiding community life.[31]

Only if such programs are developed will it be possible to overcome the present weaknesses of our corrective and penal system which are so destructive to human life and dignity. Within such programs, recreation must play an increasingly strong role, in contributing to the rehabilitation process, and in helping offenders return successfully to their communities.

Recreation and the Treatment of Drug Addicts

The problem of drug addiction has increased tremendously in the United States over the past decade. There has been an explosion of drug experimentation and addiction, particularly among the young. While estimates vary greatly, there is evidence that a majority of the students in many schools and colleges are at least occasional users of marijuana.[32] When the Gallup college drug survey was initiated in 1967, only 5 per cent of all college students said they had tried marijuana. By 1972, the percentage was over 50 per cent.

Accurate statistics are not available for other forms of drugs, but it is evident that this has become a major problem of American youth, on all levels of society. Heroin, once used chiefly by blacks in urban ghettos, has now made inroads in fashionable suburban communities. It is being used at an increasingly early age. In New York City alone—where experts estimate that roughly half the nation's heroin addicts live—over 200 teen-agers died from overdoses or heroin-related infections in a recent year. At the California-based Synanon self-help centers for addicts, the teen-age population has risen from zero in the mid-1960s to 400 by 1970. A San Francisco drug authority called heroin:

. . . the most readily available drug on the streets. In my wildest nightmares, I never dreamed of what we are seeing today . . .[33]

By the early 1970s, drug addiction had reached "epidemic" proportions in Vietnam. Military authorities were concerned about the easy flow of heroin to American soldiers, and the soaring numbers hooked on this deadly narcotic—not only because

---

[31] "A Nickel for Rehabilitation." *New York Times,* September 30, 1971, p. 46.

[32] Peter Kihss: "Gallup Finds Rise in Marijuana Use." *New York Times,* February 6, 1972, p. 52.

[33] "Kids and Heroin: The Adolescent Epidemic." *Time,* March 16, 1970, p. 16.

of their immediate medical problem, but also because of the danger to American society when addicted soldiers return to the mainland with a craving for a drug that costs many times more than it did in Asia.

On all levels, the drug problem poses a challenge to educational, medical and social authorities in the United States.

Although most adults tend to be shocked by the growing statistics of drug use among children and youth, the fact is that adults themselves are extremely heavy users of tranquilizers and other legal, or prescribed, stimulants. Many millions of adults are "hooked" on cigarettes or alcohol, and teen-agers frequently comment that for them, "pot" is no different from their parents' martini cocktails. Indeed, it seems clear that for many, drug-taking represents a form of leisure activity, a way of having fun, of avoiding boredom. One mental health authority suggests that "for people who are chronically unhappy, drugs bring some relief from a world without purpose." Corry writes:

> Students themselves are not particularly articulate about why they take drugs. For kicks, they say, or because they are bored, or because drugs are easy to get or because drugs offer them deep personal insights. . . . They offer an illicit pleasure that is almost entirely without sanction in the adult world and they open an immense gap between parent and child.[34]

Hechinger suggests that among middle-class youth, drug experimentation is the "chain reaction of a combination of permissive homes with the speed-up of youth's experiences in an affluent society." The early onrush of adolescence encourages youth to experiment with partying, dating, sex, smoking, drinking and, before long, glue-sniffing and marijuana. "As old thrills wear off, the search is on for new ones."[35] In the armed forces, it

has been concluded that alcoholism among senior noncomissioned officers and drug abuse among young draftees stem from boredom.[36]

Resistance to constructive, organized programs, and the choice of escape through drugs frequently stem from social attitudes that "put down" the "establishment" and prefer instead, the illicit lure of narcotics or alcohol. Realistically, the sensation gained from drug use provides pleasure that is far more overwhelming than that which other activities might yield. One sociologist who has examined hundreds of marijuana users comments that a variety of reasons have been advanced for its growing popularity. These include such explanations as: (a) it is an "escape from reality;" (b) kids today are frightened and insecure, and "grass" is a misplaced effort at solving problems; (c) marijuana is an "ego-boost for youngsters with low self-esteem;" (d) it is a product of a too "permissive" society; (e) it is a result of social pressure from peers; and (f) it is a form of rebellion against one's parents or the society at large, or a means of doing something daring and dangerous.

However, Goode concludes:

> The simple fact is, marijuana is fun to smoke. . . . In my own study of marijuana users, pleasure emerged as the dominant motive for continued use. Almost 70 per cent said that sex was more enjoyable high. Almost 90 per cent said that the simple act of eating became more fun. Almost 90 per cent said that listening to music was a richer, more exciting adventure. . . . Marijuana has become, and will continue to be, increasingly, a *recreational* drug, and for larger and larger numbers of young (and not so young) people. This will not disappear, and it will not abate; drug "education" campaigns are doomed to failure. . . . Outlawing fun has always been a tough job.[37]

There continues to be considerable controversy about the actual effects of mari-

---

[34] John Corry: "Drugs a Growing Campus Problem." *New York Times*, March 21, 1966, p. 27.

[35] Fred Hechinger: "Drugs: Threat on Campus." *New York Times*, April 10, 1966, p. E-7.

[36] David Binder: "A Dangerous Foe: Boredom of G.I.'s." *New York Times*, March 14, 1972, p. 7.

[37] Erich Goode: "Turning on for Fun." *New York Times*, January 9, 1971, p. 27.

juana. A growing body of experts have concluded that this form of drug use is nonadditive and actually less dangerous than many other stimulants, including alcohol. On the other hand, evidence has been gathered of numerous psychotic reactions stemming from marijuana use. There appear to be marked behavioral changes associated with the use of marijuana among some subjects. Wikler writes of a group of subjects involved in a pharmacological experiment that:

> During the first few days, they exhibited euphoria, bursts of spontaneous laughter, silly behavior, and difficulty in concentrating. Later, they showed loss of interest in work, decreased activity, indolence, nonproductivity, and neglect of personal hygiene. . . .[38]

There is also considerable evidence that many young people move from experimentation with marijuana, glue-sniffing, pills and other soft drugs, to involvement with harder and more dangerous narcotics. Without question, it is essential that every effort be made to stem the tide of drug use in American society.

Recreation in Drug Treatment Centers

Obviously, there are a number of different forms of care for drug addicts. One method is the so-called British system, based on the premise that heroin addiction is a sickness, not a crime. This approach makes drugs available, by prescription, to formally registered addicts, and is intended to meet the needs of those who are unwilling to undergo a cure or enter an institution—thus minimizing the commercial exploitation of the drug addict's needs.

A second approach to the problem of heroin addiction is the methadone maintenance program. This involves switching an addict from heroin, which can cost $50 or more a day, obtained illegally, to methadone, a synthetic substitute that costs about 15 cents for a day's dosage. Methadone eases heroin withdrawal and blocks heroin's euphoric effects. However, it is addictive in itself, and many legal and medical authorities resist substituting one form of addiction for another. On the other hand, methadone is much less dangerous than heroin, and permits the addict to lead a relatively normal life.

The most popular approach to working with drug addicts has become the small, controlled therapeutic community, like Synanon, begun in California and extended throughout the country, or New York's city-run Phoenix and Horizon House. Such residential centers are run largely by former addicts; they first detoxify and then attempt to rehabilitate the drug user by restructuring his ego and life pattern. They accept only those who have proved their determination to kick the habit, and they strive to increase the addict's self-understanding and self-regard through frequently brutal group-encounter sessions.

The traditional method of institutional care has been the special hospital, or hospital unit, such as the two federal narcotics hospitals at Lexington, Kentucky, and Fort Worth, Texas. Most of these programs are more conservatively run. Having been ordered there by the courts, their patients are less highly motivated for change, and records indicate that over 90 per cent of those discharged from such institutions eventually return to heroin.[39]

Finally, there are a variety of treatment centers connected to mental health hospitals or outpatient programs, part of state mental health systems, or municipal or voluntary hospitals. Many of these are residential, while others provide a variety of "crisis" or continuing treatment services for addicts living in the community. In almost all cases, they use a variety of treatment approaches, including individual and group therapy, remedial education, vocational training and placement and other social services—including recreation.

---

[38] Abraham Winkler: "Marijuana *Is* Dangerous." *New York Times,* April 3, 1971, p. 29.

[39] "How Addicts Are Treated." *Time,* March 16, 1970, p. 20.

The nature of recreation service in drug addiction centers is heavily influenced by the typical personality patterns of drug users. Characteristically, they tend to have extremely low self-esteem, to be overly dependent on others and to have a very weak capacity for frustration. Their defense and adjustment mechanisms are often juvenile; they demand immediate gratification, have little sense of time and are unable to plan effectively for the future.

Like other social deviants, drug users typically engage in few organized, constructive recreational activities. While they may have been involved in sports or social programs at an earlier point, they usually relinquish such interests when they become heavily addicted. Their lives revolve about the drug culture. They associate with other addicts; getting and using drugs becomes their chief preoccupation. Those who work with addicts in drug treatment programs comment that they tend to be extremely passive in their use of free time, and that they usually resist structured programs.

The goals of recreation in treatment centers for drug users should therefore be:

1. To contribute to the overall rehabilitation of the addict, in terms of his developing more varied interests and talents for the constructive use of leisure time that may lessen the need for him to turn to drugs for pleasure or release.
2. To encourage personality changes that will strengthen his self-concept and ego controls and give him a sense of personal worth and accomplishment.
3. To contribute to the overall therapeutic environment by providing a relaxed, tension-free atmosphere, and by encouraging enjoyable group activities which can break down barriers among participants, and between participants and staff members.

The specific forms that therapeutic recreation service may take in programs for drug addicts may depend heavily on the particular setting. In state treatment centers, programs tend to be of a traditional type, depending heavily on organized sports and arts and crafts. In community-based facilities, they are usually much less formally organized, and involve more casual and relaxed activities.

Young and Hutchison suggest that a key factor in such programs is the need for the recreation specialist to establish a relationship of mutual trust and respect with the addict under treatment. It may take days or weeks for this to develop, and it is essential that he become accepted as a trustworthy person who is not going to "put down" the addict in any verbal or nonverbal way. Gradually, he must come to be seen—not as a representative of the establishment—but simply as a friend and helper. They write:

> The therapeutic recreation program revolves around a "core" of planned group activities. Enough variety is provided in group programming to give each individual patient a chance to find his sphere of interest and to function at his particular level of comfortable interaction with others. Because the attention and interest span of the post-addict tends to be limited, specific recreative activities are provided in periods of from thirty minutes to one hour in length. The number of activities per day, and the number of times an individual patient is involved in a given activity per day or per week depend on the center's population at a given time. Activities that allow for various combinations of patient-staff ratio are scheduled according to the individual patient's current level of dependency.[40]

Young and Hutchison stress that it is important not to place too much pressure on the addict during the initial stages of his treatment. Although he has passed through the physiological trauma of withdrawal, he is still fighting a psychological battle to remain off drugs. The specific rules related to attendance and behavior at the center involve a degree of pressure

---

[40] Elliott G. Young and Ira Hutchison: "Prescription Recreation: A Bridge to Community Living for the Narcotics Addict." *Recreation in Treatment Centers,* September, 1964, p. 60.

which many addicts find difficult to accept. Until they can comfortably handle these basic responsibilities, it is useless—and can be damaging—to exert additional pressures.

Gradually, patients are encouraged to develop sustained interest in specific forms of recreative activity. Among the special interest activities suggested by Young and Hutchison as appropriate for such groups are: instrumental "combos," listening to music, vocal groups, weightlifting, dramatics, newspaper work, social dancing, cooking and such hobbies as stamp clubs and model railroading. Other program activities found in addict rehabilitation programs include: bingo, table tennis, billiards, table games like chess and checkers, crafts like ceramics and weaving, movies, gardening, work parties and discussion groups.

At this phase of involvement, there is usually a shift in the addict's level of participation. When this is observed, leadership approaches are changed:

> . . . a gradual increase of pressure from the staff, and involvement in situations where the post-addict takes more responsibility—and risks greater chance of failure—are introduced into the individual program plan. At this point, the recreation specialist becomes primarily a supportive figure. He spares no effort to ease the transition from a dependent attitude and existence to a semi-independent or independent level of functioning.[41]

LEADERSHIP RESPONSIBILITIES.
Throughout this process, the recreation leader working with addict groups must operate much less as a direct, authoritarian leader of activities, and much more as a nondirective counselor and friend, a catalyst who gently encourages and makes changes in behavior and attitudes possible.

The recreation specialist must function as a professional member of the treatment team. He should be fully involved in interdisciplinary staff meetings, and should work closely with psychiatrists, psychologists, unit counselors, vocational rehabili-

tation specialists and other personnel to exchange information and share in planning to meet the needs of each patient. Furthermore, he should be active in promoting community programs designed to serve addicts and discharged patients. Some of his functions may include:

1. Conducting community meetings and orientation sessions to assist civic groups or the professional staffs of other agencies in serving addicts.
2. Providing continuing consultation services to such groups, and demonstrating specific techniques useful in involving addicts in community recreation programs.
3. Scheduling special events, such as carnivals, open houses, dances, lectures and workshops, in order to encourage community involvement in the work of the rehabilitation center.
4. Encouraging work by community volunteers in the center's program.
5. Providing individual and group recreation-counseling sessions with postaddicts, both before and after discharge, and accompanying post-addicts to community recreation programs, especially in the early stages of their return to community life.
6. Periodically checking with community recreation personnel and offering assistance in solving problems which may inevitably be expected to arise.
7. Joining in community task forces designed to attack the problem of addiction, and emphasizing the role of recreation in this overall program. His emphasis should be on educating other professionals and the public at large on the objectives and techniques of therapeutic recreation service for narcotics addicts.

These responsibilities suggest a major area of concern for all recreation personnel who have a special responsibility for working with the socially deviant—the need to promote more effective community-based services to serve such groups.

---

[41] *Ibid.,* p. 61.

Community Recreation Programs and Delinquency

As indicated, since its inception in the early decades of this century, the recreation movement has had as a major purpose the prevention and "cure" of juvenile delinquency. The slogans of "keep kids off the streets," or "give them something useful to do," have been the basis for funding many public recreation agencies, particularly in large cities, where youth problems have been severe. However, few recreation departments have been successful in this area of concern. The reasons for this failure have been several:

1. Most obviously, delinquency is the result of a variety of factors, such as family instability, slum housing, poor education, limited vocational opportunity or the lack of other vitally needed social services. Within this context, it is unrealistic to believe that recreation, by itself, can significantly deter delinquent activity. However, it can and should be an important part of total community efforts to serve the socially deviant.
2. Most recreation departments and agencies do *not* make a special attempt to serve delinquent or predelinquent youths. Often they view this as a difficult task which they are not equipped to handle. In many cases they bar disruptive and antisocial youth from their facilities, thus making it impossible to serve them meaningfully.
3. Usually, antisocial and gang youth reject organized activities and are unwilling to become part of the formal structure of community agencies. In part this is because they do not wish to be controlled, or because their high-impulse, hedonistic values are unwilling to conform to the rules and limitations inherent in youth programs, team sports and the like.

In some cities, gangs may use community centers as hangouts—often discouraging other participants from entering. However, it is rare for them to be meaningfully involved in such programs. Instead, in most communities, special youth boards or commissions, or anti-poverty organizations—where these exist—have been the only formal agencies to work with delinquent youth.

Guidelines for Working with Problem Youth

How *can* the public recreation department or voluntary agency that is concerned about working with delinquent or pre-delinquent youth gangs do so effectively?

1. It is essential to view recreation, at the outset, as a positive and meaningful form of community service. Unless it is seen and supported in this light, it cannot be successful in any form of significant social programming.
2. In working with problem youth, it is not possible to plan programs at a high level of authority and simply present them with the results. Instead, it is essential to involve youth *fully* in the planning and development of programs. This may be done by having representatives from various gangs or neighborhoods join together in a recreation center council, to plan programs and formulate agency policies.
3. Gangs generally are thought of negatively—and it is true that they often are responsible for various forms of crime in urban slums. However, gangs also represent an understandable need for group affiliation, for status and even for self-protection in ghetto areas. In some cases, minority-group gangs have taken on the task of driving drug pushers out of their neighborhoods, or similar desirable goals. It is essential to recognize their existence, and attempt to work with them positively rather than simply to try to wipe them out.
4. Recreation programs designed to serve antisocial youth often fail to at-

tract them because they are not interesting or challenging enough. Therefore, such programs *must* be well planned and staffed, and should involve exciting goals and experiences. They may include trips, cultural programs, activities that have career-development potential, or—when possible—activities that have a degree of risk or danger about them. Activities like skiing or tobogganing, horseback riding or underwater exploration, which are in a sense a "testing" of manhood, have been used successfully with such youth. Their particular value is that they may sublimate the urge to take part in dangerous, unlawful activities, by providing an equally challenging, but socially acceptable leisure outlet.

5. Community center programs designed to meet the needs of delinquent youth *must* provide more than recreation. They should also include educational or remedial educational programs, vocational training and placement, psychological counseling services, drug abuse programs, and similar activities. Whenever possible, job opportunities should be provided for youth in their middle and later teens, to strengthen their work orientation, and to help them develop a sense of self-discipline and commitment. All this can be woven into the overall program of an agency that is primarily geared to offer recreation services.

6. In any long-range program intended to reduce delinquency, it is essential to reach children in the elementary school age range, between six and 12. Often, the patterns of antisocial behavior are set at the age of as low as six or seven, and children, by eight or nine, are involved regularly in criminal activity and antisocial gang affiliation. Therefore, every effort must be made to work regularly with children at this age, to reduce antisocial group involvement, and to recognize and refer to appropriate agencies those children who have severe individual problems of adjustment.

As much as possible, parents should be drawn into this effort.

7. Programs in centers need to be more carefully organized and structured. In many community centers in low-income areas, there is a constant flow—in and out—of unregistered participants. Often activities are carried on in a completely casual way, with informal games and music being the heart of the program. Instead, it is desirable to have a registration system so that only center members may enter, with rules set by the youth council itself as to the basis for membership. Programs should be scheduled and carefully directed to encourage the maximum participation in organized activities.

8. A final guideline applies to those youth who are *not* willing to enter community centers at all, and who have no regular contact with adult leaders or youth workers. These are unaffiliated gang youth, who hang out in the neighborhoods, are frequently school dropouts, and are often responsible for incidents of gang violence or sporadic criminal activity. The only solution to working with such youth is through the "out-reach" approach, under which recreation departments assign so-called roving workers to make contact with gangs, and to attempt to guide them in constructive channels.

The Roving Leader Approach

A number of cities have adopted an approach under which special youth workers—usually individuals who have themselves grown up in slum neighborhoods and may have been involved in gangs—are assigned the task of making contact with unaffiliated youth. They are usually detached from organized programs, and go out into the street, neighborhood hangouts or other places where problem youth may be found.

Typically, in Washington, D.C., where the Roving Leaders Program of the Recreation Department has been in operation since 1956, roving leaders work directly with several hundred gang youth, as well as others who are sporadically associated with gangs. They receive on-the-job training in group-work techniques, streetcorner contact methods, community resources and psychological counseling. The goals of these workers are both short-range and long-range.

Their short-range objectives are to: (a) reduce the severity and frequency of offenses, such as gang warfare, murder and theft; (b) redirect behavior into more desirable channels; and (c) help adolescents make use of available community resources. Their long-range goals are to help gang youth become more fully integrated in the "major culture," and to change their social values and life patterns in more constructive directions, in terms of becoming responsible, law-abiding and gainfully employed citizens. They have the following specific tasks:

1. To help gang youth make use of available community resources.
2. To encourage drop-outs to return to school.
3. To intervene on their behalf with school authorities.
4. To make court appearances in support of the youth, and provide assistance in hearing or correctional procedures.
5. To help boys and girls develop a more favorable understanding of adults and the total society.
6. To help them understand the consequences of their antisocial acts.[42]

Since they are often attempting to reach extremely hostile and alienated individuals, who come from broken homes, have arrest records or have been confined to correctional institutions and are wary of adult contact, leaders must often work for months and years to establish favorable rapport with target gangs. They seek to get to know them, gain their confidence, counsel and assist them and ultimately guide them in the constructive directions previously described.

While this may be seen primarily as a social-work function, it has been assigned to the Recreation Department in Washington and other cities, simply because the recreation program has the broadest capability for reaching and involving the large mass of youth in the community. In addition, recreation *is* an important aspect of the Roving Leader program. For example, programs offered by Washington's detached workers have included trips to such places as amusement parks, theatres and art galleries, and soccer, football, baseball and basketball games; also, picnics, fishing, nursing aide and census-taking projects, bowling, skating, talent shows, camping, and boat and airplane rides are offered.

The roving leader approach is being used in an increasing number of large cities. It has been encouraged by the U.S. Office of Education's Division of Manpower Development and Training, which has funded the Office of Recreation and Park Resources at the University of Illinois, in cooperation with the National Recreation and Park Association, to promote and research the roving leader concept.

Over a three-year period, between 1968 and 1971, project personnel researched examples of roving leader programs throughout the country, developed guidelines for the training of roving leaders and conducted— with assistance from the Office of Education—a series of workshops, in large cities throughout the country, for Roving Leader trainers. Efforts are now being made to promote programs of Roving Leader training, in two-year community colleges throughout the country, as part of manpower leadership development to meet social needs.[43]

Such programs are examples of how recreation may serve preventative as well as treatment needs—in community settings as well as in institutions. Obviously, the problem of working with deviant groups is much less costly, both in human and financial terms, if it can be done be-

---

[42] *Roving Leader Program.* Manual of Washington, D.C., Recreation Department, 1970, pp. 4–5.

[43] Joseph J. Bannon: "The Roving Leader: A New Look." *Parks and Recreation,* February, 1972, pp. 23–24.

fore patterns of serious antisocial behavior are clearly established. The treatment process in institutions is too often ineffective when antisocial attitudes and behavior patterns have become deeply ingrained.

Therefore, a major thrust of therapeutic recreation service must be to prevent antisocial behavior at its inception. Programs like those described here are essential in this effort.

Suggested Topics for Class Discussion, Examinations or Student Papers

1. What are some of the basic factors underlying juvenile delinquency, as a major form of social deviance, that make the provision of constructive and well-planned recreation programs an essential in correctional institutions?
2. How can recreation serve both as a preventative and as a form of treatment in community and institutional programs for drug addicts?
3. Describe the use of the roving leader approach as a technique used by recreation departments to combat socially deviant gang behavior. What are its strengths and limitations as a form of community service?

Chapter 9

Community Services
for the Disabled

This chapter focuses on the role of community organizations in providing special programs to serve the needs of the disabled in noninstitutional settings. It describes the scope and focus of such agencies—both public and voluntary—and presents guidelines for expanding their efforts.

Focus of Community-Based Therapeutic Recreation

Obviously, it is the purpose of community-based recreation or social service agencies to serve disabled persons who are not housed in institutions, but live with their families or in other settings where they have a degree of social independence. The great majority of aging or mentally retarded persons, for example, are not institutionalized. However, they may require modified or specially designed programs or environments to meet their recreational needs.

While the goal of therapeutic recreation service is to integrate the disabled with the nondisabled wherever possible, this is not always a feasible objective. Essentially, the disabled may be divided into three categories, whatever the nature of their particular limitation:

1. Those whose limitations are so severe that they require completely separate

and segregated programs and social groupings. This may be because they are unable to participate successfully in activities carried on by the nondisabled, or because they are rejected by the nondisabled or excluded by sponsoring authorities.

2. Those whose disabilities prevent them from taking part in integrated programs in some areas of activity, but who can readily share in other programs. To illustrate, children with severe physical impairments might not be able to engage in sports leagues with nondisabled children, as part of a summer playground program, but might engage successfully in arts and crafts or dramatic activities, on an integrated basis.

3. Those who are able to take part with a considerable degree of success in varied activities with the nondisabled. Efforts should be made to integrate such individuals as fully as possible with the overall population.

For many individuals, it is possible to go through a process of gaining social and physical skills and self-confidence, and thus move from segregated programs into integrated group membership. As an example, disabled children may become involved first in a day camp serving those with impairment on a segregated basis.

Gradually, they may become able to attend a sleep-away camp and, ultimately, to take part in camping programs that serve both the disabled and the nondisabled.

In the case of illness which involves a process of recovery and rehabilitation, the issue of segregated versus integrated grouping should be seen as a continuum of service. The mentally ill patient, for example, engages initially in recreation programs in the hospital setting, on a segregated basis (see pages 80–93). He may become involved more fully in integrated programming by attending community activities that serve both types of clientele, and ultimately should move into participation in such programs on a completely integrated basis.

According to the degree of integration which is possible, various types of programs may be provided. Usually, their sponsors fall into the following categories.

Sponsors of Community Services for the Disabled

PUBLIC RECREATION AGENCIES. These include public recreation or recreation and park departments, school districts, youth service agencies, community service departments in housing projects, publicly sponsored libraries, museums or other agencies which provide recreation for the public at large.

ORGANIZATIONS CONCERNED WITH DISABILITY. As described earlier, a considerable number of national organizations with local or regional chapters promote programs designed to meet the needs of individuals with special disability. If they do not provide such services directly, often they cooperate with other agencies that do, by providing funding, technical advisement, volunteers or other forms of support.

SERVICE ORGANIZATIONS. In most American communities, there are a variety of service organizations or civic clubs that are committed to providing or assisting programs that meet social needs. Fraternal or service organizations such as the Elks, Moose, Kiwanis or Oddfellows, or veterans' organizations, such as the Veterans of Foreign Wars or the American Legion, are frequently involved in sponsoring programs serving disabled children and youth.

SPECIAL AGENCIES. In a few cities, special agencies have been established that have as their primary purpose the provision of recreation to varied groups of disabled persons. One such agency, the San Francisco Recreation Center for the Handicapped, is described later in this chapter.

COMMUNITY COUNCILS OR BOARDS. In order to develop systematic recreation services to meet the leisure needs of disabled persons, special community councils or boards have been formed in a number of major cities. Such councils usually serve to promote public awareness of the needs of the disabled, to identify existing programs and to make recommendations for, develop support and coordinate new services.

The range of services offered is extremely wide. It may include any or all of the following:

Social clubs for mentally retarded or physically disabled youth and adults.

Day camps or special residential vacation camps for those with varied disabilities, including the aging.

The sponsorship of special facilities, such as playgrounds, parks or community centers, designed to be suitable for those with physical handicaps.

After-care programs for discharged mental patients, former drug addicts or other persons who require sheltered social settings in their transition to community life.

Volunteer services for homebound individuals with severe disability.

Public Recreation Programs for the Disabled

In a number of major cities around the United States, as well as in many smaller communities, public recreation or recreation and park departments offer comprehensive programs to serve the leisure needs of the physically and mentally disabled.

Similarly, in a number of Canadian cities, interest has grown in providing rec-

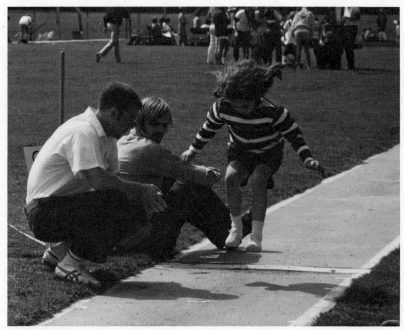

Example of municipally sponsored recreation for special groups: children take part in a state-wide Olympics track meet funded by the Kennedy Foundation and conducted by the Eugene, Oregon Department of Parks and Recreation.

reation for the ill and disabled. In Vancouver, British Columbia, for example, the number of elderly persons served in municipal recreation activities departments expanded from 21,414 in 1963 to 108,269 in 1970, while participation figures for disabled children in summer programs rose from 781 to 2519 during the same period. The city park and recreation department offers "meals on wheels" services to shut-ins, serves disabled elderly persons in community center day-care programs, and offers weekly recreational activities to mental health patients living in city-licensed boarding houses. In Winnipeg, Manitoba, and in the city of Montreal, similar programs have been initiated to serve mentally retarded children, the physically disabled, and aging persons.

In Seattle, Washington, an extensive program of services is offered under the direction of a full-time therapeutic recreation specialist employed by the Recreation Division of the municipal Park Department. The schedule of special programs in Seattle includes such elements as:

1. Monthly meetings for disabled children in various recreation centers around the city, usually on Friday or Saturday afternoons. These are continued throughout the year and involve varied club and recreational activities.
2. Special swimming lessons for disabled children, given in ten-week series during the fall. These are specially designed so that there is at least one instructor for every two or three children. Beginners, or those who cannot support themselves in the water, are taught individually.
3. A summer day camp for disabled children six years of age or older. These are held in three three-week sessions at several camp and park locations in Seattle and King County. Activities include nature crafts, music, games, singing, creative dramatics, sports, cookouts and hiking.

Other programs in Seattle include special groups organized by the Cerebral Palsy Workshop and the Washington Association for the Retarded. There is a special bowling league for the retarded, and wheelchair basketball for the orthopedically disabled, as well as a basketball league for adult deaf participants. A major portion of the leadership is provided through the use of volunteers, with the assistance of a central volunteer bureau and a number of service agencies in the community.

Many other cities offer comparable programs. For example, the Los Angeles Park and Recreation Department provides programs for blind adults, multiply-disabled youth, the physically disabled and the mentally retarded.

The Chicago Park District has special programs for the disabled in 15 of its major centers, providing assistance to Alcoholics Anonymous, to the mentally retarded or perceptually handicapped, to the deaf and blind and to discharged mental patients and their families.

The Ill and Handicapped Division of the Greensboro, North Carolina Parks and Recreation Commission provides 18 different programs for the mentally retarded, cerebral palsied, blind, orthopedically handicapped, emotionally disturbed and other disabled individuals. Special programs are provided for nursing homes, and a six-week summer day camp serves a substantial number of disabled children with music, nature activities, games, sports and crafts.

Based on a study of recreation services for the ill and disabled in selected public recreation departments, Miller has presented a number of basic recommendations for community organization in this field.

It is her view that, while voluntary organizations or inter-agency councils may be extremely effective in arousing public awareness of needs, or providing advice or technical assistance, it is the public recreation department that should carry the major responsibility in this area. She recommends that:

1. Local public recreation systems recognize and assume responsibility for making recreation opportunities available to the ill and disabled in their communities.

2. Public recreation administrators assume the initiative and leadership in developing such programs.
3. Established principles for community recreation be used, in carrying on non-institutional recreation programs for the ill and disabled.
4. The resources of those agencies familiar with working with the ill and disabled be used in planning, cooperating, and evaluating such programs.
5. Such programs represent "community efforts," from their initial planning, to the developmental phase and finally the execution of the program.
6. Primary responsibility for administering the program be centered in the local, public recreation managing authority.
7. Financial support be established on a continuing basis, through the contributions of both public and private agencies.
8. An advisory committee be established, representing various community groups, with definite duties and responsibilities outlined in a written charter, and consistent with the administrative policies of the local public recreation system.
9. Appropriate professional consultation be utilized, especially in the initial stages of planning and development of community recreation services for the ill and disabled.[1]

Organizations Concerned with Specific Forms of Disability

Many voluntary community organizations which are concerned with specific disabilities, such as blindness, mental retardation, cerebral palsy or orthopedic disability, provide recreation service as a part of their total program of rehabilitation and social assistance. A list of the national offices of such organizations and federations is provided elsewhere (see p. 223). In many cases, the national organization carries on research, or develops guidelines or materials in this area, or provides other forms of funding assistance. Usually, when direct programs of recreation sponsorship are offered, it is by local chapters or organizations in the cities themselves.

[1] Betty Miller: "Re-Count for Recreators." *American Recreation Journal*, November-December, 1963, p. 19.

While it is not possible to provide examples drawn from each of these organizations, an excellent illustration may be found in the work of the Lighthouse, a service center operated by the New York Association for the Blind. This voluntary, nonsectarian, nonprofit agency serves legally blind, visually impaired persons (many of whom are multiply disabled), with a year-round program. Its clientele consists of approximately 3300 persons ranging in age from six months to 90 years, of all races, creeds and socio-economic backgrounds.

Its overall services include the following:

1. Medical, including a Low Vision Clinic.
2. Rehabilitation, including evaluation of needs, orientation and individual training in mobility.
3. Social services: admission, referral consultation and case work, with respect to personal and economic problems, welfare status and similar problems.
4. Music school.
5. Library service.
6. Recreation and camping.
7. Transportation.
8. Men's and women's residences.
9. Lighthouse Industries, including a sheltered workshop.
10. Craft shop.
11. Child development center.
12. Nursery school.
13. Reader's service.
14. Food service.

The objectives of the Recreation and Camping Division include the following: (a) providing recreational counseling, in order to help clients develop a personal philosophy of recreation that meets their needs and skills for participation; (b) providing information as to available community opportunities for recreation; (c) using recreation to assist in the personal development, social adjustment, health and appearance of participants; and (d) promoting participation in independent, self-directed programs.

Activities are offered for five different age groups or categories of visually disabled persons, ranging from children of nursery school age to a recreation program for older adults. They include a wide range of both active and passive activities, such as arts and crafts, bowling, trips, table games, dancing, dramatics, swimming, newspaper work, and such special events as parties, festivals, carnivals, and fairs and similar programs. The Lighthouse operates its own 14-story building, with such recreation facilities as bowling alleys, a swimming pool, social hall, auditorium, lounges, crafts shops, a play roof for younger children and two summer camps for residential camping.[2]

Similar programs for the blind are offered by voluntary agencies in such cities as San Francisco, California; Duluth, Minnesota; Jackson, Mississippi; Newark, New Jersey; Raleigh, North Carolina; and Cleveland, Ohio. A number of these organizations sponsor excellent summer camping programs, using their own camps and lodges, which are specially adapted for those with visual disability.

Service Organizations

Fraternal, civic and service organizations like the Elks, Moose, Lions, Oddfellows or Kiwanis have traditionally taken a strong responsibility for providing special programs for the disabled. In the past, with comparatively few services offered by public recreation departments, these organizations cooperated closely with health and welfare agencies to co-sponsor recreation programs of this type. As a single illustration, the Lions of North Carolina have joined together with the North Carolina Association for the Blind, to develop Camp Dogwood, a camp and vacation facility for visually handicapped residents of that state, at a projected cost of approximately a half million dollars.

There are numerous other examples of such organizations, along with civic groups and youth associations, such as the Boy

---

[2] *Program Report of Recreation and Camping Department.* New York Association for the Blind, 1972.

and Girl Scouts, that assist or sponsor programs for the disabled.

Special Agencies for Therapeutic Recreation

In a limited number of cities, special centers have been established to provide recreation for the mentally and physically disabled.

A leading example is the Recreation Center for the Handicapped, Inc., in San Francisco, California.[3] This nonprofit corporation has pioneered in providing therapeutic recreation service in the San Francisco Bay Area since 1952, when it was founded as a demonstration project to meet the needs of the disabled. It provides year-round recreation and camping programs for children, youth and adults. Most are severely handicapped—many in wheelchairs, on crutches or even bedfast. Others have severe speech impediments, visual handicaps or hearing loss. This program, directed by Janet Pomeroy, a noted authority in the field of therapeutic recreation service, serves over 550 children, youth and adults. In a recent year, over 15,000 program hours each month were provided, with supervision by over 20 full-time recreation professionals and a large number of volunteers.

The bulk of the Center's programs is carried on in the Fleishhacker Pool Building on the Great Highway, in San Francisco. The building has been converted to include two large social halls, a craft room, music room, library, multipurpose rooms, stage, offices, kitchen, gymnasium, indoor swimming pool and four activity rooms. Outdoor activities are also provided on a day camp site adjacent to the Center and at Lake Merced—a nearby zoo, playground and beach. Resident camping is provided at La Honda, approximately 60 miles from San Francisco.

FUNDING. The Center began with completely private funding, and still relies heavily on contributions. Its Board of Di-

rectors raises a major portion of the budget through solicitations from individuals, civic and fraternal organizations, fund-raising campaigns, shows, benefits and rummage sales. However, the San Francisco Recreation and Park Department, the Community Mental Health Service and the Department of Social Services subsidize a portion of the Center's budget on a contractual basis. It has also received as many as five federal grants at a time to provide care for previously institutionalized, mentally retarded participants, children receiving day care services, and to support a physical fitness program serving all participants. The San Francisco Recreation and Park Department donates the use of the Fleishhacker Pool Building, and fees are paid by the families of participants who are able to afford them.

TRANSPORTATION. Participants of all ages are transported from their homes to the Center and back each day, including those in wheelchairs, on crutches and on portable cots. Nine specially equipped buses are in operation six days a week, from 8 A.M. to 11:30 P.M., with transportation planned by a full-time coordinator, and 14 bus drivers—specially selected for their skill in working with severely retarded and disabled participants—working on day and evening shifts.

Whenever possible, parents of disabled children provide transportation for their children; furthermore volunteer aides assist in accompanying children on the daily bus trips. In addition to traveling to and from the Center, many special trips are scheduled throughout the year to nearby sites of interest.

PROGRAM SPONSORSHIP. The immense effort required to plan and carry out this program would not be possible without the help of an active Board of Directors, composed of both lay and professional persons representing public and private institutions, and such fields as recreation, education, medicine, welfare and business. The Board works through committees that deal with: finance and budget, program, personnel, publicity, speakers' bureau, transportation, parent auxiliary, building construction, equipment and supplies and by-laws.

[3] "San Francisco Has 'Model Recreation Program.'" *Information Center, Recreation for the Handicapped, Newsletter,* June, 1970, pp. 1, 4.

STAFF. The paid staff includes three recreation program supervisors, a co-ordinator of volunteer services, a social worker and a number of recreation leaders and specialists in varied activity areas—along with a business manager, clerical staff and other dietary and housekeeping personnel. This staff is assisted by approximately 225 volunteers throughout the year. Each year, a number of graduate and undergraduate college students serve full-semester internships at the Recreation Center for the Handicapped, along with a number of classes from various California colleges whose students carry out field work assignments there.

Program participants are separated into small groups, according to such factors as age, degree of retardation or physical impairment, social independence and mobility. A substantial proportion of the participants are multidisabled children and youth who have not been accepted in any school. During a recent five-year period, almost half of these participants improved so markedly that they were able to be accepted in city schools for the retarded, or in special classes in regular schools. In addition to this group, many previously institutionalized teen-agers and adults have gained sufficient confidence and leisure skills to be able to "graduate" into community-sponsored recreation and park programs.

The activities provided cover a broad range of recreation services, including arts and crafts, music, dance, games, sports, drama, trips and a variety of special events and trip programs. Increasingly, camping and nature-oriented activities have been introduced. Special programs for integrating even the most severely disabled with nondisabled children, teens and adults are offered regularly at the Center. In addition, integrated programs are conducted at other community recreation and camping facilities under the direction of the Center's staff.

The Recreation Center for the Handicapped is unique, in terms of its variety and scope, in the United States. While it owes much of its success to the energy and interest of its founder, Janet Pomeroy, it should be possible for other cities through-out the nation to develop similar centers, through large-scale citizen support and the development of the kinds of recreation opportunities for the disabled that are now available in San Francisco.

Community Councils or Boards

A final type of administrative structure for programs serving the disabled is the formation of a special council or board with representation from a variety of agencies and professional disciplines, and with a primary concern for providing programs for the disabled. The author has described in another text the unique work of the Greater Kansas City Council on Recreation for the Handicapped.[4] He repeats that description here, because it provides an excellent model for other communities to follow.

The Recreation Division of the Welfare Department of the Kansas City municipal government has for a number of years conducted special summer programs for the orthopedically disabled, diabetic, cardiac and cerebral palsied children. In the early 1950s, it established day camp programs for the deaf and hard of hearing and orthopedically disabled.

In 1955, a Supervisor of Special Recreation was appointed with the purpose of establishing a year-round comprehensive program of recreation service—initially for the orthopedically disabled, of whom there were estimated to be about 14,000 within the Kansas City metropolitan area. Before developing the program, the following agencies were approached for consultation and advice: the United Cerebral Palsy Association, the National Foundation for Infantile Paralysis, the Jackson County Society for Crippled Children, the Kansas City Board of Education, Goodwill Industries, the Muscular Dystrophy Association, the Arthritis and Rheumatism Foundation, the Multiple Sclerosis Association and others.

---

[4] See description of Kansas City plan in Richard Kraus: *Recreation Today: Program Planning and Leadership.* New York, Appleton-Century-Crofts, 1966, pp. 337–339.

It was found that 11 different day and overnight camping, Scouting, club and swimming programs were already being sponsored for the disabled by various organizations in the metropolitan area. However, the following important needs were revealed:

1. The majority of orthopedically disabled youth and adults in the city were not being served by the programs offered.
2. There were many adults who were able to leave their homes, but who felt they were too disabled to join regular social groups, as well as teen-agers who had gone as far as they could in school, but could not find work and therefore had lost all meaningful social involvement.
3. Many homebound children and adults were completely left to their own resources in terms of recreational pursuits.
4. Existing programs were so limited in terms of budget and staff that they could not satisfactorily meet the needs of those they attempted to serve.

In an effort to meet these needs, a Greater Kansas City Council of Recreation for the Handicapped was formed— to serve not only the physically disabled, but also those with emotional or social limitations. Encouragement and support came from a nearby Veterans Administration hospital which sought to improve opportunities in the community for its discharged patients. Other organizations which joined the Council—in addition to those first involved—included the YWCA, American Red Cross, the Junior League, the Boys' Clubs, the Visiting Nurses' Association and others. This Council worked closely with the Recreation Division in establishing policies and procedures, planning programs, helping to recruit and train volunteers, stimulating interest and participation in the program by referring disabled persons to appropriate groups and providing clerical and office assistance. Among its first steps was the establishment of a comprehensive insurance plan to protect program participants and sponsors.

Through the years that followed, the Greater Kansas City Council on Recreation for the Handicapped developed a program which included the following elements:

1. A visiting program for homebound children and adults, to help them discover new interests and abilities in such areas as games, crafts, puppetry, collections, instrument playing or other hobbies. This was based heavily on the use of volunteers.
2. A club program for orthopedically disabled adults, with stress on their taking over leadership responsibility themselves. Activities included weekly meetings, parties for holidays and special occasions, square dancing, group singing, movies, hobbies, dramatics and games.
3. A similar program for orthopedically disabled teen-agers, with activities suited to their interests.
4. A training program in home recreation activities for orthopedically disabled children, which was given to parents of such children or to other interested adults. In a series of ten sessions, workshops and discussions were held, dealing with ways of minimizing disability, modifications of recreational activities, and other forms of assistance.
5. Television programs which were directed to the orthopedically disabled. These served both to encourage them by presenting "write-in" tournaments and contests, interviews with disabled persons who had special hobbies, and the teaching of craft projects and games, and also to educate the public in general, with respect to the needs and capabilities of the disabled.

In addition, special outdoor programs were initiated during the summer months, including overnight camping for children with cardiac conditions, diabetes, cerebral palsy or blindness, and day camping for children who were deaf or hard of hearing, orthopedically disabled or mentally retarded.

Overall, the Kansas City Council on Recreation for the Handicapped serves a valuable coordinating function by: (a) making surveys of community needs for therapeutic recreation and carrying on other research projects; (b) acting as a referral agency for disabled individuals; (c) stimulating public interest; (d) enlisting the help of community groups and the public at large; and (e) recruiting and training professional and volunteer workers in this field.

Guidelines for Agencies Providing Therapeutic Recreation Service

Community agencies that seek to provide recreation services for the disabled must function within several areas of administrative concern. These include the following: (a) determining needs, priorities and capabilities; (b) developing programs; (c) providing trained leadership; (d) maintaining an effective public relations and community relations program; (e) financing programs; (f) operating needed transportation services; and (g) planning and developing facilities to serve the disabled.

Each of these is described in the following section of this chapter.

Surveying Needs, Priorities and Capabilities

It is essential to get a clear picture of the existing need for therapeutic recreation service within a given community before attempting to plan programs. In general, this is done by determining the number of persons with disability and then assessing the current ability of existing programs to serve these individuals.

There are three possible ways of determining the extent of disability in a given area. Allan writes:

The first is the abstract method of applying a formula based on the estimated or known national figures for specific types of disabil-

ities, or the composite figures and percentages for broad classes of disability from national or regional surveys, applied to the local population. The second is the pooling of available data from local agencies and services to form the basis for an "educated guess" on the total disability picture. The third method is the house-to-house survey or canvass type of personal contact, carried out on either a broad or limited segment of the community.[5]

The community survey is generally regarded as the most useful of these approaches, because it provides a fuller and more accurate picture of actual needs than the other methods, and also because it may serve as an important first step in developing community interest and a nucleus of individuals and agencies that will be prepared to carry the work further. As described by Warren, here are the major steps to be followed in carrying out a community survey:

1. *Determine Scope and Size of Survey.* It is important to determine in advance the size of the service area, the number of people to participate in the study, the amount of time available, and the degree of detail required in the survey.
2. *Sponsorship of the Survey.* Appropriate sponsorship not only lends prestige to the survey but also provides effective guidance, funding and authority. If no single sponsoring organization is suitable, it may be desirable to form a special sponsoring group or council.
3. *Cost of Survey.* It is necessary to estimate, in advance, the costs of the survey, including personnel needs, supplies, equipment, transportation and printing costs. This estimate should be realistic, and if different co-sponsoring groups agree to share the costs, this arrangement should be clearly spelled out.
4. *Organization.* A typical pattern is to develop an overall survey committee, which selects its own chairman, and a number of sub-committees. The survey committee should represent the major interests of the community, as well as those with

---

[5] W. Scott Allan: In *Community Planning for the Rehabilitation of Persons with Communication Disorders.* Washington, D.C., National Association of Hearing and Speech Agencies, 1967, p. 45.

special interest in therapeutic recreation, and with appropriate technical skills. In a large-scale survey, it may be necessary to hire a professional researcher, or team of experts, to head up the study.

5. *Volunteers.* In any survey which involves large-scale interviewing or canvassing, it is helpful to be able to count on volunteers. These may be drawn from interested parents, representatives of service organizations, college students, or similar groups.

6. *Survey Instruments.* Forms for the collection of data should be carefully developed, or adapted from previously used instruments. If they have not been used before, they should be pilot-tested to determine their validity, ease of administration, and general usefulness. Complete accuracy in the collection, tabulation and presentation of all data is imperative.

7. *The Survey Report.* The survey report should cover the work of the entire survey team, integrating the findings of various sub-committees. It should outline the need for therapeutic recreation service, the target populations, the existing programs, and both short and long-range recommendations both for policies and specific projects in this area.[6]

In addition to surveys of this type, it is also advisable to consult with individuals or agencies serving the disabled. Public school administrators, special educational services for the disabled, visiting nurse services, hospital-based recreation and social work personnel, doctors, public health departments, and organizations working with the disabled, all can provide much information.

If the plan is to develop program services for a specific population, inquiries may be directed at that population. Mitchell, for example, describes the planning process followed in Washington, D.C., in developing a comprehensive community-based recreation program for the mentally retarded. After an initial survey had disclosed some 7000 retardates in the District, she writes:

In order to assess the availability of persons in this group for program, 500 of the 7,000

were sent a brief questionnaire. The 500 names were selected at random and represented a cross-section of the retarded population. Other factors considered were the families' economic conditions, place of residence, and ages of the retarded children. The results of this sample indicated that the bulk of those questioned would be interested in programs in the morning and early afternoon, and those currently enrolled in other programs would be available for Saturday programs. It was evident that many of the retarded were concentrated in certain geographic regions of the District. The original 500 names, plus an additional 1,000 names were located by address on an overlay of the District. . . . the resulting map showing both postal zones and recreation regions enabled us to locate the children in terms of their accessibility to the playgrounds and community centers which could provide special programs.[7]

If information is gathered about specific individuals, Pomeroy suggests that it should include the following:

1. Name, address, age, sex, and type of disability.
2. Type of services already being received: i.e., recreational, educational, vocational, etc.
3. Formal education, past and present; social experiences.
4. Current or past membership in or association with organizations, agencies, or clubs.
5. Individual interests, hobbies, and skills.
6. Transportation needs and resources.
7. Economic status of family.[8]

In addition to such information, community surveys should examine all recreation agencies in the community—whether or not they are currently serving the disabled. This might include the numbers, ages and types of those served, the types of recreation programs offered,

[6] R. I. Warren: *Studying Your Community.* New York, Russell Sage Foundation, 1955.

[7] Helene Jo Mitchell: "A Community Recreation Program for the Mentally Retarded." *Therapeutic Recreation Journal,* 1st Quarter, 1971, p. 4.

[8] Janet Pomeroy: *Recreation for the Physically Handicapped.* New York, The Macmillan Co., 1964, p. 41.

available facilities and leadership, financial resources and funding potential, transportation capability, and similar information.

Program Development

In planning a recreation program to serve the disabled, whether it is to be for a broad range of impairments or for a single clearly defined group, several steps need to be taken:

1. A careful survey of need, as indicated in the preceding section, carried out, with both the number and type of disabled persons and the potential sponsors of programs clearly identified.
2. In order to indicate the possible directions which the program might take, programs serving similar populations in other communities should be observed, and the professional literature explored for specific guidelines and examples. In addition, consultants and authorities on therapeutic service, or on the disability itself, might be asked to make recommendations.
3. At this point, it might be advisable to call a meeting of interested parents or relatives, to answer such questions as: "What are the recreational needs of their children?" "What types of activities would be most desirable?" "Would the parents themselves be willing to assist in terms of volunteering as program aides, or providing transportation?"

The purpose and scope of the program would have to be defined. Decisions would be made with respect to: (a) whether the program would be separate from programs for the nondisabled, or linked fully or in part; (b) whether it would be open to all types of disabled persons, or designed for one or more specific disabilities; (c) whether the program would use regular community recreation facilities, or specially designed facilities for the disabled;

and (d) the time schedule that would be most suitable for the program.

When these basic guidelines are determined, it becomes necessary to plan program activities. The most suitable ones are chosen and fitted into a schedule, based on the following factors:

1. Appeal of activity: whether it would be enjoyed by participants as any group of nondisabled persons might enjoy it.
2. Suitability for age level: the activity should be one appropriate for the chronological age of participants.
3. Within range of capability: the activity should be one that can be carried on by disabled persons with a reasonable degree of success and accomplishment.
4. Therapeutic benefits: where possible, activities should be chosen that are valuable in terms of the particular disability or disabilities of the participants.
5. Suitability in terms of other factors: number of participants in group, needed facilities and equipment, staff numbers and leadership skills available.

In general, it is desirable to provide certain regular activities that are familiar and require little new instruction. At the same time, each session should involve some opportunity for new creative development or learning. There should be a reasonable balance between physical, mental, creative, social and other activities. As much as possible, disabled children should be treated like those with no physical or mental impairments and encouraged to help themselves, rather than rely on adult leaders or volunteers for assistance. Older participants should be drawn into planning and leadership whenever possible.

Providing Trained Leadership

Wherever possible, it is desirable to have professionally educated leaders with a background in therapeutic recreation service in key supervisory and leadership position. Pomeroy, for example, provides a detailed statement of the duties, training and experience requirements for three levels of leadership personnel (Center Director, Program Director and Senior Leader) as they have been developed at the San Francisco Recreation Center for the Handicapped.[9] These include such elements as graduation from a recognized college or university with a degree in recreation, group work or a related field, and minimum number of years of experience in responsible leadership or supervisory positions in recreation.

However, she also points out that as a general rule, recreation leaders who are successful in working with the nondisabled are able to work effectively with the disabled. In her view, it is not necessary for therapeutic recreation leaders to have specialized training in psychotherapy or medical aspects of disability, in order to work effectively with the physically disabled in the community. While this is generally the case, leaders or program supervisors who are knowledgeable about the causes of disability and the needs, behavior patterns and capabilities of the disabled, are likely to be more successful in designing and carrying out special programs than those who are not. A realistic compromise may be to work with leaders who have not had special training, in order to provide them with ongoing supervision and counseling by experts on the disability or other rehabilitation specialists.

The traits that are expected of leaders in therapeutic recreation are similar to those expected of all leaders in this field. They are expected to be emotionally stable, secure, patient, imaginative, enthusiastic, fair and responsible. Pomeroy also outlines several other important qualifications for therapeutic recreation leaders:

1. They must accept disabled persons fully as individuals who have the same basic needs, desires and problems as all other people.
2. They must be sympathetic to each participant's disability, but must not permit themselves to indulge in pity.

3. They must be patient and ingenious in helping adapt activities so that the severely disabled can take part in them, and must be able to inspire and encourage them to persevere.
4. They must recognize and be able to meet the specific, immediate social and recreational needs of participants, setting goals that allow a reasonable degree of achievement and pleasure.
5. They must be willing to help the disabled participants help themselves, rather than do everything for them.
6. They must be willing to do menial tasks such as feeding and lifting the disabled, assisting with toileting, and handling wheel chairs and portable beds. Pomeroy indicates that in many settings, "matrons" or "orderlies" are used for such tasks, but that when it is necessary to carry them out in community recreation programs, they are best handled by recreation staff members, with the help of additional staff and volunteers.[10]

As indicated elsewhere, the ratio of staff to participants must necessarily be much higher in community programs for the disabled than in programs for the general population. It is therefore essential that, in addition to trained professional leadership, substantial numbers of nonprofessional aides or volunteers be involved in such programs.

Public Relations and Community Relations

This is one of the key areas of responsibility in planning and carrying out community recreation programs for the disabled. The goals of public relations include the following:

1. To arouse concern and public awareness of the need for recreation for disabled persons in the community.
2. To encourage volunteers to provide service in existing and new programs, and to stimulate financial support for programs.
3. To create a climate in which municipal government and other voluntary

[9] Janet Pomeroy: *Personnel Handbook, Recreation Center for the Handicapped.* San Francisco, California, 1970, pp. 5–22.

[10] *Ibid.,* pp. 14–16; see also Janet Pomeroy: *Recreation for the Physically Handicapped. Op. cit.,* pp. 52–69.

agencies will support programs of therapeutic recreation.

4. To inform disabled persons and their families of recreation opportunities, in order to encourage their registration and participation.
5. To report program accomplishments and development to the community at large.
6. To share information regarding therapeutic recreation with other health, welfare and social agencies that provide services to the disabled.

Depending on the specific public that must be reached, the following types of public relations media are useful:

Printed materials: newspaper stories and special features; magazine articles; newsletters and brochures; annual reports and other printed reports.

Visual and other outlets: television and radio programs; special exhibits and displays; bulletin boards; speeches, motion pictures and slide talks.

Special events: open houses, tours, special programs to which the press and public are invited.

A well-designed public relations program makes use of each of these methods.

Newspaper stories are obviously most useful in reaching the public at large with timely information, particularly publicity designed to encourage attendance at events, or to provide information about special functions, fund-raising drives or other newsworthy matters. It is important to develop favorable contacts with newspaper editors and feature writers, and to prepare professionally designed releases and articles for their use. Such releases should be simple, clear, factual, and should emphasize the human relations aspect of programs and special projects.

Newsletters and brochures are useful in reaching more specific audiences of parents, disabled youth and adults, other professionals or municipal officials. Usually, they describe the total range of therapeutic recreation services in the community, and encourage participation in specific activities, day camps, clubs or other programs. They may range from inexpensive and brief mimeographed one-

or two-page leaflets, to carefully printed and attractive full-color brochures.

Annual reports are important in summing up the total accomplishments of a therapeutic recreation program. They usually include full details of those served, budgets, facilities and staffing arrangements, cooperating organizations, special projects and similar information.

Visual media, such as television, motion pictures, slide talks or radio programs, are more difficult to arrange than printed publicity but can provide effective public relations results. Therapeutic recreation program directors should constantly be alert to the possibility of getting television or radio news coverage of interesting events, or of scheduling panel programs or other informational "spots" on the mass media. As in the case of newspaper and magazine editors, it is important to cultivate the interest and support of radio station or television program directors. They will best be able to judge the newsworthy quality of events or possible features that are brought to their attention.

Speeches, slide talks or similar presentations are useful in reaching audiences of high school or college students, Parent-Teacher Associations, service and civic clubs and similar groups.

It is not enough to publicize the existing program, in the hope that it will receive adequate coverage in the media. The program director who is alert to public relations possibilities will deliberately *plan* events of an unusual nature, which lend themselves to promotion. These may include displays, exhibits, performances, open houses, tours, field days and similar ventures which are particularly newsworthy and of interest to the public.

Since the preparation of releases, radio or television scripts, brochures or films involves highly specialized expertise, it is important to get competent staff assistance on such efforts. Frequently, volunteer assistance may be obtained from skilled members of the community who are willing to contribute their services. A professional writer or film-maker who is not able to contribute in other ways, may be willing to assist in preparing releases or articles, radio or television features, or even in the making of informational films about the program. College and university departments of film-making or television may also include such projects as class assignments.

Community relations are obviously associated with the need for developing community support for therapeutic recreation programs. However, they involve developing community relationships, in the form of advisory councils and planning groups, neighborhood teams, task forces and similar efforts. It is essential to get citizen input in planning, and to obtain the cooperation of all interested individuals and organizations, if a community-based therapeutic recreation program is to receive the fullest possible support.

Financial Support

The process of fiscal management is a complicated one and is handled in detail in books on recreation and park administration. It includes the process of budget planning and approval, maintaining fiscal controls and auditing procedures and similar functions, and is not dealt with here in detail.

However, it is important to recognize the unique problem of community-based recreation programs in obtaining adequate financial support. Such programs are inevitably much more expensive than programs that serve the nondisabled. They require a more intensive level of staffing, specialized equipment, transportation facilities and other costly services if they are to be effective. How can the needed funds be raised? Pomeroy suggests the following sources:[11]

VOLUNTARY GROUPS. Service clubs, parent auxiliaries, Parent-Teacher Associations, United Chest or United Crusade and similar organizations may all contribute funds to programs serving the disabled.

FOUNDATIONS. National or local foundations often are willing to provide funds for developing facilities, or for establishing demonstration projects. Usually, they will support an ongoing program for a limited period of time—such as two or three years—and will then expect other sources of funding to be found. In some cases, they may be willing to provide a portion of continued funding year after year, for a special program.

INDIVIDUAL GIVING. Many organizations conduct their own funding drives annually. These may include mail solicitations of individuals, companies or organizations, door-to-door campaigns or fund-raising solicitation through churches or similar organizations. They may be carried on for a limited period of weeks at Christmas time or another appropriate season, or may include a variety of fund-raising events, such as carnivals, cake sales, bazaars, charity balls, dinners or theatre parties spaced throughout the year. In addition, some organizations make a concentrated effort to encourage large-scale individual gifts, legacies and bequests among wealthy donors or families.

GOVERNMENT CONTRACTS AND GRANTS. Some agencies, like the San Francisco Center for the Handicapped, have been successful in negotiating contracts with municipal government to provide needed services for the disabled. Such contracts may be with recreation and park departments (which in effect subcontract this particular function to a voluntary agency), or may be provided by a department of welfare, youth services or aging. Other grants may be obtained from county or state welfare departments, social rehabilitation agencies for the blind or mentally ill and similar sources. Federal funding, as in the case of day care programs, may be obtained on a matching basis through the Department of Health, Education and Welfare (Title IV of the Social Security Act) or other sections of recent federal legislation supporting special education programs.[12]

---

[11] Janet Pomeroy: *Recreation for the Physically Handicapped. Op cit.,* pp. 98–107; see also Janet Pomeroy: "The San Francisco Center for the Handicapped: A Brief Description." *Therapeutic Recreation Journal,* 4th Quarter, 1969, p. 17.

[12] Janet Pomeroy: *Recreation for the Physically Handicapped. Op. cit.,* pp. 127–129.

FEES AND CHARGES. A final important source of funding may be through fees charged to the families of participants. Reasonable fees may be established for day-camping, residential camping and similar services. However, it is essential that scholarships be provided for those unable to pay such fees, to avoid excluding participants from low-income families.

Whether the sponsoring department is a public or voluntary agency, it is essential that fund-raising be recognized as a high-priority concern, and that every possible avenue of obtaining grants and needed subsidies be explored. This function also represents a responsibility in which volunteer assistance may be obtained. A financial or fund-raising subcommittee may be established, which systematically develops a financial plan, does research on possible grants and subsidies, develops proposals and sponsors fund-raising events. Businessmen, bankers and other financial experts are useful on such committees, partly because of their personal expertise, and partly because they have the contacts in the business and government world that are essential in fund-raising.

Transportation Services

This area of concern often represents the chief stumbling block that prevents large numbers of individuals from taking part in community-based programs. Thompson describes a number of major problems encountered in transporting homebound adults to a special recreation demonstration project:

1. Untrained or uncooperative drivers.
2. Uncomfortable vehicles (with unpadded seats, for example).
3. Vehicles late for pick-ups.
4. Jostling of patients.
5. Lack of portable steps.
6. Overcrowding of vehicles.
7. Poor planning by transportation management.
8. Lack of ramp for wheelchairs.
9. Unheated vehicle (winter).
10. Improper handling of wheelchairs.[13]

Private vehicles can be used in transporting the mentally retarded, mentally ill or aging persons who do not have serious physical disabilities. In some cases, volunteers are used to man such programs through car-pool arrangements. However, this approach tends to be somewhat unreliable. Proper insurance coverage is essential, and it is necessary to have additional volunteers to go along with the disabled persons being transported. Buses and taxicabs may also be used on a contract basis, to provide transportation and, while expensive, this may offer a more reliable solution to the problem.

In some communities, service organizations, such as the Kiwanis, Lions or Elks, provide transportation services; in others, the American Red Cross Motor Corps provides cars and trained drivers. Whenever commercial services are used, drivers must have appropriate licenses and should be fully aware of the responsibilities involved in carrying the disabled. Drivers must understand the special needs of the disabled, and it is important for them to know first aid procedures and be able to handle emergencies that may occur.

The task of transporting those who are severely physically impaired, and who wear heavy braces, and are on crutches or in wheelchairs or portable cots, is obviously much more difficult. Special vehicles must be provided, with fuller space, special steps to assist the ambulatory, ramps for wheelchairs or lifting devices to assist loading and unloading. A number of car manufacturing companies have designed special vehicles for this purpose.

Whatever form of special transportation is provided, the role of the driver is extremely important. Pomeroy describes the responsibilities and needed qualities of

---

[13] Morton Thompson: *Meeting Some Social-Psychological Needs of Homebound Persons Through Recreative Experience.* Project Report. New York, National Recreation Association, 1962; see also Morton Thompson: *A Program of Recreation for the Homebound Adult.* National Recreation Association, pp. 13–14.

such drivers, as outlined in the job description code of the Recreation Center for the Handicapped. Drivers must have:

1. *Knowledge of:*
    The California State Motor Vehicle Code and the Education Code, particularly as they relate to the operation of vehicles in transporting children.
    Geography of the local area.
    Safe driving practices.
    Basic preventive maintenance of automotive equipment.
2. *Ability to:*
    Operate a large and small bus with patience and skill.
    Make minor mechanical adjustments of automotive equipment.
    Understand and carry out oral directions.
    Get along well with children.
    Maintain a calm, even disposition.
    Exercise mature judgment in relation to driving and child care.
    Maintain a semblance of order on the bus.
    Handle large children and adults with heavy braces.
3. *License:*
    A valid Class "B" chauffeur's license.
    Red Cross first aid certificate.
4. *Experience:*
    Two years of successful full-time paid experience in driving commercial or heavy-duty vehicles. Experience with children. Safe driving record and current driver's license.[14]

Precise policies should be established for all aspects of the transportation program, and schedules for pickup and delivery should be worked out in full detail and maintained as accurately as possible. Generally, this is easier to do in small towns or suburban areas than in large cities where congested traffic conditions and parking difficulties make the transportation problem even more difficult to solve.

Planning Facilities for the Disabled

In general, the facilities used by recreation programs for the disabled are of the same type as those used for the population at large. Parks, playgrounds, community centers, day camps and similar facilities are widely available and, in most cases, are able to accommodate the disabled with comparatively little modification being required. As a general policy, it is desirable for programs serving the disabled to use such facilities, since they enable disabled participants to mingle with the nondisabled.

When programs involve severely disabled persons, it is obviously necessary to make sure that halls, rest rooms, entrances and similar locations are constructed so that they can readily be used by those in wheelchairs, on crutches and in braces. A number of recommended standards for outdoor recreation facilities and community centers are described in Chapter Six (see pages 139–140).

In some communities, elaborate playgrounds and day camp sites have been constructed for special use by the disabled. While these may facilitate participation by the most severely impaired, Pomeroy questions their basic value:

> The concept behind this type of area implies that the severely handicapped should grow up in a special world which isolates and protects them from the realities of everyday living. This theory is not only at odds with modern-day philosophy of the handicapped, but its implications that special facilities are needed would certainly tend to discourage community recreation leaders from establishing programs for the handicapped. A sound procedure is to use the same facilities as other people whenever and wherever feasible, rather than to build special facilities for them.[15]

In general, effective leadership and carefully planned programs are more vital to the operation of recreation activities for the disabled than specially designed facilities and equipment.

This chapter has outlined a number of examples of community-based recreation programs for the disabled, which supplement other examples provided throughout this text. The final chapter deals with the role of research and evaluation in programs for the disabled.

[14] Janet Pomeroy: *Recreation for the Physically Handicapped. Op. cit.,* p. 140.

[15] Janet Pomeroy: *Recreation for the Physically Handicapped. Op. cit.,* p. 140.

Suggested Topics for Class Discussion, Examinations or Student Papers

1. Develop a model program of therapeutic recreation service as it might be developed by a municipal recreation and park department. Indicate the ways in which this program would be linked to institutions and voluntary agencies serving the disabled.
2. Carry out a direct analysis of a community-based agency providing comprehensive services within a specific category of disability—such as a voluntary organization serving the mentally retarded or cerebral palsied. Show how recreation service is provided or assisted by this agency, and make recommendations for its improvement.
3. What is the rationale for having a nonpublic agency, such as the San Francisco Recreation Center for the Handicapped, assume major community leadership in this area? What are the advantages and weaknesses of such an administrative approach?

Chapter 10

Evaluation and Research in Therapeutic Recreation

Within any field of social service or professional practice, it is essential that efforts be made to determine the effectiveness of programs and to develop a foundation of knowledge that will buttress both the ongoing performance and the general image of the field. The two terms that are generally applied to such efforts are *evaluation* and *research*.

These processes are quite similar, in that both rely on the use of standardized instruments or investigative procedures to gather information that will be useful in improving professional practice. They differ, however, in the following respects.

MEANING OF EVALUATION. Evaluation is usually regarded as the process of determining the effectiveness of programs, leadership or other elements of professional service, in terms of achieving predetermined goals. It is generally concerned with the examination of specific agencies or situations, and it makes use of a number of research techniques, both of a quantitative and qualitative nature.

In the field of therapeutic recreation, a secondary use of the term evaluation applies to the examination of patients or other disabled persons. They are examined, through interviews, observations or the use of check-lists and rating scales, to determine their interests, disabilities, capabilities and needs.

MEANING OF RESEARCH. Research is usually thought of as an organized search for knowledge. Its objective is to discover answers to questions through the application of scientific procedures of measurement. It generally falls into two major categories: (a) so-called *pure* research, which is concerned with conceptual or theoretical questions which do not have immediate practical value; and (b) *applied* research, which is pragmatic in nature, and is intended to provide useful information.

Like evaluation, research may gather both quantitative and qualitative information. While it may involve a wide variety of measurement procedures or patterns of design, customarily it includes the following steps: (a) a concise formulation of a problem or hypothesis; (b) the development of an investigative procedure (usually referred to as a study design) appropriate to this problem; (c) the carrying out of the study, including the gathering of data; (4) scoring, analyzing and interpreting the data; and (e) presentation of conclusions and possible recommendations for action or further study.

Importance of Evaluation and Research

Why are these two processes of importance to the field of therapeutic recreation service? The most obvious reason is that they provide information which can be directly useful in developing recreation programs and services.

Beyond this practical need, however, it is obvious that any field of professional service *must* rely on more than the judgment or common sense of its practitioners as a basis for operation. The entire field of recreation service demands a fuller understanding of the dynamics of play, the meaning of leisure in society, the attitudes and expectations that underlie participation and the significance of recreation as a form of social service or government responsibility. Specifically, within the more specialized area of therapeutic recreation service, the role of recreation *as* therapy, and its relationship to other rehabilitative functions, is an issue that demands thoughtful and intelligent analysis.

During the early decades of the development of the recreation profession, it was commonplace to comment that no significant research was being carried on in recreation, and that its evaluative procedures were lacking in validity or meaning. Today, this is not the case. With the assistance of government and foundation grants, the growth of recreation curricula in colleges and universities, and increased efforts being made by professional organizations in this field, remarkable strides have been made in developing meaningful programs of research.

Evaluation in Therapeutic Recreation

Evaluation in therapeutic recreation may be carried on in the following areas: (a) determination of effectiveness in reaching goals and objectives; (b) evaluation of patient needs and interests; (c) evaluation of patient participation; (d) evaluation of specific program elements; (e) evaluation of staff performance; (f) evaluation of facilities; and (g) evaluation of program structure, and administrative and supervisory practices.

Determination of Effectiveness in Reaching Program Goals

This area of evaluation assumes that goals have been clearly stated. Assuming

that they have, and that [...] tain distinct and meas[...] it should be possible to [...] scale through which eff[...] measured.

Ratings might be mad[...] cellent, very good, good, fair and poor, for each question, with each response being given a number value. Or they might be couched in terms of descriptive phrases like: "Places heavy emphasis on acquiring new skills," "Gives moderate emphasis on acquiring new skills" or "Seldom encourages children to learn new skills." In general, each institution or program must develop its own evaluative instruments, since no standardized tests of this kind have been widely developed to cover the broad range of programs in therapeutic recreation.

A key element in such evaluative procedures is the ability of the observer to make intelligent judgments. There are four possible types of raters:

SELF-EVALUATION BY PRACTITIONER. While it is certainly valuable to encourage self-evaluation, usually the person who is responsible for a program is not able to examine his program in a completely objective light. In any case, it is usually desirable to get other viewpoints and critical reactions.

EVALUATION OF PARTICIPANTS. Those who take part in a program may be asked to judge whether its goals are being met, in their view. Often such reactions may be extremely helpful in an evaluation process. Certain groups, such as the mentally retarded or the mentally ill, may not be able to make effective judgments in their area, although their opinions or wishes may be helpful in other ways.

EVALUATION BY OTHER PROFESSIONAL PERSONNEL. Other staff members in the same institution, who are thoroughly familiar with the work of the recreation department, may be asked to evaluate its effectiveness in reaching goals. This might include nurses, doctors, social workers or other personnel.

EVALUATION BY OUTSIDE EXPERTS. Outsiders, such as leading therapeutic recreation specialists from other institutions, college teachers, professional consultants in his field or state department officials, might carry out this type of evaluation.

Evaluation of Patient Needs and Interests

A second aspect of evaluation is the process of gathering information about patients that provides the basis for counseling them in the selection of program activities, or actually prescribing group involvement for them. This may be done by having patients or other potential participants fill out check-list questionnaires which indicate the kinds of recreational experiences they have enjoyed in the past, their skill level in program areas and the kinds of activities they would like to take part in.

Evaluation of Patient Participation

Customarily, this is done by staff members, who rate patient progress over a period of time in terms of such elements as socialization, interest, level of involvement or voluntary participation. Patients may also evaluate their own participation; this may be useful both in considering the effectiveness of the program, and in assisting the rehabilitation team in reviewing their individual cases.

Evaluation of Specific Program Elements

Here, each aspect of a program—whether it be in the area of sports and games, arts and crafts, social activities or other events—may be evaluated by asking such questions as:

"Does it contribute to overall program goals of the institution?"

"Does it attract participation and regular attendance; is it popular with patients?"

"Is it administratively feasible—that is, can it easily be provided in terms of schedule, staff and facility demands?"

"Does it contribute to specific treatment needs of individual patients?"

Again, an evaluation of this type should be carried on with instruments that pro-vide a continuum of response rather than a "Yes" or "No."

Evaluation of Staff Performance

Customarily, in large institutions, it is the practice to carry out regular evaluation of staff personnel by their supervisors. These evaluations are normally based on formal records which rate the employee on such elements as: attendance, appearance, leadership qualities, organizing ability, control and discipline, initiative, judgment and responsibility.

This tends to be a fairly mechanical procedure, although it is a useful way of getting a numerical picture of staff performance. Another method is to rely on anecdotal records, in which a supervisor will observe a leader or therapist at work over a period of time, and will write a descriptive account of his performance, including both strengths and weaknesses. This case record becomes the basis for supervisory conferences. Thus, the evaluation leads to improvement of performance, which should be the main justification for carrying it out.

Evaluation of Facilities

This may be carried out with a pre-established list of desirable facilities for a particular type of rehabilitative or therapeutic recreation setting, such as: gymnasium, swimming pool, outdoor sports facilities, lounges, arts and crafts rooms and meeting rooms. While institutions vary widely, certainly it would be feasible to develop a *minimal list* as a standard for institutions.

Another way to evaluate facilities might be to establish questions that relate to their quality and usefulness. A checklist could be developed applying to various types of facilities, such as the playground: Does it offer varied pieces of equipment for creative and active physical play? Is it aesthetically designed? Are health and safety guidelines followed? Does it permit participation by children on crutches, in wheelchairs or in braces? Does it meet the needs of various age groups? Has it been effectively maintained, and is maximum use being made of it?

Evaluation of Programs

Frequently, an evaluation may be made of a total therapeutic recreation program, either a continuing program, or one which has been set up on an experimental or demonstration basis. Customarily, when this is done, the program would be evaluated on the basis of all the criteria just suggested: its effectiveness in meeting objectives, satisfying patient needs and interests, the extent of patient participation, staff performance and facilities.

A useful set of standards for the evaluation of recreation services in residential institutions has been developed by Berryman as part of a three-year study of therapeutic recreation service supported by a grant from the Children's Bureau of the U.S. Department of Health, Education and Welfare.[1] This document provides a systematic means of looking at a total program, based on 55 different standards grouped under several major categories, and supported by illustrative criteria. Examples of several standards and illustrative criteria follow:

PHILOSOPHY AND GOALS
Standard 1. The therapeutic recreation services offered are based on a written philosophy of recreation as it applies to the residential treatment center.
Criteria
a) The statement is in accord with the philosophy, purpose, and policies of the agency and has been approved by its administrative authority.
b) Within the department, provisions are made to acquaint all recreation staff members and volunteers with this statement.

ADMINISTRATION
Standard 5. Structure. Recreation services are administered by a professional department as an integral part of the in-

---

[1] Doris L. Berryman, Project Director: *Recommended Standards with Evaluative Criteria for Recreation Services in Residential Institutions.* New York, New York University School of Education, 1971.

stitution's overall functional structure.
Criteria
a) Administrative authority and responsibilities are clearly delineated in writing.
b) Responsibility for recreation services is assigned to professionally qualified staff.
c) The department administrator participates in interdepartmental meetings.

PERSONNEL
Standard 13. Personnel Practices. The institution has written personnel policies and practices which are periodically reviewed by its governing body and revised as necessary.
Criteria
a) There is a written statement of personnel policies and practices.
b) A copy of the statement is given to each employee as well as kept on file in the department.

PROGRAMMING
Standard 37. Needs and Interests of Residents. Recreation Services are designed to meet the needs, competencies, capabilities and interests of individuals and groups and take into account individual treatment objectives.
Criteria
a) There is an established method for assessing the needs, interests, competencies and capabilities of residents which includes:
 1) an interview with each resident; and/or
 2) access to pertinent medical, psychiatric and other information concerning each resident.
b) Resident committees are utilized in planning the activities program where feasible.

AREAS, FACILITIES, AND EQUIPMENT
Standard 45. Design and Layout. Recreation areas and facilities are designed and constructed or modified to permit all recreation services to be carried out to the fullest possible extent in pleasant and functional surroundings accessible to all residents regardless of their disabilities.
Criteria
a) Recreation staff and appropriate outside consultants are consulted in the designing or modification of all recreation areas and facilities.
b) Recreation areas and facilities meet local legal requirements concern-

ing safety, fire, health, sanitation, etc., codes.

EVALUATION AND RESEARCH

Standard 54. Evaluation of Recreation Services. The recreation department has established procedures for evaluating recreation services in relation to stated purposes, goals and objectives.

Criteria

a) The recreation department maintains adequate records concerning the residents. These records include:
1) periodic surveys of their interests;
2) periodic surveys of their attitudes and opinions of the recreation services;
3) extent and level of each individual's participation in the activities program;
4) where appropriate, progress reports are maintained

b) An appropriate time schedule is established for each type of evaluation. (Some aspects of recreation services will be evaluated annually, some periodically, some after each event, etc.)[2]

It should be noted that this is only a *partial* list of the standards and criteria developed by Berryman and a panel of experts. For example, the separate standards under the heading of Personnel include the following: personnel practices; job descriptions and classification system; salary ranges; hours of work; fringe benefits; hiring, assignment and promotion of employees; recruitment; evaluation of performance; workload; staffing; supporting services; orientation program; staff development; responsibilities of director; supervision; contribution to the profession; consultation; use of volunteers; and statements of suggested qualifications on several job levels.

Research in Therapeutic Recreation

The field of research in therapeutic recreation service is broader than evaluation, both in its possible focus and in the methods employed. For example, research may deal with the dynamics of patient behavior in hospitals, and the contributions of recreational experience to recovery. In a workshop on Research in Therapeutic Recreation in 1961,[3] a number of questions and problems of this type were formulated:

"What are the relative contributions of recreation activity, the relationship of the therapist to the patient, and patient activity per se?"

"What is the comparative effectiveness of free versus forced choice of recreation activities?"

"Does the personality profile of an individual determine the type of career he chooses and the recreation activity he selects?"

"How can recreation further a patient's ability to meet reality?"

"Does recreation encourage fantasy?"

"How do patients' recreational needs compare with those of the average person outside of the hospital?"

"Do psychotic patients in mental hospitals tend to have had impoverished recreational lives before their illness?"

The problems suggested at this workshop fell into four major categories: (1) What is the intrinsic value in a specific recreational activity? (2) What types of leadership are helpful in working with patients? (3) What should be the basis and values of "prescribed" over "voluntary" selected activity? (4) Is there a relationship, not necesarily cause and effect, between the recreational experiences of people and mental illness?

Professional publications and research compilations provide typical examples of research studies in this field. They fall into several broad classifications indicated by the headings.

Examination of Organized Programs

THERAPEUTIC PLAY SERVICES IN CHILDREN'S HOSPITALS IN THE U.S. (1969). This study examined a sampling of children's general hospitals in the United States, in an effort to determine the following: which hospitals provided supervised play; under what kinds of leadership; using what kinds of activities, materials

---

[2] *Ibid.*, pp. 11, 12, 17, 33, 37, 43.

[3] Martin W. Meyer: "Report from the Workshop on Research in Therapeutic Recreation." *Journal of Health, Physical Education and Recreation,* February, 1962, p. 8.

and equipment; and with what degree of program evaluation and interpretation.[4]

RECREATION SERVICES FOR THE MENTALLY RETARDED IN THE STATE OF KANSAS (1969). This study involved a large-scale survey intended to determine the scope and nature of recreation programs for mentally retarded children and youth in the state of Kansas and to develop a set of recommendations designed to improve programs and services.[5]

A STUDY OF THERAPEUTIC RECREATION SERVICES IN KENTUCKY NURSING HOMES (1970). This study examined the extent, nature and administrative arrangements of recreation programs provided for older persons in extended care facilities in the state of Kentucky. As in similar reports, in addition to providing a statistical picture of existing services, the study concluded with recommendations for improved and expanded services.[6]

AVAILABILITY AND UTILIZATION OF RECREATION RESOURCES FOR CHRONICALLY ILL AND DISABLED CHILDREN AND YOUTH IN THE UNITED STATES (1970). This survey sought to determine the extent of recreation services offered to disabled children in a cluster sampling of nine Standard Metropolitan Statistical Areas and one Consolidated Metropolitan Statistical Area in the United States. It identified a variety of existing and potential recreation resources for children and youth, as well as major needs for development in this field.[7]

Studies of Professional Development

Typically, many research studies have been concerned with professional development in the field of therapeutic recreation service. The following are a few illustrations.

THERAPEUTIC RECREATION EDUCATION: 1969 SURVEY. This report gave findings of a major curriculum study carried out by the Society of Park and Recreation Educators. It identified specialized curricula in therapeutic recreation service in colleges and universities in eight regions of the United States, and examined such elements as faculty, number of student majors, degrees offered and similar aspects of these programs.[8]

RELATIVE IMPORTANCE OF COLLEGE COURSES IN THERAPEUTIC RECREATION (1970). This study examined the degree of importance assigned to undergraduate and graduate college courses in nine major categories by a panel of 15 national leaders and 15 educators in therapeutic recreation service. Courses were placed in rank order, and conclusions were drawn that would lead to the improvement of such curricula.[9]

THE CENTRAL LIFE INTERESTS OF ACTIVITY THERAPY LEADERS IN THERAPEUTIC RECREATION (1970). This study was concerned with the basic interest patterns of individuals working in activity therapy programs in medically oriented settings. It contrasts their interests and values with those of professionals and nonprofessionals in other areas of service, and represents an example of critical examination of the membership of a professional group.[10]

Studies of Special Groups

Many recent studies have been concerned with the leisure characteristics or recreational needs of specific population groups.

[4] Yvonne Barnthouse Williams: "Therapeutic Play Services in Children's General Hospitals in the U.S.," *Therapeutic Recreation Journal,* 2nd Quarter, 1970, pp. 17–21, 46.

[5] Gene A. Hayes: "Recreation Services for the Mentally Retarded in the State of Kansas." *Therapeutic Recreation Journal,* 3rd Quarter, 1969, p. 13.

[6] Martha Peters and Peter. J. Verhoven, Jr.: "A Study of Therapeutic Recreation Services in Kentucky Nursing Homes." *Therapeutic Recreation Journal,* 4th Quarter, 1970, pp. 19–22.

[7] John E. Silson, et al: "Availability and Utilization of Recreation Resources for Chronically Ill and Disabled Children and Youth in the U.S." *Therapeutic Recreation Journal,* 4th Quarter, 1970, pp. 1, 36.

[8] Thomas A. Stein: "Therapeutic Recreation Education: 1969 Survey." *Therapeutic Recreation Journal,* 2nd Quarter, 1970, pp. 4–7, 25.

[9] Donald Lindley: "Relative Importance of College Courses in Therapeutic Recreation." *Therapeutic Recreation Journal,* 2nd Quarter, 1970, pp. 8–12.

[10] Gus Zaso: "The Central Life Interests of Activity Therapy Leaders in Therapeutic Recreation." *Therapeutic Recreation Journal,* 4th Quarter, 1970, pp. 15–18.

RECREATION, LEISURE AND THE ALCO-HOLIC (1969). This study examined the alcoholic's use of leisure time prior to commitment to an alcoholic rehabilitation center, and its relationship to his drinking problem. A sample of 129 patients was compared to study data on the use of leisure time by the general population which had been gathered by the Outdoor Recreation Resources Review Commission.[11]

A COMPUTERIZED ANALYSIS OF CHARACTERISTICS OF DOWN'S SYNDROME AND NORMAL CHILDREN'S FREE PLAY PATTERNS (1971). This study examined the free play patterns of a group of four- to eight-year-old Down's syndrome (mongoloid) children, and four groups of normal children of preschool chronological age. The range in play and the use of special pieces of apparatus were recorded by a ceiling-mounted camera, and the data gathered in this way were carefully analyzed by computer.[12]

A COMPARISON OF ACTIVE AND PASSIVE RECREATIONAL ACTIVITIES FOR PSYCHOTIC PATIENTS (1971). This study examined the effects of a program of active and passive recreation on two groups of long-term schizophrenic patients in a state mental hospital, as measured by pulse rate and a 16-item Behavioral Adjustment Scale. Information was gathered in areas of mood, cooperation, communication and social contact, over a six-month period of involvement, and at a later stage.[13]

THE LEISURE ACTIVITIES AND SOCIAL PARTICIPATION OF MENTAL PATIENTS PRIOR TO HOSPITALIZATION (1971). This study used data gathered from interviews of a sample of psychiatric patients at a state mental hospital to determine what the leisure activities and social participation of these patients were before hospitaliza-tion, as a basis for policy-making in the area of hospital and community recreation programs, and to initiate conceptualization in certain areas of rehabilitation practice.[14]

Approximately fifty entries in a bibliography of theses and dissertations dealing with recreation, parks, camping and outdoor education apply specifically to therapeutic recreation and the leisure needs of special groups.[15] These research studies, carried out at colleges and universities, usually to meet Master's or Doctoral requirements, cover such topics as:

"The Determination of the Course Areas for a Graduate Curriculum in Hospital Recreation."

"Integrative Aspects of Therapeutic Recreation."

"A Study of Adapted Equipment for the Use of the Orthopedically Handicapped in Sports and Games."

"The Effect of an Active Recreation Program on Selected Mentally Ill Female Patients at Cambridge State Hospital."

"Developmental Dance in the Education of the Educable Mentally Handicapped Child."

"The Effects of a Program of Balance Activities on Cerebral Palsied Children."

"The Effects of a Selected Recreation Activity on the I.Q. Scores, Social Adjustment, and Physical Coordination of the Educable Mentally Retarded Child."

Types of Research Studies

Studies in the field of therapeutic recreation service tend to fall into one of the following categories of research design.

CASE STUDY. This is generally used to examine a single program, institution or culture, and involves intensive study, mak-

[11] H. Douglas Sessoms and Sidney R. Oakley: "Recreation, Leisure, and the Alcoholic." *Journal of Leisure Research,* Winter, 1969, pp. 21–31.

[12] A. G. Linford, et al.: "A Computerized Analysis of Down's Syndrome and Normal Children's Free Play Patterns." *Journal of Leisure Research,* Winter, 1971, pp. 44–52.

[13] Grant W. Bigelow: "A Comparison of Active and Passive Recreational Activities for Psychotic Patients." *Therapeutic Recreation Journal,* 4th Quarter, 1971, pp. 145–151.

[14] Irvin Babow and Sol Simkin: "The Leisure Activities and Social Participation of Mental Patients Prior to Hospitalization." *Therapeutic Recreation Journal,* 4th Quarter, 1971, pp. 161–167.

[15] Betty Van der Smissen and Donald V. Joyce: *Bibliography of Theses and Dissertations in Recreation, Parks, Camping and Outdoor Education.* Washington, D.C., National Recreation and Park Association, 1970.

ing use of a variety of data-gathering techniques. It may be of a comparative or cross-sectional type, in which two or more cases or subjects are compared.

EVALUATIVE DESIGN. This involves the analysis or appraisal of an existing program, process or service, in an effort to determine how effective it is in meeting goals.

EXPERIMENTAL DESIGN. This usually involves the testing of a new type of program or service, or establishing new environmental conditions and determining their effect. It requires careful sampling procedures, or the establishment of experimental and control groups, although, when carried on as a demonstration project, the conditions of testing need not be as rigorous.

HISTORICAL-PHILOSOPHICAL DESIGN. This approach is usually employed in studying events that occurred in the past, or in analyzing theoretical concepts or systems.

LONGITUDINAL DESIGN. This usually involves the study of quantifiable data over a period of time, and differs from historical research in that it is not as concerned with the context and interpretation of change, as in the analysis and interpretation of evidence.

The specific techniques that are employed in therapeutic recreation research tend to fall into the following categories:

SURVEY ANALYSIS. This is the most common form of research tool used in this field, as in the broad field of social research. It represents an attempt to determine current conditions, with respect to such elements as practices, participation, recreational choices and attitudes, employment, program content or a host of other subjects. Generally it is concerned with examining a number of programs, communities or organizations, or with information about a class of people, or a region or even the entire country. It may make use of such tools as the mailed questionnaire, structured interview, check lists, rating scales, opinion polls or similar data-gathering procedures.

EXPERIMENTAL ANALYSIS. This involves the application of new services, treatment procedures, equipment or other types of environmental changes, and the careful measurement of the outcomes of such changes. Usually, it is carried on in an attempt to determine whether certain pre-existing hypotheses are correct, and whether they can be supported by statistically treated data. Experimental analysis may be carried on in an actual service situation or in a community, or in a carefully controlled laboratory situation. It may involve the comparison of two or more groups that have been subjected to different treatment or program procedures, or it may involve the examination of a single group of subjects over a period of time.

In the field of recreation service, comparatively little research of an experimental nature has been carried on, chiefly because of the difficulty in controlling the environmental conditions and excluding other factors or influences that make for change.

Other research techniques may involve *documentary analysis,* which consists of the careful study of documents, reports or other written information; *critical-incident method,* which is based on the in-depth study of one or more significant episodes or incidents: *field study,* a technique widely used in both sociology and anthropology, in which the researcher immerses himself in an ongoing situation or environment and gathers information about it, using a variety of methods; *judge's appraisal,* a method of utilizing the expert judgment of a group of authorities; and *tests of behavior or performance,* which are normally used in experimental research.

As indicated earlier, research may gather either quantitative or qualitative data, or both. When it gathers the former—that is to say, information which can be measured and put in terms of numbers—it normally must be analyzed statistically. This might consist of simply grouping and reporting responses by percentages or simple frequencies, or may involve the use of more sophisticated statistical procedures and formulas, including computer analysis.

Customarily, research may be carried on by a number of different types of sponsors or investigators. These include:

Institutions and agencies. Many hospitals, rehabilitation centers or other agencies or departments conduct research studies more or less frequently, to determine their own effectiveness, establish needs and outcomes or provide a basis for program development.

Colleges and universities. A substantial amount of research is carried out by graduate students working on theses or dissertations, or by faculty members with student assistants.

Governmental agencies. Government, on its various levels, is a major sponsor of research. In the field of therapeutic recreation service, this may be carried out in government hospitals or treatment centers, or, more commonly, by government funding of research projects that are then carried on by research teams in universities or other settings.

Professional organizations. National or state organizations may carry on research, usually directed toward determining needs and trends in the field rather than toward the development or evaluation of existing programs.

Increasingly, research of an interdisciplinary nature is being carried on, with the collaboration of two or more such sponsors. For example, in some recent studies, collaboration consists of the government approving and funding a research project, which is manned and carried on by researchers drawn from a university faculty, and which is actually carried out in an institutional setting. Thus all three sponsors have a part in the research effort. Similarly, although the initiative for such research may come from therapeutic recreation educators, other faculty personnel or research specialists, such as psychologists, sociologists, physicians or statisticians, might be drawn into the research process.

In developing proposals for research in therapeutic recreation, the following kinds of questions should be asked:

"Am I—as the researcher—genuinely interested in the problem, and free from strong biases that might imperil my objectivity?"

"Is the problem an important one, in the sense that research related to it is likely to be helpful to my institution or program, or to advance knowledge in the field or be of value to other professionals?"

"Has similar research already been carried on, or will the proposed investigation yield substantially new information?"

"Can the needed administrative support and cooperation be obtained, in order to carry out the study successfully?"

"Do I have, as an individual, or does my department or agency have the needed expertise to carry on the study? If not, can assistance be obtained?"

"Will access to the needed subjects, informants or other resources necessary to carry out the study be available?"

"Will it be possible to gather accurate data in sufficient scope required to validate findings?"

Encouragement Given to Research

Within any major department or large-scale institutional program, both evaluation and research should be consistently encouraged and supported. Obviously, it must not represent a diversion from the primary objective of providing service. However, the most meaningful programs are those that are intelligently evaluated, and the most successful professions are likely to be those that have a solid basis of scientifically gained knowledge underlying their practices. Therefore, therapeutic recreation specialists should be encouraged to:

1. Use a scientific and systematic approach at all times in gathering information on program needs and services, or solving on-the-spot recreation programs.
2. Attempt to gain skill in the application of research instruments and the use of research results.
3. Cooperate with personnel in colleges and universities or in other organizations or departments, to carry on jointly sponsored research projects.
4. Be alert to the possibilities for foundation or government-sponsored grants for research or demonstration projects.

5. Assist in identifying problems in the field that require research that might be carried on by professional colleagues or experts in a better position to follow up on them.
6. Press for the allocation of both funds and staff time to carry out research and evaluation studies.

Research and Evaluation: Concluding Statement

It should be made clear that research does not automatically provide the solution to all problems of professional development or program enrichment in therapeutic recreation service. Although rehabilitation authorities may be convinced of the value of activity therapies in general, and although medical practitioners may strongly support therapeutic recreation programs, it may not be possible to derive statistical evidence as to its value in many cases.

However, it should be clearly understood that this limitation is not peculiar to the field of therapeutic recreation. The author has pointed out elsewhere how major educational programs or experiments in social innovation have yielded disappointing results, when carefully evaluated. The value of Head Start, for example, a major federally sponsored educational program designed to counteract the effects of poverty and cultural deprivation for pre-school children, which was highly praised in its early stages, has been shown to be only temporary and to have no lasting benefits.[16] Intensive group work therapy programs for teen-agers, or casework services for families with multiple problems, have shown no measurable benefits. Indeed, in the latter case, it was indicated that the more often a problem family saw its caseworker, the less progress was shown.[17] A heavily financed program of performance contracting by educational firms that were funded to provide specially designed educational programs in both rural areas and large cities has been shown to be no more effective than traditional classroom instruction.[18]

Therefore, it should not be expected that research will automatically yield supportive evidence that will assist therapeutic recreation personnel in developing their programs, and that will consistently support their professional status and importance.

However, it is essential nonetheless that every effort be made to explore, as systematically as possible, both the theoretical and practical questions underlying this field. One major conference on physical education and recreation for disabled children identified the need to carry out meaningful research within the following areas:

1. The contributions, values and effects of participation.
2. The design of programs, and their underlying rationale.
3. The extent and nature of current services, on a geographical or demographic basis, or in terms of the needs of specific disabled groups in the population.
4. The development of effective instruments and tools to assess performance or measure program outcomes.
5. The development and application of meaningful program standards for evaluation.

Finally, it is essential that new and more effective means of storing, disseminating and using research findings be developed. Often there is a marked gulf between college or university researchers and the practitioner in the field who might be able to use their findings.

Linford and Kennedy comment that the researcher is often wrongly accused of failing to communicate his results to workers in the field. In their view, this criticism is unjustified:

. . . the role of the researcher is to solve problems. The transmission of information

---

[16] Robert B. Semple, Jr.: "Head Start Value Found Temporary." *New York Times,* October 23, 1966, p. 1.

[17] "Casework Found No Poverty Cure." *New York Times,* September 19, 1968, p. 55.

[18] "Result of a Test: F." *Time,* February 4, 1972, p. 42.

to others is the role of the teacher and communications expert—not the researcher. While they are perhaps not too well qualified as researchers themselves, any college lecturer should be at least able to read research literature and interpret it for students. The communication and dissemination problem is a major one. . . .[19]

This problem of dissemination can be materially aided by national "data banks" or other comprehensive collections of research reports, which can systematically organize findings and make them available to the field. A beginning step has been made in this direction by the establishment of TRIC (Therapeutic Recreation Information Center), a literature and document storage and retrieval center for the field of therapeutic recreation service. Founded at Teachers College, Columbia University, in 1970, this valuable project has now been shifted to the University of Waterloo, in Ontario, Canada.

Coordinated by Fred W. Martin, TRIC acquires published and unpublished articles, books, conference proceedings and reports. It abstracts them, and indexes them for storage in a computer-based information retrieval system. Information requests are accepted from educators, professionals, students, practitioners and others seeking information concerning therapeutic recreation service. TRIC includes references gained from such primary sources as *Parks and Recreation; Journal of Health, Physical Education and Recreation; Research Quarterly; Journal of Leisure Research; Recreation for the Ill and Handicapped;* and *Therapeutic Recreation Journal.* Secondary sources, such as *Psychological Abstracts; Sociological Abstracts; Mental Retarda-*

tion Abstracts; Hospital Abstracts; Education Index; Rehabilitation Literature; and *Educational Resources Information Center (ERIC)* are also used, along with other information systems, particularly the *Medical Literature Analysis and Retrieval System (MED-LARS)*, in gathering data and developing abstracts keypunched within computer formats for convenient and economical storage.

Martin writes:

> TRIC can be used to assist the preparation of course bibliographies by educators offering these courses, students engaged in term projects, as well as for surveys of the literature for master's theses and doctoral dissertations. Researchers both within our field and in other fields and disciplines can save valuable research time and avoid wasteful duplication of effort. Research gaps may become more clearly defined with systematically stored and retrievable data available. Reducing the effort of the practitioner in obtaining research results and other information may increase the utilization of such material in programs removed from the academic sphere and ultimately improve on the delivery of service to clients.[20]

Such progress is making a positive contribution to the scientific development of the field of therapeutic recreation service, and to the quality of college programs of professional preparation in it. In the years ahead, improved and expanded efforts in both evaluation and research will support and strengthen this field. They deserve major priority by all therapeutic agencies and institutions, in terms of university curriculum development, government funding and allocation of staff energies and time.

---

[19] Anthony G. Linford and Dan W. Kennedy: "Research—The State of the Art in Therapeutic Recreation." *Therapeutic Recreation Journal,* 4th Quarter, 1971, p. 169.

[20] Fred W. Martin: "TRIC—A Computer-Based Information Storage and Retrieval Center for the Field of Therapeutic Recreation Service." *Therapeutic Recreation Journal,* 4th Quarter, 1971, p. 173.

Suggested Topics for Class Discussion, Examinations or Student Papers

1. Define and compare the two related processes of evaluation and research, and show how they are vital to upgrading the field of therapeutic recreation service and meeting its goals.

2. Develop a statement of a specific problem or area of needed information in therapeutic recreation service. Prepare a preliminary research proposal intended to investigate this problem, including each of the elements mentioned in the text.
3. Why is the interdisciplinary cooperation of government, institutions of higher education and agencies serving the disabled necessary to promote effective research in this field? Give an example of how such cooperation might be developed.

Bibliography

I. General References on Recreation and Rehabilitative Services

W. Scott Allan: *Rehabilitation: A Community Challenge.* New York, John Wiley and Sons, 1958.

Doris L. Berryman, Annette Logan, and Dorothy Lander: *Enhancement of Recreation Service to Disabled Children,* and *Recommended Standards with Evaluative Criteria for Recreation Services in Residential Institutions.* New York, New York University School of Education, Report of Children's Bureau Project, 1971.

Charles K. Brightbill: *Man and Leisure, A Philosophy of Recreation.* Englewood Cliffs, New Jersey, Prentice-Hall, 1961.

George D. Butler: *Introduction to Community Recreation.* New York, McGraw-Hill Book Co., 1967.

Roger Caillois: *Man, Play and Games.* London, Thames and Hudson, 1961.

Reynold Carlson, Theodore Deppe, and Janet MacLean: *Recreation in American Life.* Belmont, California, Wadsworth Publishing Company, Inc., 1963.

Frederick Chapman: *Recreation Activities for the Handicapped.* New York, Ronald Press, 1960.

Bryant J. Cratty: *Psychology and Physical Activity.* Englewood Cliffs, New Jersey, Prentice-Hall, 1968.

Virginia Frye, and Martha Peters: *Therapeutic Recreation: Its Theory, Philosophy and Practices.* Harrisburg, Pennsylvania, Stackpole Books, 1972.

Paul Haun: *Recreation: A Medical Viewpoint.* New York, Teachers College, Columbia, Bureau of Publications, 1965.

Johan Huizinga: *Homo Ludens: A Study of the Play Element in Culture.* Boston, Beacon Press, 1950.

Valerie Hunt: *Recreation for the Handicapped.* Englewood Cliffs, New Jersey, Prentice-Hall, 1960.

Richard Kraus: *Recreation and Leisure in Modern Society.* New York, Appleton-Century-Crofts, 1971, and *Recreation Today: Program Planning and Leadership.* New York, Appleton-Century-Crofts, 1966.

Richard Kraus and Joseph E. Curtis: *Creative Administration in Recreation and Parks.* St. Louis, Missouri, C. V. Mosby, 1973.

Eric Larrabee, and Rolf Meyersohn: *Mass Leisure.* Glencoe, Illinois, The Free Press, 1958.

Janet MacLean, (ed.): *Therapeutic Recreation in the Community.* Bloomington, Indiana, Conference Report, University of Indiana, 1962.

Harold D. Meyer, Charles K. Brightbill, and H. Douglas Sessoms: *Community Recreation: A Guide to its Organization.* Englewood Cliffs, New Jersey, Prentice-Hall, 1969.

Susanna Millar: *The Psychology of Play.* Baltimore, Penguin Books, 1968.

Norman Miller, and Duane Robinson: *The Leisure Age.* Belmont, California, Wadsworth Publishing Company, Inc., 1963.

Martin Neumeyer, and Esther Neumeyer: *Leisure and Recreation.* New York, Ronald Press, 1958.

Gerald S. O'Morrow: *Administration of Activity Therapy.* Springfield, Illinois, Charles C Thomas, 1966.

Janet Pomeroy: *Recreation for the Physically Handicapped.* New York, The Macmillan Company, 1964.

Josephine L. Rathbone, and Carol Lucas: *Recreation in Total Rehabilitation.* Springfield, Illinois, Charles C Thomas, 1970.

Howard Rusk: *Basic Concepts of Hospital Recreation.* Washington, D.C., American Recreation Society, 1953.

Allen V. Sapora, and Elmer Mitchell: *The Theory of Play and Recreation.* New York, Ronald Press, 1961.

Hans Selye: *The Stress of Life.* New York, McGraw-Hill Book Company, 1956.

Jay Shivers: *Principles and Practices of Recreational Service.* New York, The Macmillan Company, 1967.

Samuel Slavson: *Recreation and the Total Personality.* New York, Association Press, 1946.

Ralph Slovenko, and James A. Knight, (eds.): *Motivations in Play, Games and Sports.* Springfield, Illinois, Charles C Thomas, 1967.

Anne Marie Smith: *Play for Convalescent Children.* New York, A. S. Barnes, 1961.

II. Recreation and the Mentally Retarded

American Association for Health, Physical Education and Recreation: *Physical Activities for the Mentally Retarded: Ideas for Instruction,* and *Guidelines for Programing in Recreation and Physical Education for the Mentally Retarded.* Washington, D.C., 1968.

American Association for Health, Physical Education and Recreation, and Sex Information and Education Council of the United States: *A Resource Guide in Sex Education for the Mentally Retarded.* Washington, D.C., 1971.

American Association on Mental Deficiency: *Manual on Terminology and Classification in Mental Deficiency.* Washington, D.C. 1961.

Elliott M. Avedon: *Recreation and Mental Retardation.* Washington, D.C., Public Health Service, Division of Mental Retardation, U.S. Department of Health, Education and Welfare, 1966.

Elliott M. Avedon, and Frances B. Arje: *Socio-Recreative Planning for the Retarded: A Handbook for Sponsoring Groups.* New York, Teachers College, Columbia, Bureau of Publications, 1964.

Norman R. Bernstein, (ed.): *Diminished People, Problems and Care of the Mentally Retarded.* Boston, Little, Brown and Company, 1970.

La Donna Bogardus: *Camping with Retarded Persons.* Nashville, Tennessee, Cokesbury, 1970.

Charlotte A. Buist, and Jerome L. Schulman: *Toys and Games for Educationally Handicapped Children.* Springfield, Illinois, Charles C Thomas, 1969.

Bernice Wells Carlson, and David R. Ginglend: *Recreation for Retarded Teenagers and Young Adults.* Nashville, Tennessee, Abingdon Press, 1968.

James H. Humphrey, and Dorothy D. Sullivan: *Teaching Slow Learners Through Active Games.* Springfield, Illinois, Charles C Thomas, 1970.

Samuel A. Kirk: *Educating Exceptional Children.* Boston, Houghton-Mifflin Company, 1962.

Edward L. Meyen: *Planning Community Services for the Mentally Retarded.* Scranton, Pennsylvania, International Textbook Co., 1967.

Helen Jo Mitchell, et al.: *The Young Retarded Child at Play: A Guide for Pre-School Play Centers.* Washington, D.C., Program for the Mentally Retarded, Washington Recreation Department, 1969.

William K. Murphy, and R. C. Scheerenberger: *Establishing Day Centers for the Mentally Retarded.* Springfield, Illinois, Department of Mental Health, Division of Mental Retardation Services, 1967.

Larry L. Neal: *Recreation's Role in the Rehabilitation of the Mentally Retarded.* Eugene, Oregon, University of Oregon, 1970.

President's Panel of Mental Retardation: *A Proposed Program for National Action to Combat Mental Retardation.* Washington, D.C., U.S. Government Printing Office, 1962.

III. Recreation and the Aging

Nancy N. Anderson: *Senior Centers: Information from a National Survey.* Minneapolis, Minnesota, Institute for Interdisciplinary Studies, American Rehabilitation Foundation, 1969.

Juliette K. Arthur: *How to Help Older People.* Philadelphia, J. B. Lippincott Co., 1954.

Edward Bortz: *Creative Aging.* New York, The Macmillan Company, 1963.

Gertude Cross: *Program Ideas for Senior Citizens,* and *Senior Citizens Travel Manual.* Flint, Michigan, Recreation and Park Board, 1970.

Elaine Cumming, and William E. Henry: *Growing Old: The Process of Disengagement.* New York, Basic Books, 1961.

Joan M. Cutter, Edna B. Russell, and Elizabeth A. Stetler: *An Activity Center for Senior Citizens.* Washington, D.C., Administration on Aging, U.S. Department of Health, Education and Welfare, 1961.

Wilma Donahue, et al., (eds.): *Free Time—Challenge to Later Maturity.* Ann Arbor, Michigan, University of Michigan Press, 1958.

Robert J. Havighurst, and Ruth Albrecht: *Older People.* New York, Longmans, Green, 1953.

Langdon Hooper, Dorothy Mullen, and Irene J. Kennedy: *Recreation Service in Connecticut Nursing Homes for the Aged.* Hartford, Connecticut, State Department of Health, 1968.

Robert Kleemeier: *Aging and Leisure.* New York, Oxford University Press, 1961.

Carol Lucas: *Recreational Activity Development for the Aging in Hospitals and Nursing Homes.* Springfield, Illinois, Charles C Thomas, 1962.

Toni Merrill: *Activities for the Aged and Infirm, A Handbook for the Untrained*

Worker. Springfield, Illinois, Charles C Thomas, 1967.

Dorothy G. Mullen: *Recreation in Nursing Homes*. Arlington, Virginia, National Recreation and Park Association Management Aids, No. 88, 1971.

Virginia O'Neill: *Hodson Day Center: A Community Center Program for Persons in a Public Agency*. Washington, D.C., Office of Aging, U.S. Department of Health, Education and Welfare, 1962.

President's Task Force on Aging: *Toward a Brighter Future for the Elderly*. Washington, D.C., Report of the Task Force, 1970.

Suzanne Reichard, Florine Livson, and Paul Peterson: *Aging and Personality*. New York, John Wiley and Sons, 1962.

Esther Smith: *The Dynamics of Aging*. New York, W. W. Norton and Company, Inc., 1956.

Social Rehabilitation Service, Administration on Aging: *Aging*. Washington, D.C., U.S. Department of Health, Education and Welfare, 1969.

Bernard Stotsky: *The Nursing Home and the Aged Psychiatric Patient*. New York, Appleton-Century-Crofts, 1970.

Claire Townsend: *Old Age: The Last Segregation*. New York, Grossman Publishers, Inc., 1971.

White House Conference on Aging: *Retirement Roles and Activities*. Washington, D.C., Report of Conference, 1971.

Arthur Williams: *Recreation in the Senior Years*. Washington, D.C., National Recreation Association, 1962.

IV. Recreation and Physical Disability

Boy Scouts of America: *Scouting for the Blind, Scouting for the Deaf,* and *Scouting for the Physically Handicapped*. North Brunswick, New Jersey, Boy Scouts of America, Health and Safety Service.

Charles E. Buell: *Physical Education for Blind Children*. Springfield, Illinois, Charles C Thomas, 1966.

Bureau of Education for the Handicapped: *Physical Education and Recreation for Handicapped Children: A Study Conference on Research and Demonstration Needs*. Washington, D.C., American Association for Health, Physical Education and Recreation, and National Recreation and Park Association, 1969.

Bureau of Outdoor Recreation: *Outdoor Recreation Planning for the Handicapped*. Washington, D.C., Bureau of Outdoor Recreation, Department of the Interior, 1967.

Maurice Case: *Recreation for Blind Adults*. Springfield, Illinois, Charles C Thomas, 1966.

Hollis F. Fait: *Special Physical Education*. Philadelphia, W. B. Saunders Company, 1972.

Sheila Hewett: *The Family and the Handicapped Child: A Study of Cerebral Palsied Children in Their Homes*. Chicago, Aldine Publishing Co., 1970.

Henry H. Kessler: *Rehabilitation of the Physically Handicapped*. New York, Columbia University Press, 1953.

Frank H. Krusen, Frederick J. Kottke, and Paul M. Ellwood, (eds.): *Handbook of Physical Medicine and Rehabilitation*. Philadelphia, W. B. Saunders Company, 1971.

Edna Levine: *The Psychology of Deafness*. New York, Columbia University Press, 1968.

Louis A. Michaux: *The Physically Handicapped and the Community*. Springfield, Illinois, Charles C Thomas, 1970.

Muscular Dystrophy—The Facts. New York, Muscular Dystrophy Association of America, 1970.

Multiple Sclerosis: The Crippler of Young Adults. New York, National Multiple Sclerosis Society, 1968.

National Commission on Architectural Barriers to Rehabilitation of the Handicapped: *Design for All Americans*. Washington, D.C., Rehabilitation Services Administration, Social and Rehabilitation Service, U.S. Department of Health, Education and Welfare, 1967.

National Facilities Conference: *Planning Areas and Facilities for Health, Physical Education, and Recreation*. Chicago, The Athletic Institute and American Association of Health, Physical Education and Recreation, 1965.

Sylvia B. O'Brien: *More Than Fun: A Handbook of Recreational Programming for Children and Adults with Cerebral Palsy*. New York, United Cerebral Palsy Associations.

Janet Pomeroy: *Recreation for the Physically Handicapped*. New York, The Macmillan Company, 1964.

Frank L. Porter, (ed.): *The Diabetic at Work and Play*. Springfield, Illinois, Charles C Thomas, 1971.

George T. Stafford: *Sports for the Handicapped*. New York, Prentice-Hall, 1947.

Beatrice Wright: *Physical Disability: A Psychological Approach*. New York, Harper and Row, 1960.

V. Texts on Mental Illness and Social Deviance

Ruth Cavan, (ed.): *Readings in Juvenile Delinquency*. Philadelphia, J. B. Lippincott Company, 1969.

Richard A. Cloward, and Lloyd E. Ohlin: *Delinquency and Opportunity: A Theory of Delinquent Gangs*. New York, Free Press, 1960.

V. Cumming, and E. Cumming: *Ego and Milieu*. New York, Atherton Press, 1969.

Marshall Edelson: *Sociotherapy and Psycho-*

therapy. Chicago, University of Chicago Press, 1970.

Don C. Gibbons: *Delinquent Behavior.* Englewood Cliffs, New Jersey, Prentice-Hall, 1970.

Milton Greenblatt, and Benjamin Simon: *Rehabilitation of the Mentally Ill.* Washington, D.C., American Association for the Advancement of Science, 1959.

Julius Hoenig, and Marian W. Hamilton: *The Desegregation of the Mentally Ill.* London, Routledge and Paul, 1969.

Alfred Kahn: *Planning Community Services for Children in Trouble.* New York, Columbia University Press, 1963.

Malcolm W. Klein: *Street Gangs and Street Workers.* Englewood Cliffs, New Jersey, Prentice-Hall, 1971.

Robert M. MacIver: *The Prevention and Control of Delinquency.* New York, Atherton Press, 1966.

B. E. Phillips (ed.): *Recreation for the Mentally Ill.* Washington, D.C., Conference Report, American Association for Health, Physical Education and Recreation, 1958.

Sophia Robison: *Juvenile Delinquency, Its Nature and Control.* New York, Holt, Rinehart and Winston, 1960.

Theodore Rothman, (ed.): *Changing Patterns in Psychiatric Care.* New York, Crown Publishers, Inc., 1970.

Thomas S. Szasz: *Law, Liberty, and Psychiatry: An Inquiry into the Social Uses of Mental Health Practices.* New York, The Macmillan Company, 1963.

Treatment in the Modern Mental Hospital. Albany, New York, New York State Department of Mental Hygiene, 1966.

Alan B. Tulipan, and Saul Feldman, (eds.): *Psychiatric Clinics in Transition.* New York, Brunner-Mazel, 1969.

U.S. Task Force on Juvenile Delinquency: *Task Force Report: Juvenile Delinquency and Youth Crime.* Washington, D.C., U.S. Government Printing Office, 1967.

List of Organizations

National Organizations or Agencies Serving the Disabled

Administration on Aging, 330 C Street, S.W., Washington, D.C. 20201

American Art Therapy Association, 6010 Broad Branch Road, N.W., Washington, D.C. 20015

American Association for Health, Physical Education and Recreation, 1201 Sixteenth Street, N.W., Washington, D.C. 20036

American Association on Mental Deficiency, 5201 Connecticut Ave., N.W., Washington, D.C., 20015

American Camping Association, Bradford Woods, Martinsville, Indiana 46151

American Diabetes Association, 18 East 48th St., New York, N.Y. 10017

American Foundation for the Blind, 15 W. 16th St., New York, N.Y. 10011

American Heart Association, 44 East 23rd St., New York, N.Y. 10010

American National Red Cross, 17th and D St., N.W., Washington, D.C. 20000

American Occupational Therapy Association, 251 Park Ave. So., New York, N.Y. 10010

American Physical Therapy Association, 1156 15th St., N.W., Washington, D.C. 20005

American Psychiatric Association, 1700 18th St., N.W., Washington, D.C. 20000

Arthritis and Rheumatism Foundation, 10 Columbus Circle, New York, N.Y. 10019

Bureau of Education for the Handicapped, U.S. Office of Education, 400 Maryland Ave., S.W., Washington, D.C. 20202

Children's Bureau, Office of Child Development, 300 Independence Ave., S.W., Washington, D.C. 20201

Epilepsy Foundation of America, 733 15th St., N.W., Washington, D.C. 20005

International Society for Rehabilitation of the Disabled, 219 E. 44th St., New York, N.Y. 10017

Joseph P. Kennedy, Jr. Foundation, 1411 K St., N.W., Washington, D.C. 20005

Muscular Dystrophy Association of America, 1790 Broadway, New York, N.Y. 10019

National Association for Mental Health, 10 Columbus Circle, New York, N.Y. 10019

National Association for Music Therapy, P.O. Box 610, Lawrence, Kansas 66044

National Association for Retarded Children, 420 Lexington Ave., New York, N.Y. 10017

National Association of the Deaf, Suite 318, 2025 I St., N.W., Washington, D.C. 20006

National Council on the Aging, 375 Park Ave. So., New York, N.Y. 10010

National Easter Seal Society for Crippled Children and Adults, 2023 W. Ogden Ave., Chicago, Illinois 60612

National Foundation for Neuromuscular Diseases, 250 West 57th St., New York, N.Y. 10019

National Institutes of Health, 9000 Rockville Pike, Bethesda, Maryland 20010

National Multiple Sclerosis Society, 257 Park Ave. So., New York, N.Y. 10010

National Recreation and Park Association
  Branches: American Park and Recreation Society
            National Therapeutic Recreation Society
            Society of Park and Recreation Educators
  1601 N. Kent St., Arlington, Virginia 22209

National Tuberculosis and Respiratory Association, 1740 Broadway, New York, N.Y. 10019

President's Committee on Mental Retardation, U.S. Department of Health, Education and Welfare, Washington, D.C. 20201

Rehabilitation Services Administration (Social and Rehabilitation Service), 330 C St., S.W., Washington, D.C. 20201

United Cerebral Palsy Association, 66 E. 34th St., New York, N.Y. 10036

Veterans Administration Central Office, Washington, D.C. 20420

Other Organizations Serving Specific Groups of Disabled With Sports

American Association for the Deaf, P.O. Box 105, Talladega, Alabama 35160

American Blind Bowling Association, P.O. Box 306, Louisville, Kentucky 40201

American Junior Blind Bowling Association, 4244 Heather Rd., Long Beach, California, 90808

American Wheelchair Bowling Association, Route 2, Box 750, Lutz, Florida 33549

National Amputation Foundation (Golf), 12–45 150th St., Whitestone, N.Y. 11357

National Amputee Skiing Association, 3738 Walnut Ave., Carmichael, California 95608

National Track and Field Committee for the Visually Impaired, 4244 Heather Rd., Long Beach, California 90808

National Wheelchair Basketball Association, Rehabilitation-Education Center, Oak St. and Stadium Dr., University of Illinois, Champaign-Urbana, Illinois 61820

National Wheelchair Athletic Association, 40–24 62nd St., Woodside, N.Y. 11377

Special Olympics, Inc., 1701 K St. N.W., Washington, D.C. 20006

Films

Selected Films on Recreation for the Disabled

And So They Move. (16 mm, Black and White, Sound, 19 minutes). Use of creative play, in specially designed environment, with physically disabled children. Audio-Visual Center, Michigan State University, East Lansing, Michigan 48824.

Cast No Shadow. (16 mm, Color and Sound, 27 minutes). Shows wide range of recreation activities for physically and mentally disabled participants, at Recreation Center for the Handicapped in San Francisco. Professional Arts, Inc., Box 8484, Universal City, California.

New Concepts in Children's Play Areas. (Filmstrip, 80 frames, Sound, Color, 20 minutes, 33⅓ rpm record). Shows innovations in playground design to meet children's developmental needs. Associated Film Services, 3419 West Magnolia, Burbank, California 91505.

Paralympics, Israel, 1968. (16 mm, Color and Sound, 14 minutes). Documentary of international Wheelchair Athletic competition. U.S. Wheelchair Sports Fund, 40–24 62nd St., Woodside, N.Y. 11377.

Physical Education for Blind Children. (16 mm, Color and Sound, 20 minutes). Shows visually handicapped school children in varied physical education and recreational sports activities. Charles Buell, 4244 Heather Rd., Long Beach, California 90808.

Recreational Activities for Mentally Retarded Children. (16 mm, Color and Sound, 28 minutes). Comprehensive summer recreational program, including games, crafts, music, swimming, outings and parties, for mentally retarded. National Association for Retarded Children, 420 Lexington Ave., New York, N.Y. 10017.

Recreation and Occupational Therapy. (16 mm, Black and White, Sound, 13 minutes). Adapted activities suited for patients with limited mobility or physical disability. Audio-Visual Media Center, Washington State University, Pullman, Washington 99163.

Recreation for the Handicapped. (16 mm, Color and Sound, 23 minutes). Shows program, over several months, serving varied ages of disabled. Filmed by Stanford University film group. Recreation Center for the Handicapped, Great Highway at Sloat Blvd., San Francisco, California 94132.

Recreation Unlimited. (16 mm, Black and White, Sound, 15 minutes). Swimming, folk dancing, acting and crafts for mentally retarded children. National Association for Retarded Children, 420 Lexington Ave., New York, N.Y. 10017.

The Shape of a Leaf. (16 mm, Black and White, Color, Sound, 26 minutes). Creative approach to arts and crafts instruction with retarded children. Perkins School, Lancaster, Massachusetts 01523.

The Therapeutic Community. (16 mm, Color and Sound, 28 minutes). Milieu therapy approach in hospitalization of geriatric patients. University of Michigan Television Center and Division of Gerontology, Ann Arbor, Michigan.

Therapeutic Camping. (16 mm, Color and Sound, 28 minutes). Shows multidisciplinary approach of workers with emotionally disturbed adolescents in summer camp. Devereux Schools, Santa Barbara, California 93102.

Therapy Through Play. (16 mm, Color and Sound, 17 minutes). Adapted sports for physically disabled children. Human Resources Center, Albertson, N.Y. 11507.

To Paint is to Love Again. (16 mm, Color and Sound, 21 minutes). Art work with retarded children at Exceptional Children's Foundation in Los Angeles. Conrad Films, 6331 Weidlake Drive, Hollywood, California 90028.

You're It. (16 mm, Color and Sound, 25 minutes). Shows role of recreation in educational program for mentally retarded. MacDonald Training Center, 4424 Tampa Bay Boulevard, Tampa, Florida 33614.

Personnel Standards Developed by the National Therapeutic Recreation Society

The National Therapeutic Recreation Society, a branch of the National Recreation and Park Association, has developed the following set of minimum standards for position classification in therapeutic recreation. Based on these standards, individuals employed in the field may apply for voluntary registration with the society as a means of establishing their professional qualifications at a given job level.

1. *Therapeutic Recreation Assistant*
   a. Two years of successful full-time paid experience in therapeutic recreation field.

   or

   b. Two hundred clock hours in-service training in therapeutic recreation field.

   or

   c. A combination of a. and b. may be substituted.
2. *Therapeutic Recreation Technician*
   a. Associate of Arts degree from an accredited college or university or satisfactory completion of two years of college with major work in recreation or in other fields related to therapeutic recreation. (physical education, music, dance, drama, psychology, and sociology)

   or

   b. Diploma, certificate or other proof of satisfactory completion of two academic years of study in an art or technical field related to therapeutic recreation from an approved or recognized school.
3. *Therapeutic Recreation Worker*
   a. (Provisional) Baccalaureate degree from an accredited college or university with a major in recreation or field related to therapeutic recreation.

   or

   b. (Registered) Baccalaureate degree from an accredited college or university with a major or emphasis in therapeutic recreation.

   or

   c. (Registered) Baccalaureate degree from an accredited college or university with a major in recreation and one year of experience in therapeutic recreation field.

   or

   d. (Registered) Baccalaureate degree from an accredited college or university with a degree in a field related to therapeutic recreation and two years of experience in therapeutic recreation field.

or

    e. (Registered) Master's degree from an accredited college or university with a major in recreation or other field related to therapeutic recreation.

4. *Therapeutic Recreation Specialist*

    a. Master's degree from an accredited college or university with a major in therapeutic recreation.

or

    b. Master's degree from an accredited college or university with a major in recreation and one year of experience in therapeutic recreation field.

or

    c. Master's degree from an accredited college or university with a major in a field related to therapeutic recreation and two years of experience in therapeutic recreation field.

or

    d. Baccalaureate degree from an accredited college or university with a major or emphasis in therapeutic recreation and three years of experience in therapeutic recreation field.

or

    e. Baccalaureate degree from an accredited college or university with a major in recreation and four years of experience in therapeutic recreation field.

or

    f. Baccalaureate degree from an accredited college or university with a major in a field related to therapeutic recreation and five years of experience in therapeutic recreation field.

5. *Master Therapeutic Recreation Specialist*

    a. Master's degree from an accredited college or university with a major in therapeutic recreation and two years of experience in therapeutic recreation field.

or

    b. Master's degree from an accredited college or university with a major in recreation and three years of experience in therapeutic recreation field.

or

    c. Master's degree from an accredited college or university with a major in a field related to therapeutic recreation and four years of experience in therapeutic recreation field.

or

    d. Baccalaureate degree from an accredited college or university with a major or emphasis in therapeutic recreation and five years of experience in therapeutic recreation field.

or

    e. Baccalaureate degree from an accredited college or university with a major in recreation and six years of experience in therapeutic recreation field.

or

    f. Baccalaureate degree from an accredited college or university with a major in a field related to therapeutic recreation field and seven years of experience in therapeutic recreation field.

For further information, or to apply for voluntary registration, individuals should write: Executive Secretary, National Therapeutic Recreation Society, 1601 N. Kent St., Arlington, Virginia 22209.

Index